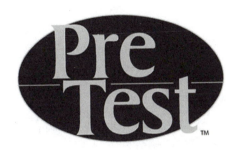

Pharmacology

PreTest™ Self-Assessment and Review

Notice

Medicine is an ever-changing science. As new research and clinical experience broaden our knowledge, changes in treatment and drug therapy are required. The authors and the publisher of this work have checked with sources believed to be reliable in their efforts to provide information that is complete and generally in accord with the standards accepted at the time of publication. However, in view of the possibility of human error or changes in medical sciences, neither the authors nor the publisher nor any other party who has been involved in the preparation or publication of this work warrants that the information contained herein is in every respect accurate or complete, and they disclaim all responsibility for any errors or omissions or for the results obtained from use of the information contained in this work. Readers are encouraged to confirm the information contained herein with other sources. For example and in particular, readers are advised to check the product information sheet included in the package of each drug they plan to administer to be certain that the information contained in this work is accurate and that changes have not been made in the recommended dose or in the contraindications for administration. This recommendation is of particular importance in connection with new or infrequently used drugs.

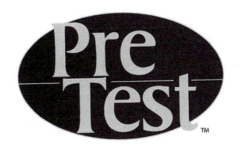

Pharmacology
PreTest™ Self-Assessment and Review
Twelfth Edition

Marshal Shlafer, PhD
Professor, Department of Pharmacology
Director of Undergraduate Medical Pharmacology Education
University of Michigan Medical School
Ann Arbor, Michigan

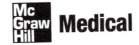

New York   Chicago   San Francisco   Lisbon   London   Madrid   Mexico City
Milan   New Delhi   San Juan   Seoul   Singapore   Sydney   Toronto

The McGraw·Hill Companies

Pharmacology: PreTest™ Self-Assessment and Review, Twelfth Edition

1 2 3 4 5 6 7 8 9 0   DOC/DOC   0 9 8 7

ISBN-13: 978-0-07-147181-7
ISBN-10:   0-07-147181-2

This book was set in Berkeley by International Typesetting and Composition.
The editors were Catherine A. Johnson and Regina Y. Brown.
The production supervisor was Sherri Souffrance.
Project management was provided by International Typesetting and Composition.
The cover designer was Maria Scharf.
Cover photo: Medication. Assorted capsules and tablets spilling from a triangular holder.
   Tek Image / Photo Researchers, Inc. (RM)
RR Donnelley was printer and binder.

This book is printed on acid-free paper.

Library of Congress Cataloging-in-Publication Data

Pharmacology : PreTest self-assessment and review.—12th ed. / [edited by] Marshal Shlafer.
   p. ; cm.
Includes bibliographical references and index.
ISBN-13: 978-0-07-147181-7 (pbk. : alk. paper)
ISBN-10:   0-07-147181-2 (pbk. : alk. paper)
1. Pharmacology—Examinations, questions, etc.   I. Shlafer, Marshal.
[DNLM: 1. Pharmaceutical Preparations—Examination Questions.
2. Drug Therapy—Examination Questions.   QV 18.2 P536   2007]
RM301.13.P475   2007
615'.1076—dc22

                                                    2006038287

Student Reviewers

Tyler James Harris
University of Washington—School of Medicine
Class of 2007

Mona Karimullah
University of Texas—Houston School of Medicine
Class of 2006

David Scoville
Kansas University—School of Medicine
Class of 2008

Contents

Local Control Substances: Autacoids and Drugs for Inflammatory Processes

The Gastrointestinal System and Nutrition

The Endocrine System, Uterine Stimulants and Relaxants

Anti-Infectives

Cancer Chemotherapy and Immunosuppressants

Toxicology

Preface

Welcome to this, the 12th edition, of *Pharmacology: PreTest™ Self-Assessment and Review*. I'm pleased to have been invited back to do this edition after doing the 11th. Whether you're studying for Step 1 of the USMLE or for a course exam that includes pharmacology content, I think you'll find this helpful.

Among the changes here you'll find are:

- Over 200 new or extensively revised questions, most based on clinical vignettes or scenarios, and nearly all pretested on hundreds of first- and second-year medical students

- Many more questions in the format you'll likely see on Step 1 of the USMLE

- A better blend of questions that integrate your basic pharmacology knowledge with clinical applications, and with information from other basic preclinical disciplines

- More integration of question content between the various areas of pharmacology and therapeutics. This is a general "build upon the base" approach in which questions in later chapters encourage you to integrate new material with content presented earlier

- Clearer explanations for why correct answers are correct and the others aren't

- Updates of cross-references to major pharmacology text cross-references in the answers so you can easily find additional information or explanations if you wish

Introduction

Each *PreTest*™ *Self-Assessment and Review* helps you evaluate and review your intensive and extensive knowledge of pharmacology and therapeutics, your expected knowledge of basic facts, and your ability to apply facts and concepts to some common (yet perhaps new, to you) clinical situations. The 502 questions you'll find here parallel the format and degree of difficulty of questions likely to be found in the United States Medical Licensing Examination (USMLE) Step 1. They should also help if you want to hone your knowledge base before USMLE Step 2 or 3, or similar licensure exams.

At the start of each chapter I provide a short list of key terms (mainly drug classes or basic concepts) to help orient you to the general scope of the question topics that follow. Each question is accompanied by several answers, only one of which is the "best choice"; explanations of a length, depth, and scope that I deem appropriate to understanding the answer; and cross-references to pages in one or more of three commonly used textbooks so you can get more information if you wish.

Study Tips, and How to Use This Book

Each of you has a study and review method that has worked best for you over the years. "Go with a winner," as they say. It has gotten you into medical school, and kept you there. But do prepare yourself to answer the questions in each chapter by reviewing first the corresponding material from your lecture notes and favorite (or, at least, assigned) text. This volume that you hold in your hands is, after all, a review and self-assessment tool, not an original source of learning information.

Each multiple-choice question in this book contains four or more possible answer options. In each case, select the ONE BEST ANSWER to the question. Mark your answer by each question, allowing yourself about a minute or so for each question, but don't be rushed. There are no negative consequences from going through this review and answering incorrectly, and no rewards for haste. The point is that you learn, or merely refresh your knowledge.

Be brave: don't skip the questions that initially stump you—and there will be a few of them—or those that test beyond the "rat facts," as there are some of those too.

I'm going to implore you *not* to do one rather tempting thing: read, or even peek, at the answers to individual questions in a chapter before you've answered all the questions in that chapter. I know this may be painful in a variety of ways ("no pain, no gain" as they say). Nonetheless, explanations for the answers to one question may give you a tip-off (if not the outright correct answer) to another question. That would be fine, ultimately, but in this review process—assessing your own knowledge, understanding, and recall— such tip-offs may lull you into arriving at the correct answer by a short-circuited approach, having just read a similar or applicable answer when you checked your responses of a previous question. There is "planned redundancy" in some of the questions and the answers.

After you finish going through all the questions in a chapter, spend as much time as you need verifying your answers and carefully reading the explanations provided. This is particularly important if you're stumped for a right answer, or even didn't have a clue about what the right answer might be.

However, the explanations I provide as answers to questions should serve as a beneficial review for all of you to reinforce concepts and facts you seem to know already. And if you got a question right, was that because you knew the answer, and understood what was going on, or just made a lucky guess?

Regardless, pay special attention to the explanations for the questions you answered incorrectly —but read *every* explanation. I have designed the explanations to reinforce and supplement the information sought by the questions, and sometimes to gently encourage you to look at (usually earlier) parts of this review book (as well as your class notes and your favorite or required pharmacology text) to see important connections—for example, those essential connections between basic autonomic pharmacology and cardiovascular, respiratory, or CNS topics.

Before you work on the questions and your studying overall, try organizing things in these ways, and aim to accomplish the following:

Be able to identify main drug classes, recognizing that sometimes we use more than one classification scheme, e.g., chemical; by main mechanism(s) of action; by clinical use; and be able to cite a prototype drug for each. Conversely, given a named prototype or otherwise representative drug, be able to work backward and know the rest of the most relevant information.

For example, you can identify a group of drugs that are nonselective cyclooxygenase (COX) inhibitors, a main chemical class of which includes acetylsalicylic acid (salicylates); the prototype drug is aspirin, and the main uses are for management of fever, inflammation, and mild pain. But also know the "special" properties of representative or unique agents in a group: for example, the use of aspirin for prophylaxis of arterial thrombosis, and something important about, say, indomethacin.

You could (if not should) take a reverse approach by identifying propranolol as the prototype nonselective β-adrenergic blocker; identifying the main actions (due to blockade of β-adrenergic receptors, which implicitly means your knowing what activating the β_1 and β_2 receptors does); and recognizing that propranolol has such uses as management of hypertension, certain types of angina pectoris, heart failure, tachycardia, and so on. You should be able to recognize the term *catecholamine* as applicable to a drug or drug group with structures and actions similar to epinephrine or norepinephrine.

Be able to recognize the most common and/or most important (e.g., serious or life-threatening) side effects or adverse responses for the main drugs or drug classes.

In my first lectures on pharmacology to every group of new students I teach, I say that if drugs did only the good and predictable things they're supposed to do, life—and learning—would be a heck of a lot simpler for you. For better or worse, however, side effects and other adverse responses happen. Then, too, there are the sometimes unavoidable and potentially disastrous consequences of polypharmacy drug-drug interactions. These are just as important, if not more important, than knowing merely what the drug does, what it's used for, or how it works.

Often you know intuitively what the side effects or adverse responses to a particular drug or drug group may be. The more common and perhaps important ones are often "extensions" of expected effects of the drug or class. For example, most antihypertensive drugs can cause hypotension (when blood levels are excessive), and many drugs cause nephrotoxicity and/or hepatotoxicity because the kidneys or liver are the main sites of elimination of the drugs, or their metabolites. However, some drugs cause effects that are, for lack of a better phrase, unique or unexpected: ototoxicity from aminoglycoside antibiotics or loop diuretics; a lupus-like syndrome from hydralazine or isoniazid; thyroid hormone and pulmonary problems from amiodarone; cyanide poisoning from nitroprusside. Learn these "unique" responses; I'll ask you about them, and I won't be the only one to do that.

Learn to recognize that intended effects or side effects that you simply should know give you a good idea of what the relevant precautions or contraindications are, even if you haven't been taught about the latter, even if your learning focus hasn't been too clinical.

For example, you no doubt learned that β-adrenergic blockers can reduce cardiac rate, contractility, and electrical impulse conduction velocity (especially through the AV node), and sometimes these drugs are used specifically to cause one or more of those effects. You should then realize that excessive doses may cause unwanted degrees of suppression of those cardiac parameters.

And, although you may not have been taught explicitly, you should realize that the effects of these drugs warrant extra caution (or contraindicate altogether) the use of a β-blocker in patients who already have bradycardia, significantly reduced ventricular contractility, or some degree of heart block. Making these associations or extrapolations is not rocket science that you must have been taught about explicitly. You should be able to use your basic knowledge of pharmacology and drug action, and of physiology and pathophysiology, to piece things together and get the correct (or most logical or likely) answer.

Breadth and Depth of Questions and Answers

Most students who have reviewed previous editions of *Pharmacology: PreTest™* found the book to be extremely useful. However, some questions were cited by a few reviewers as being "low-yield," "too basic," "too clinical," and the like.

Let me opine that, at this point in your medical education, you're not in the best position to make valid judgment calls on such matters. What students often cite as a low-yield question is actually basic but "must know" information, even though the correct answer may be blatantly obvious. Just because you automatically know or recognize the answer doesn't mean that the information isn't important, or isn't high yield, or that your ability to recognize it shouldn't be evaluated. It could well mean that you've learned the essential basics, and that's a good thing. Conversely, some students have called certain questions "low yield" simply because they haven't learned about the facts and concepts addressed in the question. It's very easy to attribute little importance to things one doesn't know or understand, and shrug-off the question as being trivial.

This is a critical, yet odd, place you find yourselves in your medical education. You are expected to be at your "peak" in terms of basic science knowledge, with enough of a foundation that you'll not only get through "the boards," but also be able to remember and carry it over to your clinical years when you hit the wards in a very short time. You should be able to do the former more easily than the latter, since knowledge fades with time, especially if you don't use that knowledge often. Borrowing from literature, you are expected to be like the cheerful Major General in Gilbert and Sullivan's *Pirates of Penzance*. You need to know "all the facts" and be able to spit them back almost reflexively. Yet you cannot be like him, whether for the Boards or upcoming years, when you are actually caring for patients and devising or interpreting treatment plans, because you need to be able to make sense of, and apply, all those facts into some more integrated and grander plan that has the greatest likelihood of success and the lowest risk of failure or harm.

The truth of the matter is that neither you—nor anyone else—will be able to answer all these questions correctly, or even correctly as far as I cite the answers. There is simply too much information presented to you in the pre-clinical years, and no matter how well you think you know your information (pharmacology or otherwise), it tends to become jumbled and incomprehensible when you're faced with the task of knowing it all at once. Much of your knowledge is important now; much more will be important later on (whether for an exam or for a patient); and some of what you've been taught is ultimately trivial and useless. But you just don't know at this time, and so I'll ask questions as fairly and forthrightly as possible and do my best to explain things in the answers in such a way that the information sticks, and you see the connections between ostensibly diverse areas of pharmacology and therapeutics. My goal is not to show you how much or how little you know. It's to help you acknowledge what you do know, and learn and understand what you don't.

It is in some ways rewarding to answer an ostensibly complicated or detailed question correctly (you possess the main positive attributes of Gilbert and Sullivan's happy Major General), but you don't want to find yourself so bogged down in knowing the details that you miss seeing the more important big picture, or how the facts apply or relate to one another (the Major General's main flaw). The simplest or most basic concepts can be overlooked with teaching or learning that is too detailed in terms of fact and focus. You have had an abundant (or excessive) amount of information about pharmacology presented to you, but that's only the foundation of a broad knowledge and experience base on which you'll build over the coming years.

Sometimes things aren't as obvious or as rational as they may seem, and knowing "too much" may not be at all sufficient once we get into a clinical situation. One example of this, which sticks out in my mind, based on years of teaching and some personal experience, has to do with a not-that-common clinical problem, hyperuricemia, gout, and their drug therapy. I've had students (and one new doc) cite every metabolic intermediate, and the responsible enzymes, in the biosynthesis of uric acid by the so-called purine degradation pathway. This is, of course, the metabolic crux of the problems in hyperuricemia and gout. They have correctly stated that allopurinol inhibits the "last two steps" in uric acid synthesis (the conversion of hypoxanthine to xanthine, and xanthine to the final product) by inhibiting xanthine oxidase.

That's great. Unfortunately, the majority of those students (and that one new MD caring for me) then stated what seemed so mechanistically rational but quite wrong: Given the role of uric acid in the pathophysiology of gout, and the efficacy of inhibiting urate synthesis with allopurinol, their first choice therapy for an acute gout attack would be (obviously, they've said) allopurinol. Oops. Wrong choice.

It's good to know many important facts, and even to be tested on them, but I don't necessarily agree that fact-based knowledge alone is sufficient. My philosophy on that point has caused initial consternation for the medical (and Pharm D, nursing, and dental) students I've taught for over 25 years. Students often expect such questions as "which of the following is a β-adrenergic blocker?" and get pumped when they correctly select propranolol out of a short list of drugs that may or may not do anything to β-adrenergic or other adrenergic receptors. I consider that knowledge as being important and essential (what you might call a high-yield fact), but rudimentary, not very challenging, and generally insufficient. That is why I may pepper my exams with a few fact-based fundamental questions, but then go on to require the student to take that fundamental and expected basic knowledge and extrapolate and apply it to new or different situations, or to state the "whys" more than the "whats." Some questions will go beyond the bounds of what most might consider to be traditionally in the domain of pharmacology and pose it in ways that require the student to recall what I'm sure they learned in some other preclinical "course" (I use quotation marks because we've long abandoned most discipline-based courses in our curriculum), such as physiology.

Practicing good medicine requires a better understanding, and rational application of basic knowledge, beyond possessing the rote memory of drugs and their mechanisms. It is, in that way, a creative and thought-provoking (and not necessarily precise) art. You have to go beyond the "use this drug for that purpose" level of knowledge.

Your experiences from the courses you've taken may be quite different from those of students in other medical schools, or the medical students I've taught. After all, there is (for better or worse) no one "standard" pharmacology curriculum for all medical schools, and points emphasized by a particular instructor that you've had can differ (sometimes markedly) in scope and orientation from those made by faculty elsewhere.

You may have had a stand-alone pharmacology course or two (at our medical school we no longer have any), perhaps with a focus on basic characteristics of drugs. That focus may have been on mechanisms of action (simple and straightforward, or quite detailed and complex), perhaps replete with such things as specific pathways of drug metabolism, structure-activity relationships, mathematical approaches to pharmacokinetics, or detailed cellular biochemical mechanisms of action. Little or no clinical relevance or application may have been presented, unfortunately.

Or, you may have had your preclinical pharmacology content integrated in some systems-based curriculum (that's what we do here), which sometimes teaches and tests on drug-related material in a very clinically oriented yet pharmacologically simplistic way. For example: "Your 50-year-old male patient has recently been diagnosed with Type 2 diabetes mellitus. He loves to eat. His liver is good. Prescribe metformin." As Homer Simpson might say, "duh-oh, ok." But why?

"You have a patient on long-term warfarin therapy. You know they shouldn't take aspirin (really?). Recommend acetaminophen." Why? Do you have a clue about the rationale, the reason why they shouldn't take aspirin (or can they?), or why they might be given acetaminophen? What problems might acetaminophen cause? Or do you simply memorize an admonition that doesn't always apply, and not understand it?

What's the magic of these drugs? How do they work? Are there any problems? What are they? How do you recognize, predict, avoid, or manage them?

For some of you it's tempting to view some of my questions as "too clinical"; others may find things "too basic or mechanistic." However, answering all the questions in this book is relatively simple if you think about the basic drug information you should have acquired; if you integrate it with what you should have learned in other courses (e.g., in a physiology or cell and molecular biology course); and if you start doing what you will have to do soon—make reasoned judgments based on applying your knowledge to a possibly new clinical picture: which is "most likely," for example.

What may be "too clinical" for some of you may be old hat for others. What may be a low-yield, no-brainer, or mere rat fact question to you might be assessing essential information overlooked or not presented to someone else who is studying just as diligently, trying to achieve the same goal on the very same exams as you.

There's another point you may be overlooking. You may know very well what you need to know when studying intensively, for example, CNS drugs. But are you able to extrapolate and integrate that information to a cardiovascular or autonomic nervous system problem? That's precisely what you'll have to do when you hit your clinical rotations, and what you may be asked to do on Step 1. I'll challenge you on that cross-disciplinary knowledge here, and so suddenly a question that seems "low yield" when considered in a discrete area becomes more challenging (and may shake your confidence) when posed in a broader perspective.

How pharmacology is presented, and what "defines" the basics or core of the discipline, vary tremendously from not only one text to another, but also from one medical school, or course, or instructor, to another. What you have learned from your lectures, or from your assigned text, inevitably reflects a bias (that is not meant in a pejorative sense), preference, or didactic style of the lecturers or the text book authors. And, just as your learning and testing experiences may vary, depending on where you are, so may the way you've prepared for a standardized exam that includes pharmacology (or any other preclinical content. There is no standardized pharmacology curriculum, nor a standardized way to present it in lecture or by way of a text. Nor are you all likely to have had questions written in a format that's common for other students. Some faculty (whether they are pharmacologists or from some other discipline) write scenario-based questions (in the so-called "board-style") and many still write questions in other formats (true-false, multiple correct answers, and so on).

Once you begin looking at my questions, and my answers to them, you may find that there is no explicit reference to one of the three cross-referenced texts I've cited. I'm sure, too, that many of you may find that the questions I ask, the way I ask them, or the answers I give, are different from what you have learned or how you learned it. They may be too clinical, or not mechanistic enough (or too mechanistic). They may address drugs you have not studied explicitly. Indeed, some questions may focus on drugs you haven't heard about at all (some drugs too new to make it into some of the older texts cited above are found below). That is, I have biases or preferences or areas I think are important to emphasize too.

Don't worry. Review, study, read, and learn as much as you can from the questions and the explanations. Keep in mind that content in an ostensibly circumscribed area (or book chapter, or lecture) can have significant ramifications on other areas. Appreciate the fact that in order to understand some concepts you have to integrate material from several disciplines or areas of pharmacology—and, of necessity, you may have to integrate material you have learned from such other basic biomedical disciplines as physiology, pathophysiology, biochemistry, molecular and cell biology, and many more.

Realize that whatever text or lecture material you have learned from, you may have to take whatever knowledge you have and apply it in new ways or in different situations.

This book is no guarantee for success on Step 1, or in your course exams. However, I humbly believe it is a great start for your study review and your ultimate success in learning the basics and being able to think about drugs in a holistic way.

Good luck.

Marshal Shlafer, PhD
Professor, Department
  of Pharmacology
Director of Undergraduate Medical
  Pharmacology Education
University of Michigan Medical School
Ann Arbor, Michigan

Cross-References to Selected Pharmacology Texts

"Brunton"—*Goodman & Gilman's the Pharmacological Basis of Therapeutics,* 11th Edition, L. Brunton, J. Lazo, and K. Parker, eds., McGraw-Hill, 2006.

"Craig"—*Modern Pharmacology with Clinical Applications,* 6th Edition, C. R. Craig and R. E. Stitzel, eds., Lippincott Williams & Wilkins, 2004.

"Katzung"—*Basic and Clinical Pharmacology,* 9th Edition, B. G. Katzung, ed., McGraw-Hill, 2004.

Explanations for the answers to the questions provided in this edition of *Pharmacology: PreTest* are cross-referenced to one or more of these pharmacology texts.

Each of these texts excels in certain respects, yet they do differ in terms of actual content and how it is presented. Look at the text cross-references in each of the Pre-Test questions and you'll see the differential focus. One text may be more mechanistic or more detailed; another may be more clinical; one may paint a discussion about certain drugs or drug groups, or a particular medical condition, with broader brush strokes than another.

Some texts address a particular point on several pages, another on one or two, and another might have no specific coverage at all. This is not surprising, and it parallels the way you were probably taught pharmacology: there is no one standard preclinical pharmacology curriculum for all the medical schools, and how the content may be presented at one school is likely to differ significantly from what one can find elsewhere.

List of Abbreviations and Acronyms

Here are some of the more common abbreviations you are likely to encounter either in this book or in your texts or lectures. I have omitted common symbols for chemical elements or their cationic or anionic forms (e.g., Ca, Cl), chemical formulae (e.g., NaCl), abbreviations of common biochemicals (ATP, ADP, DNA, etc.), units of measure (volume, weight, time), and Greek letters.

5-FU—5-fluorouracil
5-HT—5-hydroxytryptamine; Serotonin
ACE—angiotensin converting enzyme (also known as bradykininase, kininase II)
ACh—acetylcholine
AChE—acetylcholinesterase
AChEI—acetylcholinesterase inhibitor
ACS—acute coronary syndrome
ACTH—adrenocorticotropic hormone; corticotropin—adrenocorticotropic hormone
ADD/ADHD—attention-deficit (hyperactivity) disorder
ADH—antidiuretic hormone [vasopressin (VP)]
ADHD—attention deficit hyperactivity disorder
AF (AFIB)—atrial fibrillation
AFL—atrial flutter
AIDS—acquired immunodeficiency syndrome
ALG—antilymphocyte globulin
ANS—autonomic nervous system
ATPase—adenosine triphosphatase
AUC—area under the (blood concentration *vs.* time) curve
AV—atrioventricular
A-V—arteriovenous
B. fragilis—*Bacteroides fragilis*
BAL—British anti-Lewisite (dimercaprol)
BPH—benign prostatic hypertrophy
BPM—beats per minute
BUN—blood urea nitrogen
C_{av}—average (mean) plasma concentration
C_{max}—maximum plasma concentration
C_{min}—minimum plasma concentration
C_{ss}—steady-state plasma concentration
C. albicans—*Candida albicans*
C. botulinum—*Clostridium botulinum*
C. difficile—*Clostridium difficile*
C. neoformans—*Cryptococcus neoformans*
CAD—coronary artery disease
CCB—calcium channel blocker

CHD—coronary heart disease
CHF—congestive heart failure
CK—creatine kinase
Cl—clearance (of drug)
Cl^-—chloride
Cl_{total} — total body clearance
CNS—central nervous system
COMT—catechol-O-methyltransferase
COPD—chronic obstructive pulmonary disease
COX—cyclooxygenase(s); may be modified as COX-1 or COX-2
CRF—corticotropin-releasing factor
CSF—cerebrospinal fluid
CYP—cytochrome P450 (system or member of it)
D_1 or D_2—dopamine D_1 or D_2 receptor
DA—dopamine
DHT—dihydrotestosterone
DOPA—dihydroxyphenylalanine
DVT—deep venous thrombosis
ECG—electrocardiogram; EKG
E. coli—*Escherichia coli*
EDRF—endothelium-derived relaxing factor (nitric oxide)
EEG—electroencephalogram
EKG—electrocardiogram
EPI—epinephrine
ER—endoplasmic reticulum
EtOH—ethanol
FH_2—7,8-dihydrofolic acid
FH_4—5,6,7,8-tetrahydrofolic acid
FSH—follicle-stimulating hormone
FU—fluorouracil
G. lamblia—*Giardia lamblia*
G protein—guanine nucleotide-binding protein
GABA—γ-aminobutyric acid
G-CSF—granulocyte colony–stimulating factor
GERD—gastroesophageal reflux disease
GI—gastrointestinal
GM-CSF—granulocyte macrophage colony–stimulating factor
GnRH—gonadotropin-releasing hormone
GSH, GSSG—glutathione, reduced or oxidized
GU—genitourinary
H_1—histamine H_1 receptor
H_2—histamine H_2 receptor
H. influenzae—*Haemophilus influenzae*
H. pylori—*Helicobacter pylori*
Hb—hemoglobin

hCG—human chorionic gonadotropin
HF—heart failure
HDL—high-density lipoprotein
HIT—heparin-induced thrombocytopenia
HIV—human immunodeficiency virus
H^+, K^+, ATPase—hydrogen–potassium–adenosine triphosphatase; proton pump
hMG—human menopausal gonadotropin
HMG—CoA-β-hydroxy-β-methylglutaryl-coenzyme A
HRT—hormone replacement therapy
HTN—hypertension
IDDM—insulin-dependent diabetes mellitus, often called (not always appropriately) Type I diabetes mellitus
IgE, G (etc.)—immunoglobulin E, G, etc.
IL (-1, -2, etc.)—interleukin(s)-1, -2, etc.
IM—intramuscular(ly)
INH—isoniazid
IP_3—inositol-1,4,5-trisphosphate
IV—intravenous(ly)
k_e—elimination rate constant
K. pneumoniae—Klebsiella pneumoniae
L. pneumophilia—Legionella pneumophilia
L-dopa—levodopa
L-thyroxine (T_4)—levothyroxine
LDL—low-density lipoprotein
LHRH—luteinizing hormone–releasing hormone (hypothalamic)
LSD—lysergic acid diethylamide
LT—leukotriene
MAO—monoamine oxidase
MAO-A, -B—MAO type A, type B
MAOI—monoamine oxidase inhibitor
MI—myocardial infarction
mRNA—messenger ribonucleic acid
MTX—methotrexate
NE—norepinephrine
N_M receptors—nicotinic-skeletal muscle receptors (found at the skeletal-somatic neuromuscular junction)
N_N receptors—nicotinic-neural receptors (found in sympathetic ganglia and on cells of the adrenal (suprarenal) medulla)
N. gonorrhoeae—Neisseria gonorrhoeae
NADH—nicotinamide adenine dinucleotide
NADPH—nicotinamide adenine dinucleotide phosphate
Na^+, K^+, ATPase—sodium–potassium–adenosine triphosphatase
NAPA—N-acetylprocainamide
NE—norepinephrine
NIDDM—non-insulin-dependent diabetes mellitus; usually associated with Type II diabetes mellitus

NMDA—*N*-methyl-D-aspartate (glutamate channel)
NMS—neuroleptic malignant syndrome
NNRTI—nonnucleoside reverse transcriptase inhibitor
NPH—isophane (Neutral protamine Hagedorn) insulin
NRTI—nucleotide reverse transcriptase inhibitor
NSAID—nonsteroidal anti-inflammatory drug (nonopioid analgesic/antipyretic)
NTG—nitroglycerin
P450—the cytochrome P450 mixed-function oxidase system
P. aeruginosa—Pseudomonas aeruginosa
P. carinii—Pneumocystis carinii
P. falciparum—Plasmodium falciparum
P. mirabilis—Proteus mirabilis
P. vivax—Plasmodium vivax
PABA—*p*-aminobenzoic acid
PAC—premature atrial contraction
PAM (2-PAM)—pralidoxime
PAS—para-aminosalicylic acid
PDGF—platelet-derived growth factor
PG —prostaglandin
PGE_1—prostaglandin E_1 (alprostadil)
PGE_2—prostaglandin E_2 (dinoprostone)
PGI_2—prostaglandin I_2 (prostacyclin)
PNS—parasympathetic nervous system
PO—(administration route) by mouth (*per os*)
PO_2—partial pressure (tension) of oxygen, arterial
PPD—purified protein derivative of tuberculin
protein G—guanine nucleotide–binding protein
PTH—parathyroid hormone
PVC—premature ventricular contraction
RDA—recommended daily allowance
REM—rapid eye movement
6-MP— mercaptopurine
S. aureus—Staphylococcus aureus
S. haematobiu—Schistosoma haematobium
SA—sinoatrial
SAR—structure-activity relationship
SC—subcutaneous [administration route]
SH—sulfhydryl
SK—streptokinase
SR—sarcoplasmic reticulum
SRS-A—slow-reacting substance of anaphylaxis
SSRI—selective serotonin reuptake inhibitor
SVT—supraventricular tachycardia
$T_{1/2}$—half-life (e.g., biologic or plasma half-life) of a drug
T_3—triiodothyronine

T_4—thyroxine
TB—tuberculosis
TG—triglyceride(s)
TIA—transient ischemic attack
TNF—tumor necrosis factor
tPA— tissue plasminogen activator
TRH—thyrotropin-releasing hormone
tRNA—transfer ribonucleic acid
TSH—thyroid stimulating hormone
TX_{A2}—thromboxane A_2
UTI—urinary tract infection
V_d—volume of distribution
VIP—vasoactive intestinal peptide
vitamin B_1—thiamine
vitamin B_2—riboflavin
vitamin B_6—pyridoxine
vitamin C—ascorbic acid
vitamin D—calcitriol (metabolite [active form-1,25-$(OH)_2D_3$])
VLDL—very-low-density lipoprotein
VP—vasopressin (antidiuretic hormone [ADH])
VT (VTACH)—ventricular tachycardia

General Principles

Biotransformation
Development of new drugs
Dosage regimens and pharmaco-
   kinetic profiles
Dose-response relationships
Drug names and nomenclature
Drug receptor interactions

Factors affecting drug dosage
Molecular models of receptors and
   signal transduction mechanisms
Pharmacodynamics
Pharmacokinetics
Regulation by the Food and Drug
   Administration

Questions

DIRECTIONS: Each item contains a question or incomplete statement that is followed by several responses. Select the **one best** response to each question.

1. Azithromycin, an antibiotic, has an apparent volume of distribution (V_d) of approximately 30 L/kg. The best interpretation of this information is that azithromycin is which of the following?

a. Effective only when given intravenously
b. Eliminated mainly by renal excretion, without prior metabolism
c. Extensively distributed to sites outside the vascular and interstitial spaces
d. Not extensively bound to plasma proteins
e. Unable to cross the blood-brain or placental barriers

2. Experimental evaluation of the pharmacokinetics of a drug under development leads to the finding that it "undergoes significant first-pass hepatic metabolism." Which of the following administration routes was most likely used to reach this conclusion?

a. Intramuscular
b. Intravenous
c. Oral
d. Rectal
e. Sublingual (SL)

3. Two drugs act on the same tissue or organ *via* activation of different receptors, resulting in effects that are *qualitatively* the opposite of one another. An example would be the direct effects of norepinephrine and acetylcholine on heart rate. This represents which of the following types of antagonism?

a. Chemical
b. Competitive
c. Dispositional
d. Pharmacologic
e. Physiologic

4. We are repeatedly administering a drug orally. Every dose is 50 mg; the interval between doses is 8 h, which is identical to the drug's plasma half-life. The bioavailability is 0.5. For as long as we conduct the experiment no interacting drugs are added or stopped, and there are no patient-related factors (affecting such things as absorption or elimination) that might change the drug's pharmacokinetics.

Which of the following formulas gives the best estimate of how long it will take for the drug to reach steady-state serum concentrations (C_{ss})?

Abbreviations:
AUC: area under the concentration-time curve
Cl: clearance (mL/min)
D: dose (mg)
F: bioavailability (<1.0 for this drug given orally)
k_e: elimination rate constant
$t_{1/2}$: half-life (h)
V_d: volume of distribution

a. $(0.693 \times V_d)/Cl$
b. $1/k_e$
c. $4.5 \times t_{1/2}$
d. $(t_{1/2}) \times (k_e)$
e. $D/(F \times t_{1/2})$

5. We want to estimate, following drug administration, some measure that most reliably reflects the total amount of drug reaching the target tissue(s), over time. We're giving the drug orally. Which of the following would provide that measure best?

a. Area under the blood concentration-time curve (AUC)
b. Peak (maximum) blood concentration
c. Product of the V_d and the first-order rate constant
d. Time-to-peak blood concentration
e. V_d

6. Experiments show that 95% of an oral 80-mg dose of Drug X is absorbed in a 70-kg test subject. However, because of extensive biotransformation during its first pass through the hepatic portal circulation, the bioavailability was only 0.25 (25%). Assuming a liver blood flow of 1500 mL/min, which of the following is the hepatic clearance of Drug X in this situation?

a. 60 mL/min
b. 375 mL/min
c. 740 mL/min
d. 1110 mL/min
e. 1425 mL/min

7. A speaker at Grand Rounds is summarizing the literature on a very small subset of patients who develop acute hemolytic disease in response to drug therapy. The causative agents included common antimalarial drugs (chloroquine, quinine, and especially primaquine); cardiovascular drugs (hydralazine, procainamide, quinidine); and various antimicrobials (chloramphenicol, nitrofurantoin, sulfonamide antibiotics). Which of the following patient-related factors most likely accounts for their susceptibility to hemolysis?

a. Concurrently taking aspirin
b. Genetically based glucose 6-phosphate dehydrogenase (G6PD) deficiency
c. Primary renal disease
d. Recently received chemotherapy with vincristine
e. Serum cholinesterase deficiency

8. We are conducting pharmacokinetic studies on a new drug that we hope will be approved for clinical use. We insert a venous catheter to sample blood at various times after drug administration, and also take a sample for the immediate predrug blood level of the drug (which should be zero). After assaying the blood samples for the drug we make a graph that plots serum drug concentrations over time, continuing until tests reveal blood levels as undetectable. Which of the following is calculated as the ratio of the area under the curve (AUC) obtained by oral administration vs. the AUC for intravenous administration of the same drug?

a. Absorption
b. Bioavailability
c. Clearance
d. Elimination rate constant
e. Extraction ratio
f. Volume of distribution

9. We administer an acidic drug (A) with a pK_a of 3.4 orally. But pH is 1.4, and plasma pH is 7.4. Assume the drug crosses membranes by simple passive diffusion (e.g., no transporters are involved). Which of the following observations would be true?

a. Only ionized forms of the drug, A^-, will be absorbed from the gut into the plasma
b. The concentration ratio of total drug ($A + HA^-$) would be 10,000:1 (gut > plasma)
c. The drug will be hydrolyzed by a reaction with HCl, and so cannot be absorbed
d. The drug will not be absorbed unless we raise gastric pH to equal pK_a, as might be done with an antacid
e. The drug would be absorbed, and at equilibrium the plasma concentration of the nonionized moiety (HA) would be 10^4 times higher than the plasma concentration of A^-.

10. Identical doses of a drug are given orally (■) and intravenously (●), we sample blood at various times, measure blood concentrations of the drug, and plot the data (shown in the figure).

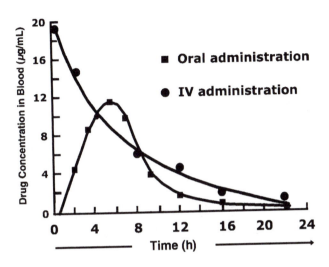

Further analysis of these data will allow us to determine which of the following?

a. Elimination route(s)
b. Extent of plasma protein binding
c. Oral bioavailability
d. Potency
e. Therapeutic effectiveness

11. The elimination of a drug is described as being heavily dependent on Phase II metabolic reactions. Which of the following is a Phase II reaction as far as drug elimination goes?

a. Glucuronidation
b. Deamination
c. Ester hydrolysis
d. Nitro reduction
e. Sulfoxide formation

12. We start intravenous infusion of a drug using a pump that ensures that the rate of drug delivery is constant over time. Which of the following factors determines how long it will take for the drug to reach a steady-state concentration (C_{SS}) in the blood?

a. Apparent volume of distribution
b. Bioavailability
c. Clearance
d. Half-life
e. Infusion rate (mg of drug/min)

13. Yee et al. (Effect of grapefruit juice on blood cyclosporine concentration; Lancet 345:955–956, 1995) examined several pharmacokinetic variables related to oral cyclosporine administration with water, grapefruit juice, and orange juice:

	Grapefruit Juice	Orange Juice	Water	p*
AUC (ng•h/mL)	7057 ± 2172	4871 ± 2045	4932 ± 1451	<0.0001
C_{max} (ng/mL)	1269 ± 381	972 ± 379	1080 ± 269	0.01
T_{max} (hr)	2.86 ± 0.77	2.57 ± 0.85	2.36 ± 0.63	0.14

The numbers listed are arithmetic means ± one standard deviation of the mean. C_{max} is the peak blood concentration, and T_{max} is the time after administration at which peak serum concentrations of the drug are reached. p values are based on analysis of variance (ANOVA) corrected for repeated measures.

These data, and what you should have learned from your basic pharmacology studies, are most consistent with the hypothesis that grapefruit juice does which of the following?

a. Acidifies the urine, favoring cyclosporine's tubular reabsorption via a pH-dependent effect
b. Activates an intestinal wall transporter for cyclosporine
c. Alters the route(s) of elimination for cyclosporine
d. Inhibits the first-pass metabolism of cyclosporine
e. Reduces binding of cyclosporine to plasma proteins, thereby raising free (active) drug levels in the circulation

14. A 60-year-old man with rheumatoid arthritis will be started on a nonsteroidal anti-inflammatory drug to suppress the joint inflammation. Published pharmacokinetic data for this drug include:

Bioavailability (F): 1.0 (100%)
Plasma half-life ($t_{1/2}$): 0.5 h
Volume of distribution (V_d): 45 L

For this drug it is important to maintain an average steady-state concentration 2.0 mcg/mL in order to ensure adequate and continued anti-inflammatory activity.

The drug will be given (taken) every 4 h.

What dose will be needed to obtain an average steady-state drug concentration of 2.0 mcg/mL?

a. 5 mg
b. 100 mg
c. 325 mg
d. 500 mg
e. 625 mg

15. We take a blood sample from a patient (baseline measurement) and then administer Drug A intravenously. We take additional blood samples periodically thereafter and measure drug concentration in each sample. We repeat the experiment, this time giving the same drug orally. Then we plot the logarithm of drug concentration vs. time with data from both administration routes, and find to comparable elimination "curves" indicative of first-order elimination. What do the slopes of the resulting concentration vs. time curves tell us best about the pharmacokinetics of Drug A?

a. Area under the curve (AUC)
b. Bioavailability
c. Elimination rate constant
d. Extraction ratio
e. Volume of distribution

16. We want to determine some important pharmacokinetic properties of a new aminoglycoside antibiotic that we're putting through preclinical testing. We give an IV dose (5 mg/kg) of the drug to a 70-kg volunteer, 19-years-old, who is healthy and taking no other drugs. After allowing time for redistribution and equilibration of the drug in various body compartments, we measure plasma concentrations at various times. The data are shown in the table and figure; assume that the drug is being eliminated at a rate that reflects typical first-order kinetics.

Time After Dosing Stopped (h)	Plasma Aminoglycoside Concentration (mcg/mL)
1.0	5.8
2.0	4.6
3.0	3.7
4.0	3.0
5.0	2.4
6.0	1.9
8.0	1.3

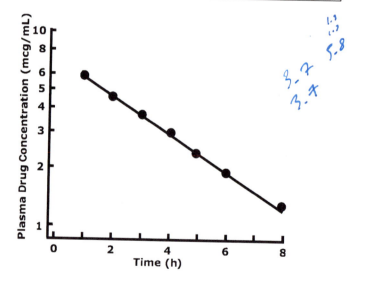

Which of the following values comes closest to the elimination rate constant (k_e) for this drug in this patient?

a. $0.15\ h^{-1}$
b. $0.22\ h^{-1}$
c. $0.33\ h^{-1}$
d. $0.60\ h^{-1}$
e. $1.13\ h^{-1}$

17. When we evaluate new drugs in preclinical testing, one of many things we'd like to know is whether it's largely confined to the vascular compartment (before it is eliminated) or distributes more widely. This is, of course, ultimately important to you, the clinician who may prescribe or administer the drug if it gets FDA approval. One way to get a handle on that is to calculate the apparent volume of distribution (V_d).

Using the data for the hypothetical aminoglycoside, shown in Question 16, which of the following values comes closest to the apparent V_d for this drug?

a. $0.62\ L$
b. $19\ L$
c. $50\ L$
d. $110\ L$
e. $350\ L$

18. When evaluating the effects of certain adrenergic agonists in a variety of *in vitro* and *in vivo* models, we find that the responses exhibit the phenomenon of tachyphylaxis. Which of the following best describes what the term tachyphylaxis means?

a. An increase in the rate of the response, for example, an increase of the rate of muscle contraction
b. Immediate hypersensitivity reactions (i.e., anaphylaxis)
c. Prompt conformational changes of the receptor such that agonists, but not antagonists, are able to bind and cause a response
d. Quick and progressive rises in the intensity of drug response, with repeated administration, even when the doses are unchanged
e. Rapid development of tolerance to the drug's effects

19. A postoperative patient will require prolonged analgesia. We choose a drug that has the following pharmacokinetic properties:

Half-life: 12 h
Clearance: 0.08 L/min
Volume of distribution: 60 L

The patient has an indwelling venous catheter with a slow drip of 0.9% NaCl, and we will use this to administer intermittent injections of the drug every 4 h. The target blood level of the drug, following each injection, is 8 mcg/mL.

With this plan in mind, which of the following comes closest to the dose that should be administered every 4 h?

a. 0.960 mg (or 1 mg)
b. 6.4 mg (or 6 mg)
c. 25.6 mg (or 25 mg)
d. 150 mg
e. 550 mg

20. A patient is experiencing severe postoperative pain, and we need to give a loading dose of an analgesic drug for prompt relief of discomfort. The drug we choose has the same pharmacokinetic properties as the one described in Question 19:

Half-life: 12 h
Clearance: 0.08 L/min
Volume of distribution: 60 L

Our target serum concentration for the drug is 8 mcg/mL. Which of the following comes closest to the correct loading dose?

a. 0.48 mg (rounded to 0.5 mg)
b. 150 mg
c. 320 mg
d. 480 mg
e. 640 mg

21. We administer a highly lipid-soluble drug and monitor its elimination *in vivo* and *in vitro*. All the data indicate that it is transformed to a variety of more polar metabolites by a group of heme proteins that activate molecular oxygen to a form that is capable of interacting with organic substrates such as our test drug. Which of the following is the most likely enzyme or enzyme system involved in the initial metabolism of our test drug?

a. Cyclooxygenase
b. Cytochrome P450s
c. Monoamine oxidase (MAO)
d. Nicotinamide adenine dinucleotide phosphate (NADPH)
e. UDP–glucuronosyltransferase

22. We measure the heart rate of a healthy subject under the folowing conditions, allowing ample time for return to baseline conditions and full elimination of drugs between each . . .

1. at rest
2. during treadmill exercise sufficient to activate the sympathetic nervous system at a time when maximum heart rate is reached
3. after administration of acebutolol, a drug with affinity for β-adrenergic receptors
4. after giving acebutolol, followed by exercise at the same level used in condition 2

Acebutolol given at rest causes a slight but consistent increase of heart rate. Give a bigger dose at rest and heart rate rises a bit more.

When the patient exercises after receiving a low dose acebutolol, heart rate rises significantly less than it did in the absence of acebutolol. With exercise after the higher dose of acebutolol, the tachycardia is blunted even more.

The figure summarizes the main findings.

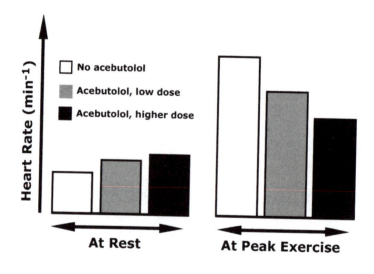

Which of the following statements best summarizes the actions of acebutolol?
a. Has higher affinity for adrenergic receptors than the endogenous agonists, epinephrine, and norepinephrine
b. Is a partial agonist for β-adrenergic receptors
c. Is activating spare receptors on myocardial cells
d. Is an irreversible or noncompetitive β blocker
e. Is changing conformation of the adrenergic receptors

23. We are planning to infuse a drug intravenously at a constant amount per unit time (rate). It has a first-order elimination rate constant (k_{el}) of 0.35 h^{-1}. No loading dose will be given. Approximately how long will it take for blood levels to reach steady state after the infusion begins?
a. 0.7 h
b. 1.2 h
c. 3.5 h
d. 9 h
e. 24 h

24. A patient who is supposed to be taking a drug once a day gets confused and for a couple of days takes excessive daily doses, leading to toxicity. The drug has a mean plasma half-life of 40 h.

Right now the patient's plasma concentration of the drug is 6 mcg/mL. Although what to do next will depend on actual blood tests for drug levels, the usual plan in this case is to have the patient skip one or several daily doses of the drug until blood levels first enter the therapeutic and nontoxic range, which in this case is 0.8 mcg/mL. How many daily doses should be withheld?
a. 1
b. 2
c. 3
d. 4
e. 5

25. We want to calculate the apparent volume of distribution (V_d) for a hypothetical drug (Drug A) that has a half-life of 4 h. All (100%) of an absorbed dose of this drug undergoes Phase I oxidation, followed by conjugation (Phase II reaction).

We rapidly inject a known dose, and 30 min later begin taking serial blood samples (30 min apart) and quantifying drug concentration in each sample. Which of the following information must we measure or otherwise determine to calculate V_d in the easiest possible way?

a. Area under the drug concentration-time curve (AUC)
b. Bioavailability
c. Clearance
d. Elimination rate constant (k_{el})
e. Maximum blood concentration immediately after the bolus injection (C_0)

26. A patient with a bacterial infection requires intravenous antibiotic therapy. The chosen drug has a clearance (*Cl*) of 70 mL/min. The apparent volume of distribution (V_d) is 50 L. The plan is to administer the drug intravenously every 6 h and achieve a 4-mg/L steady-state blood level of the drug. No loading dose strategy is to be used. Which of the following maintenance doses is needed to achieve this?

a. 14 mg
b. 24 mg
c. 100 mg
d. 300 mg
e. 1200 mg

27. We are working with a pharmacologically inert but easily measured substance, X. Its elimination shows linear kinetics (first-order plot of log drug concentration vs. time during elimination is a straight line). The plasma half-life is 30 min. Bolus IV doses well in excess of 100 mg must be given in order to saturate the enzymes responsible for metabolizing the drug, which will then lead to zero-order elimination kinetics.

We infuse a solution of X intravenously. The concentration of the solution is 2 mg/mL; the infusion rate is 1 mL/min and is kept constant at that. We continue the infusion for 24 h.

After allowing ample time for the drug to be eliminated completely, we repeat the administration. This time the concentration of the solution of X is 4 mg/mL, and we infuse it at a rate of 2 mL/min.

Which of the following other variables will also be changed as a result of the stated changes to the infusion protocol?

a. Elimination rate constant
b. Half-life
c. Plasma concentration when C_{ss} is reached
d. Time to reach steady-state concentration (C_{ss})
e. Total body clearance
f. Volume of distribution

28. A new drug, Drug A, undergoes a series of Phase I metabolic reactions before its metabolites ultimately are eliminated. Which of the following statements best describes the characteristics of Drug A, or the role of Phase I reactions in its metabolism or actions?

a. Complete metabolism of Drug A by Phase I reactions will yield products that are less likely to undergo renal tubular reabsorption
b. Drug A is a very polar substance
c. Drug A will be biologically inactive until it is metabolized
d. Phase I metabolism of Drug A involves conjugation, as with glucuronic acid or sulfate
e. Phase I metabolism of Drug A will increase its intracellular access and actions

29. Dopamine, epinephrine (or norepinephrine), and histamine are important neurotransmitter agonists. When these ligands interact with their cellular receptors, how do they mainly elicit their responses?

a. Activating adenylyl cyclase, leading to increased intracellular cAMP levels
b. Activating phospholipase C
c. Inducing or inhibiting synthesis of ligand-specific intracellular proteins
d. Opening or closing ligand-gated ion channels
e. Regulating intracellular second messengers through G protein–coupled receptors

30. The FDA assigns the letters A, B, C, D, and X to drugs approved for human use. To which of the following does this classification apply?

a. Amount of dosage reduction needed as serum creatinine clearances fall
b. Amount of dosage reduction needed in presence of liver dysfunction
c. Fetal risk when given to pregnant women
d. Relative margins of safety/therapeutic index
e. The number of unlabeled uses for a drug

31. The Food and Drug Administration has regulatory authority over prescription drugs, OTC drugs, and nutritional supplements (herbals and other so-called nutriceuticals). Such authority includes approval, marketing (advertising), and withdrawal of drugs from the market. Which of the following statements about these regulatory matters is correct?

a. Drugs approved for sale OTC first received FDA approval for sale and marketing "by prescription only"
b. If a pharmaceutical manufacturer provides data sufficient to obtain FDA approval for sale by prescription, the manufacturer is then allowed to sell the drug over-the-counter (OTC)
c. If the FDA approves a prescription drug for sale (prescribing), the MD can prescribe the drug only for the FDA-approved indication (use)
d. Nutritional supplements can be marketed without providing proof of efficacy or safety to the FDA
e. Phase III testing of prescription drugs that have been approved by the FDA gives complete information about adverse responses and pertinent drug-drug interactions

General Principles

Answers

1. The answer is c. (*Brunton, pp 14–16; Craig, pp 28–29, 51–52; Katzung, pp 34–38.*) For a 70-kg individual, total body water is about 40 L (0.6 L/kg); interstitial plus plasma water occupies about 12 L (0.17 L/kg).

Azithromycin, with a V_d of 30 L/kg, would be distributed in an apparent volume of about 2100 L in a typical 70-kg person.

Use simple logic to answer this question, but look at the answer to Question 17, if you wish. Even if you don't remember what total body water is (about 40 L or 0.6 L/kg), or the approximate value for interstitial plus plasma water (about 12 L or 0.17 L/kg), do the quick math. If you take the stated 30 L/kg and compute the total (and very hypothetical) apparent volume for a 70-kg individual, you would arrive at 2100 L. That number not only reflects distribution into a hypothetical volume far in excess of vascular and interstitial volumes, but is also far beyond what could be physically real. After all, 2100 L of water equals 2100 kg; you won't find human beings weighing that much!

Without more information, you cannot make definitive conclusions about the other properties listed as answer choices.

2. The answer is c. (*Brunton, pp 4, 11, 18; Craig, p 25; Katzung, pp 42–43.*) The first-pass effect is commonly considered to involve the biotransformation of a drug during its first passage through the portal circulation of the liver. Drugs that are administered orally enter the hepatic portal circulation first and can be biotransformed there, extensively, before reaching the systemic circulation. Typically, and sometimes significantly, this can reduce bioavailability and systemic blood concentrations of the drug. The net therapeutic consequence of first-pass metabolism depends on the drug. If hepatic metabolism inactivates a drug (as it often does), then serum levels and the magnitude of the effects will be reduced accordingly. However, if the orally administered drug is a prodrug (one that is inactive in the form administered, but is metabolized to one or more active metabolites), then the outcome will be greater activity due to greater bioavailability of the biologically active metabolite.

Administration by the intravenous, intramuscular, and sublingual routes usually allows the drug to attain effective concentrations in the systemic circulation, and to be distributed throughout the body before hepatic metabolism has had much of an impact on the administered dose "going in." Rectal administration also avoids the problems to a great degree since, for example, the inferior rectal vein flows into the inferior vena cava, bypassing the liver initially.

Finally, the lungs can subject some inhaled drugs to a significant "first-pass" effect, but such a situation is uncommon in the grander scheme of things.

3. The answer is e. (*Brunton, pp 35–38; Craig, pp 16–18; Katzung, pp 14–17.*) Physiologic, or functional, antagonism occurs when two drugs produce opposite effects on the same physiologic function by interacting with different types of receptors. A practical example of this, in addition to what is described in the question, is the use of epinephrine as a bronchodilator to counteract the bronchoconstriction that occurs when the parasympathetic nervous system releases ACh or when we administer bethanechol or an acetylcholinesterase inhibitor to a patient with asthma. ACh constricts airway smooth muscle by acting as an agonist on muscarinic receptors. Epinephrine relaxes airway smooth-muscle cells and dilates the bronchi, through its agonist activity on β_2-adrenergic receptors.

Chemical antagonism (a) typically is said to occur when two drugs combine with each other chemically and the activity of one or both is reduced or abolished. For example, dimercaprol chelates lead and reduces the toxicity of this heavy metal; and calcium in certain foods or beverages (e.g., milk) interacts with tetracycline antibiotics and reduces bioavailability.

Competitive antagonism (b) is one of the two main types of pharmacologic antagonism (d). It occurs when two compounds (drugs) compete for the same receptor site—both having affinity for the receptor, only one having efficacy (or one having much more efficacy than another with partial agonist activity). With competitive antagonism this is a reversible interaction (because both the agonist and the antagonist can dissociate from the receptor sites)—and a surmountable ("overcomeable") one. It is certainly the most common form of drug-drug antagonism when we think of often-used therapeutic agents. Thus, atropine (the prototype muscarinic receptor antagonist) antagonizes the effects of ACh on the S-A node by competing for the same population of receptors. Propranolol does the same with respect to antagonizing the β_1-stimulatory effects of epinephrine, norepinephrine, and such other β agonists on the heart.

Irreversible antagonism, the other main type of pharmacologic antagonism (d), generally results from the binding of an antagonist to the same receptor site as the agonist by covalent interaction or by a very slowly dissociating noncovalent interaction. An example of this antagonism is the blockade produced by phenoxybenzamine on α-adrenergic receptors, resulting in a long-lasting reduction in the ability of norepinephrine, epinephrine, or other sympathomimetics to activate the α-adrenergic receptors.

Dispositional antagonism (c) is a term sometimes used to describe the ability of one drug to enhance the elimination (and so reduce the serum levels and intensity of responses to) of another drug. Thus, it is mainly a pharmacokinetic interaction. Its most common basis involves one drug enhancing the metabolic inactivation and elimination of another drug. For example, phenytoin (anticonvulsant/antiepileptic drug) or rifampin induce the hepatic metabolic inactivation of warfarin, reducing (antagonizing) warfarin's anticoagulant activity by reducing its serum levels.

4. The answer is c. (*Brunton, pp 16–17; Craig, pp 49–51; Katzung, pp 44–46.*) This question, with its many variables and equations, was written intentionally to see whether you would take a needlessly complicated approach to a very straightforward concept. If you give doses of a drug repeatedly (and this works best when the dosing interval is identical to the drug's half-life) and hold every other pertinent variable constant (dose, route, elimination status, etc.) constant, you simply multiply the half-life by 4 or 5 (hence, our use of 4.5) to arrive at the approximate time until C_{ss}—the time at which "drug in = drug out"—is reached.

You can see in the figure that with repeated administration of a drug at intervals equal to the drug's half-life. Note that the *average serum concentration* (C_{av}) does not appear to "flatten-out," or reach a plateau, until at least four doses have been given.

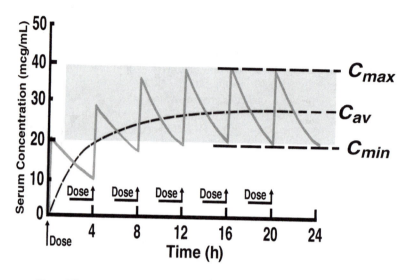

Note: The equation $(0.693 \times V_d)/Cl$ (answer a) is the equation for calculating the half-life.

5. The answer is a. (*Brunton, pp 17–21; Craig, pp 49–50; Katzung, pp 41–42.*) We obtain the AUC orally and compare that value with the AUC obtained with giving the same drug intravenously (where bioavailability is, by definition, 1.0). The fraction of a drug dose absorbed after oral administration is affected by a variety of factors that can strongly influence the peak blood levels and the time-to-peak blood concentration. The V_d and the total body clearance also are important in determining the amount of drug that reaches the target tissue. Only the area under the blood concentration-time curve, however, reflects absorption, distribution, metabolism, and excretion factors; it is the most reliable method of evaluating bioavailability overall.

6. The answer is d. (*Brunton, pp 17–21; Craig, pp 49–50; Katzung, pp 41–42.*) Bioavailability is defined as the fraction or percentage of a drug that becomes available to the systemic circulation following administration by any route. This takes into consideration that not all of an orally administered drug is absorbed and that a drug can be removed from the plasma and biotransformed by the liver during its initial passage through the portal circulation. A bioavailability of 25% indicates that only 20 mg of the 80-mg dose (i.e., 80 mg × 0.25 = 20 mg) reached the systemic circulation. Organ clearance can be determined by knowing the blood flow through the organ (Q) and the extraction ratio (ER) for the drug by the organ, according to the equation:

$$Cl_{organ} = Q \times ER$$

The extraction ratio is dependent on the amounts of drug entering the organ (arterial side; C_A) and leaving it on the venous side (C_V).

$$ER = \frac{(C_A \times C_V)}{C_A}$$

In this problem, the amount of Drug X entering the liver per unit time was 76 mg (80 mg × 0.95) and the amount leaving was 20 mg. Therefore,

$$ER = \frac{76 \text{ mg} - 20 \text{ mg}}{76 \text{ mg}} = 0.74$$
$$Cl_{liver} = (1500 \text{ mL/min}) (0.74) = 1110 \text{ mL/min}$$

7. The answer is b. (*Brunton, pp 85–88, 101–102; Katzung, p 1102.*) Keep the list of drugs/drug groups noted in the question on your short list of agents that can cause acute hemolysis/hemolytic anemia in patients with G6PD deficiencies, which is an X-linked monogenic trait that is present in about 10% of African-Americans and Caucasians with Mediterranean or Middle-Eastern origin. All the offending drugs can be considered pro-oxidants, and erythrocytes are particularly vulnerable to oxidative stress. Normal activity of G6PD normally protects against such damage by regulating levels of reduced glutathione (GSH), a main intracellular "antioxidant." Impair antioxidant mechanisms (such as via G6PD deficiency) and erythrocyte membranes become more fragile and prone to damage. G6PD deficiency is important to recall not only because of the prevalence of the polymorphism, and the clinical consequences of that for many drugs, but also because it is one of the first to be discovered and studied in the realm of genetically based differences in drug effects (pharmacogenomics).

Aspirin (a), *via* inhibition of cyclooxygenases and thromboxane A2 synthesis, obviously has antiplatelet effects (beneficial or deleterious, depending on the situation) and so can increase bleeding risks. It is not typically associated with acute hemolytic disease, however. There is no reason to suspect renal disease (c) as a cause of the described condition. At first glance chemotherapy using a variety of drugs that can cause bone marrow depression might be considered as a reasonable answer, but in reality it is not a good choice here: chemotherapy-induced bone marrow toxicity mainly affects leukocyte counts; and vincristine (d) is a cancer chemotherapeutic agent noteworthy for its lack of bone marrow toxicity. Serum cholinesterase activity (e), clearly genetically variable, is not responsible for metabolism of the drugs listed in the question. You should, however, recall that cholinesterase deficiencies are important clinically in terms of excessive and excessively prolonged responses to such substrates as succinylcholine.

8. The answer is b. (*Brunton, pp 12–22; Craig, pp 50–51; Katzung, pp 41–42.*) Among other things, knowing the AUC of a drug given intravenously (which, by definition, is associated with a bioavailability of 1.0, or 100%) is a prerequisite for knowing the bioavailability of the same drug given by any other route; bioavailability is calculated as the ratio of AUC for any non-IV route and the AUC_{IV}.

9. The answer is e. (*Brunton, pp 2–3; Craig, pp 20–22; Katzung, pp 7–8.*) Recall the two Henderson-Hasselbach equations, which apply to how local pH affects the ionization of molecules in an aqueous environment. And, recall, that all other things being equal, that we assume membranes are permeable only to nonionized (and lipid-soluble) forms of a drug:

For acidic drugs: $pH = pK_a \log [A^-]/[AH]$

For basic drugs: $pH = pK_a = \log [B]/[BH^+]$

Our drug was an acid with $pK_a = 3.4$. In the stomach (assume pH = 1.4 as noted) the ratio of nonionized to ionized molecules will be about 1:0.01. The nonionized molecules will diffuse across the membrane. Once in the plasma, pH 7.4, the ratio of HA:A⁻ will become 1:10,000. And the concentration ratio of total drug across the membrane will be 10:000:1, but with the larger amount being in the plasma, not the gut.

You might also want to look at the following figure to get a "big picture" of how changing pH changes the ionization of acidic and basic drugs.

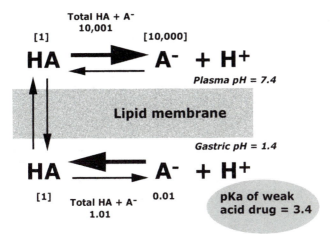

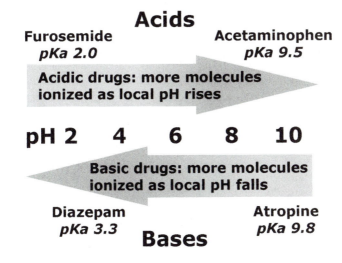

10. The answer is c. (*Brunton, pp 3–7; Craig, pp 50–51; Katzung, p 41.*)
We are making this data comparison to determine the drug's bioavailability. We define the bioavailability of a drug given intravenously as 1.0 (100%), since with IV administration we avoid all the applicable barriers

to drug absorption. But, of course, it's important to know how much total drug, over a period of time, gets into the bloodstream with other administration routes that we might want to use clinically. Drugs given by routes other than IV must be absorbed (and be exposed to all the barriers that limit or slow or otherwise affect absorption); and because they might not be absorbed from their administration site, or might be susceptible to such processes as hepatic first-pass metabolism, they usually have a bioavailability < 1.0.

The calculation of bioavailability is based on the ratio of the area under the concentration-time curve (AUC) for the administration route being considered (oral, IM, etc.) and the AUC obtained with IV administration:

Measurement of blood levels of a drug at a single time point will not give us the information we need to determine bioavailability.

Note that with oral absorption there is a delay until there is some detectable drug in the blood, which reflects both the time needed for absorption of the drug and, in most cases, the sensitivity of the assay to measure the drug (which may be present, but at undetectable levels). With IV administration blood levels rise instantaneously. With oral administration you should also note that as blood levels of the drug rise toward the peak the rates of drug entry into the blood exceed rates of elimination (whether by metabolism, excretion, or both, depending on what the drug is) because blood levels are rising. Once blood concentrations start to fall the amount of drug entering the system becomes less than the amount being eliminated, per unit time. That is, "amount in < amount out."

Finally—and although you can't tell precisely from the graph—the half-lives for the drug, measured under different experimental conditions, are identical: in general (and it depends on the drug and its blood level), the drug will be eliminated at the same rate (based on usual kinetic influences, such as first-order kinetics) regardless of administration route.

None of the other choices in the question (i.e., potency, effectiveness, or plasma protein binding) can be evaluated using this type of comparison.

11. The answer is a. (*Brunton, pp 71–80; Craig, pp 37–38; Katzung, pp 52–56.*) Biotransformation reactions involving the oxidation, reduction, or hydrolysis of a drug are classified as Phase I (or nonsynthetic) reactions; these reactions may result in either the activation or inactivation of a pharmacologic agent. There are many types of these reactions; oxidations are the most numerous. Phase II (occasionally called synthetic) reactions, which almost always result in the formation of an inactive product, involve conjugation of the drug (or its derivative) with an amino acid, carbohydrate, acetate, sulfate—or glucuronic acid as noted in the question. The conjugated form(s) of the drug or its derivatives may be more easily excreted than the parent compound.

12. The answer is d. (*Brunton, pp 12–18; Craig, pp 48–49; Katzung, pp 39; 44–46.*) With intravenous infusions of a drug, only the drug's half-life determines how long it will take for blood levels to reach a steady state (on average, neither rising nor falling thereafter) so long as the infusion rate is not changed. By definition, when steady state is reached, the amount of drug entering the blood per unit time is equal to the rate at which drug is being eliminated, whether by excretion, metabolism, or a combination of both (depending on the drug).

The apparent volume of distribution has no impact on time to C_{SS}. Bioavailability does not, either, because with intravenous drug administration the bioavailability is 1.0 (100%). Clearance, a parameter that relates elimination rate of a drug to the drug's concentration [Cl = rate of elimination (mg/h)/drug concentration (mg/mL)]. Because clearance considers a rate of drug elimination, it affects the C_{SS}, but it is not a determinant of it.

The infusion rate clearly affects the blood concentration reached at steady state, but it does not affect the time needed to reach C_{SS}. For example, if we had a drug with a half-life of 4 h, infused it at a rate of x mg/min, and then repeated the experiment with the same drug at an infusion rate of $2x$ mg/min, blood concentrations at steady state would clearly be different. However, it would still take the same amount of time (roughly 4–5 half-lives), to reach steady state.

13. The answer is d. (*Brunton, pp 78, 88; Craig, p 36; Katzung, p 62.*) Grapefruit juice (but not most other citrus juices) contains compounds (e.g., naringin, furanocoumarins) that can inhibit the metabolism of several drugs, one of which is cyclosporine, specifically *via* inhibitory effects on CYP3A4. The effect is especially important for hepatic metabolism of oral drugs that are susceptible to the first-pass effect and on CYP3A4. (Other drugs involved in this interaction include verapamil, some of the statin-type cholesterol-lowering medications; most of the second generation anti-histamines, including fexofenadine; and several antidepressants and antihypertensives.) The result is increased bioavailability of an orally administered dose and increased AUC. Peak and total (integrated over time) plasma levels of the interactant typically are increased, and one potential (if not likely) outcome is excessive (toxic) effects.

The "grapefruit juice effect" does not alter the main route(s) of drug absorption or elimination, nor affect plasma protein binding capacity, because those are properties related to the drug, not how—or how well or quickly—it enters the circulation. Note that these data are consistent with the hypothesis that grapefruit juice does not statistically significantly slow entry of cyclosporine entry into the blood; it is mainly an effect on "how much," not on "how fast."

14. The answer is d. (*Brunton, pp 14–22; Craig, pp 52–53; Katzung, pp 45–46.*) Here is how you solve the problem.

Note: It's easy to be misled by inconsistent use of units of measurement (mcg vs. mg, mL vs. L), so be sure you convert units as necessary.

First calculate the drug's elimination rate constant:

$$k_e = 0.693/t_{1/2} \quad \text{or}$$
$$k_e = 0.693/0.5 \text{ h} = 1.386/\text{h}$$

Then calculate the clearance:

$Cl = k_e \times V_d, \quad \text{or} \dots$

$Cl = 1.386/\text{h} \times 45 \text{ L}$, which equals 62.37 L/h, or 62,370 mL/h

Recall that $C_{ave} = (F/Cl) \times (\text{Dose}/t)$, where t represents the dosing interval (time; given as 4 h).

Rearrange to solve for the dose.

$$\text{Dose} = (C_{ave} \times Cl \times t)/F, \quad \text{or}$$
$$\text{Dose} = [(2 \text{ mcg/mL}) \times (62,370 \text{ mL/h}) \times 4 \text{ h}]/1.0$$

Thus, Dose = 499,000 mcg, or 499 mg (close enough to 500 mg).

15. The answer is c. (*Brunton, pp 14–22; Craig, pp 49–50; Katzung, pp 34–47.*) Regardless of which administration route has been used, if we plot the log of serum concentration of a drug vs. time (and assuming first-order kinetics, which applies to the elimination of most drugs when blood levels are therapeutic after initial redistribution), we get a straight line. It is described by the equation

$$\ln C = \ln C_0 - kt$$

The slope of this line, k, is the elimination rate constant.

An arguably more useful (and familiar) measure of the rate at which a drug is eliminated is the half-life ($t_{1/2}$). It is equal to $0.693/k$, and is defined as the time it takes for the concentration of a drug in the blood to fall to precisely one half of what it is now (or at any specified time).

The area under the curve (AUC) is the integration of a time vs. concentration plot for a drug. It is a linear—not a logarithmic or semilog—plot. One use for plots of AUC is to estimate one's "total exposure" to a drug, usually from "time zero" (instantaneously upon administration) until blood concentrations of drug are no longer reliably detectable or further measurements are impractical. The AUC can be used to estimate total body clearance of a drug, without the need to know the drug's volume of distribution or its half-life, since

$$\text{Clearance} = \frac{\text{Dose}}{\text{AUC}}$$

Determining AUC also enables us to calculate a drug's bioavailability. Bioavailability (F) is a measure of the fraction of an administered dose that is absorbed systemically and is detectable in the plasma. Note that when a drug is given intravenously, bioavailability is, by definition, 1.0 (100%), since there are no barriers that might prevent the absorption of drug from the administration site. So by administering a drug intravenously, and also giving it by another route, we can calculate bioavailability. For example, assume the other route we use is oral (PO).

$$\text{Bioavailability} = \left(\frac{\text{Dose}_{IV}}{\text{Dose}_{PO}}\right) \times \left(\frac{\text{AUC}_{PO}}{\text{AUC}_{IV}}\right)$$

If we do our bioavailability determinations by giving the same dose of the drug, the dosage units in the above equation cancel out, and so

$$\text{Bioavailability} = \frac{\text{AUC}_{PO}}{\text{AUC}_{IV}}$$

The extraction ratio (E) is a measure of a drug's removal from the blood as it passes through an organ (e.g., the liver) that can metabolize (or otherwise extract) it, for example, from the arterial to the venous side of that organ.

The rate of drug entry to an organ is the product of blood flow (Q) and the arterial concentration of the drug (C_A). The rate at which the drug leaves is flow × the venous concentration (C_V). If flow into and out of an organ are identical (as it often is), then the extraction ratio can be expressed as

$$E = \frac{(C_A - C_V)}{C_A}$$

We can also use the extraction ratio to calculate the organ clearance of a drug—i.e., the volume per unit time from which an organ removes a drug

Organ clearance = Blood flow × Extraction ratio

The volume of distribution (V_d) relates the amount of drug in the body to its concentration in the blood (or plasma). It is typically calculated as the administered dose divided by the concentration of drug in the blood

$$V_d = \frac{D}{C}$$

To simplify the assessment of the kinetics we typically give the drug intravenously (so we know how much drug enters the system—the entire dose, since bioavailability = 1.0) and measure the concentration immediately thereafter (or use a plot of the log of drug concentration vs. time), then extrapolate to find drug concentration at "time zero" (the y-axis intercept).

16. The answer is b. (*Brunton, pp 14–16; Craig, pp 48–50; Katzung, pp 40–41.*) The fractional change in drug concentration per unit of time for any first-order process is expressed by k_e. This constant is related to the half-life ($t_{1/2}$) by the equation $k_e t_{1/2} = 0.693$.

The units of k_e are time^{-1}, while the $t_{1/2}$ is expressed in units of time.

You need to know the half-life for this drug, and for the purpose of answering this question (remember, I asked you to pick the "closest to the correct value") you can see by inspection of either the table or the graph that the $t_{1/2}$ is about 3 h. Put that into the above equation; rearrange to solve for k_e, and get the answer:

$$k_e = \frac{0.693}{t_{1/2}} = \frac{0.693}{3.0 \text{ h}} = 0.23 \text{ h}^{-1}$$

$$k_e = 0.23 \text{ h}^{-1}$$

There are other mathematical approaches to arriving at the same answer. We showed an easy one here, but acknowledging the possibility that someone might expect a more sophisticated approach:

$$\log (A) = \log (A_0) - (k_e/2.303) \, (t)$$

where (A_0) is the initial drug concentration, (A) is the final drug concentration, t is the time interval between the two measurements of A, and k_e is the elimination rate constant. For example, by solving for k_e using the plasma concentration values at 2 and 5 h,

$$\log (2.4 \text{ mg/mL}) = \log (4.6 \text{ mg/mL}) - (k_e/2.303) \, (3 \text{ h})$$

k_e will equal 0.22 h^{-1}.

17. The answer is c. (*Brunton, pp 14–16; Craig, pp 51–52; Katzung, pp 40–42.*) The apparent V_d is defined as the volume of fluid into which a drug appears to distribute with a concentration equal to that of plasma, or the volume of fluid necessary to dissolve the drug and yield the same concentration as that found in plasma. By convention, we use the value of the plasma concentration at (or extrapolated to) zero time. In this problem, that is about 7 mcg/mL. Therefore, the apparent V_d is calculated as:

$$V_d = \frac{\text{Total amount of drug in the body}}{\text{Drug concentration in plasma at time zero}}$$

The total amount of drug in the body initially is the dose we gave (100% bioavailability, since we gave it IV), 350 mg (i.e., 5 mg/kg × 70 kg). The estimated plasma concentration at zero time is 7 mcg/mL (0.007 mg/mL). Putting these numbers in the equation yields the apparent V_d:

$$V_d = \frac{350 \text{ mg}}{0.007 \text{ mg/mL}} = 50,000 \text{ mL} = 50 \text{ L}$$

18. The answer is e. (*Brunton, pp 31, 162–163, 170–171.*) Tachyphylaxis is defined as rapidly developing tolerance to the effects of an agonist that is administered repeatedly, even if the subsequent dosages are not changed or they may actually be progressively increased. It is sometimes also called desensitization or down-regulation of the receptor(s). The mechanism behind the phenomenon varies, and to a degree depends on which drug (or agonist) is being used, and what the target (effector) is. For example, frequent and repeated exposure of receptors to a drug may change (at least temporarily) the conformation of the receptor to one that is less able to bind further drug. In systems that require quick synthesis of new receptors, repeated exposure to agonist may occur at such frequent intervals that there is inadequate time for new receptors to be made. Two good examples are the diminished response (of a variety of cells/tissues) to repeated administration of amphetamine, which acts by releasing neuronal norepinephrine. Challenge the system repeatedly and the amount of intraneuronal NE available to be released—which is essential for causing the ultimate response—goes down. Another example, with more clinical relevance, is the rapid development of "tolerance" of airway smooth muscles, and their ability to relax (i.e., cause bronchodilation) in response to repeated administration of β-adrenergic agonists, such as albuterol, arguably the most widely used adrenergic bronchodilator for asthma. This tolerance—often developing quickly enough to be called tachyphylaxis—is one of the pitfalls of managing asthma mainly with adrenergic bronchodilators, particularly if they are administered too often and at increasing dosages.

(Note: There is no "magical" number—hours or days, for example—that distinguishes between tachyphylaxis and "regular" tolerance. The brevity which the tolerance develops is the key point.)

19. The answer is d. (*Brunton, pp 12–29; Craig, pp 52–53; Katzung, pp 44–50.*) The dose to give equals the product of the target blood concentration and the drug's clearance.

$$D = C_{desired} \times Cl$$

To simplify things, let's get the units of volume the same for both clearance and concentration. The clearance of 0.08 L/min = 80 mL/min.
Therefore

$$D = 8 \text{ mcg/mL} \times 80 \text{ mL/min} = 640 \text{ mcg/min}$$

The stated dosing interval is 4 h, so

$$640 \text{ mcg/min} \times 60 \text{ min/h} \times 4 \text{ h} = 153{,}500 \text{ mcg}$$

which (rounded) is closest to 150 mg.

20. The answer is d. (*Brunton, pp 12–22.*) Here the loading dose (D) equals the product of the target blood concentration ($C_{desired}$) and the volume of distribution (V_d).

$$D = C_{desired} \times V_d$$

As always, convert units to make things consistent. The volume of distribution, 60 L, is, of course, 60,000 mL

$$D = 8 \text{ mcg/mL} \times 60{,}000 \text{ mL}$$
$$= 480{,}000 \text{ mcg}$$
$$= 480 \text{ mg}$$

21. The answer is b. (*Brunton, pp 72–78; Craig, pp 34–37; Katzung, pp 52–56.*) There are four major components to this *mixed-function oxidase* system: (1) cytochrome P450, (2) NADPH, or reduced nicotinamide adenine dinucleotide phosphate, (3) NADPH–cytochrome P450 reductase, and (4) molecular oxygen.

Cytochrome P450s catalyze a diverse number of oxidative reactions involved in drug biotransformation; it undergoes reduction and oxidation during its catalytic cycle. A prosthetic group composed of Fe and protoporphyrin IX (forming heme) binds molecular oxygen and converts it to an activated form for interaction with the drug substrate. Similar to hemoglobin, cytochrome P450 is inhibited by carbon monoxide. This interaction results in an absorbance spectrum peak at 450 nm, hence the name P450.

NADPH gives up hydrogen atoms to the flavoprotein NADPH-cytochrome P450 reductase and becomes NADP. The reduced flavoprotein transfers these reducing equivalents to cytochrome P450. The reducing equivalents are used to activate molecular oxygen for incorporation into the substrate, as described above. Thus, NADPH provides the reducing equivalents, whereas NADPH-cytochrome P450 reductase passes them on to the catalytic enzyme cytochrome P450.

Cyclooxygenase (a) involves two enzymes, I and II (COX-1 and 2) that metabolize endogenous arachidonic acid to prostaglandins, prostacyclins, and leukotrienes. Its substrate specificity is largely limited to the arachidonic acid cascade, not xenobiotics.

Monoamine oxidase (MAO; c) is a flavoprotein enzyme that is found on the outer membrane of mitochondria. It oxidatively deaminates short-chain monoamines only, and it is not part of the drug-metabolizing microsomal system. ATP is involved in the transfer of reducing equivalents through the mitochondrial respiratory chain, not the microsomal system.

UDP–glucuronosyltransferase, along with such enzymes as glutathione-S-transferase, methyltransferases, and N-acetyltransferases, are important in Phase II metabolism of various drugs. Substrates for these enzymes generally are drugs or xenobiotics that were previously transformed by Phase I reactions, such as the actions of the CYP450 mixed-function oxidases. These enzymes add a functional group to a substrate, rather than chemically modifying the original substrate via oxidation, reduction, deamination, and the like—all of which are responsibilities of the mixed-function oxidase systems.

22. The answer is b. (*Brunton, pp 24–26, 33–38, 272, 274t, 285; Craig, pp 113–114; Katzung, pp 16–17.*) Partial agonists have both the ability to bind to receptors (affinity), and the ability to evoke a response by activating those receptors (efficacy), albeit weakly, under basal conditions. Thus, when acebutolol is administered at rest (a condition under which endogenous catecholamine levels are low), heart rate rises slightly due to β_1-receptor activation via weak agonist activity. However, the occupation of adrenergic receptors by this weak agonist reduces the number of receptors available to bind and respond to stronger agonists (epinephrine, norepinephrine). As a result, the magnitude of the response to stronger agonists in the presence of the partial agonist is lower than in the absence of it (all other things being equal).

23. The answer is d. (*Brunton, pp 14–17; Craig, pp 48–50; Katzung, pp 40–47.*) With first-order elimination of a drug, we get a straight line if we plot the log of drug concentration in the blood vs. time. The slope of the line is the elimination rate constant (k_{el}). The drug's half-life—a value we will need to use momentarily—is related to k_{el} as follows: $t_{1/2} \times (k_{el}) = 0.693$. So, for the drug noted in the question, $t_{1/2} = 0.693/0.35$, or approximately 2 h. It takes approximately 4–5 half-lives to reach a steady-state blood concentration. Do the simple math and you will see that the time for this drug to reach steady state is approximately 8–10 h, and the answer given is therefore the best answer.

24. The answer is e. (*Brunton, 14–17; Craig, pp 48–50; Katzung, pp 38–41, 47.*) After a 40-h drug-free interval passes (about 1.67 days) the serum concentration of the drug will fall, as predicted by the half-life, to 3 mcg/mL to 1.5 mcg/mL 40 h after that; and to 0.75 mcg (now in the nontoxic range) after yet another 40 h passes. Thus we have to wait 120 h, or five daily doses skipped, to achieve our goal.

25. The answer is e. (*Brunton, pp 14–17; Craig, pp 48–52; Katzung, pp 40–47.*) You should recall that V_d = Dose/C_0. We know what the dose is. What we must calculate is the initial drug concentration (C_0)—the peak drug concentration that is reached "instantaneously" after giving the IV bolus dose. Unfortunately, we've waited 30 min before taking our first blood sample, but that is not a significant problem: plot the log of drug concentration vs. time and extrapolate to where the line intercepts the log-concentration axis (t_0). This gives us a good estimate of C_0. Plug the extrapolated C_0 into the equation and you have your answer.

Note that bioavailability is not a factor in this instance, because with IV administration bioavailability is 1.0 (100%). Knowing or calculating the elimination rate constant won't help either, because it is inextricably linked to the half-life, which we already know as $k_{el} = 0.693/t_{1/2}$ (and you can rearrange the equation easily).

Calculating the AUC (concentration vs. time integral) with a bolus injection will give us no information more useful than what we already have. Clearance (generally referring to renal clearance) is irrelevant in this situation: we've stated that the drug is completely metabolized to other products; thus, there is no Drug A to measure in the urine.

26. The answer is c. (*Brunton, pp 18–22; Craig, pp 52–53; Katzung, pp 35, 41–47.*) The scenario above makes calculations relatively straightforward, particularly because no loading dose therapy will be used.

Steady-state blood levels occur when the rate of "drug in" equals the rate of "drug out." The volume of distribution, given in the question, is irrelevant for the calculations.

The rate of drug out is given as a $Cl = 70$ mL/min.

Recall that the Dose $(D) = Cl \times C_{SS}$

Therefore, with a little rearranging, the dose can be computed as: Desired plasma level (4 mg/L) $\times Cl$ (70 mL/min).

Convert the units so they're consistent for both variables, and don't forget to calculate how many minutes there are in the dosing interval, 6 h. Now, the rest of the math:

The target blood level of 4 mg/L is the same as 4 mcg/mL, and this is a reasonable change of volume units to make for subsequent calculations, since clearance is given in units of mL/min.

$$4 \text{ mcg/mL} \times 70 \text{ mL/min} = 280 \text{ mcg/min} = 0.28 \text{ mg/min.}$$

And since the drug will be given every 6 h:

0.28 mg/min $\times$ 60 min/h $\times$ 6 h = 100.8 mg (closest answer is 100 mg) every 6 h.

27. The answer is c. (*Brunton, pp 18–22; Craig, pp 48–52; Katzung, pp 34–43.*) Only the drug concentration at steady state will change (it will be greater with this altered protocol). Do not be misled by the numbers. The time to reach C_{SS} with a constant drug infusion is a function of half-life (or the elimination rate constant, which is related to it: $k_{el} = 0.693/t_{1/2}$), and that will not change under the conditions stated. Likewise, with the vast majority of drugs eliminated by first-order kinetics, there will be no change of total body clearance or of volume of distribution. (Note: We described Substance X as being pharmacologically inert simply so you didn't conjure up confounding but largely irrelevant issues, such as an active drug that is able to cause residual or long-lasting effects on its elimination or elimination rate, for example, a drug that caused long-lasting induction of hepatic drug-metabolizing enzymes.)

28. The answer is a. (*Brunton, pp 72–77; Craig, pp 34–37; Katzung, pp 52–56.*) Phase I metabolic reactions generally convert (via addition or unmasking of such polar functional groups as $-NH_2$ or $-OH$ through, say, oxidations, reductions, or deamination) very nonpolar (i.e., very lipid-soluble) drugs into more polar (more water-soluble) metabolites. Among other things, polar metabolites of drugs in general are less likely to undergo tubular reabsorption; thus, it can be said that Phase I reactions play a role in forming metabolites that are "more easily excreted." If Drug A, the parent drug, was already very polar (answer b), there would be little need for Phase I metabolism. There is no reason to assume that Drug A will lack intrinsic biological activity (answer c); and because it is quite lipid-soluble to begin with, once in the circulation it should have good ability to diffuse across membranes and reach intracellular sites (hence, e is incorrect). Finally, note that those reactions described as Phase II are the ones that further increase polarity (water-solubility) of some drugs via forming conjugates with glucuronic acid or sulfate.

29. The answer is e. (*Brunton, pp 28, 49–56, 323–326, 334; Craig, pp 11–12, 98–100; Katzung, pp 16–27.*) The key concept is that these very important agonists, and many others, "transduce" their signals and eventually change a characteristic of cell function (cause a response) through G proteins—a family of guanine nucleotide-binding proteins. These ligands bind to the extracellular face of the transmembrane protein. The various G proteins (e.g., Gi, Gq, Gs) bind to intracellular portions of the receptor. They then couple the initial ligand interaction to the eventual response through a series of effector enzymes or enzyme systems that are G protein-regulated.

For example, adenylyl cyclase can be activated, catalyzing the formation of cAMP that then activates one or several kinases that phosphorylate specific intracellular proteins. But the actual steps that occur after ligand binding depend on what the ligand is, what specific G protein is involved, and which kinases are activated and what proteins they phosphorylate. And what happens (i.e., what the response is) depends on all of the above and, of course, which cell type is being affected.

Activation of adenylyl cyclase and increased cAMP levels may occur in one system, but the opposite may occur in another. Some signal transduction pathways involve phospholipase C, others do not. A calcium channel may be affected in one system and a potassium channel (or no ion channel) in others.

By way of review, recall that there are three other main mechanisms or pathways for signal transduction about which we have reasonable knowledge.

One mechanism or pathway uses a receptor protein that spans the cell membrane, but G proteins are not involved. On the inner membrane face it possesses enzymatic activity that is regulated by the presence or absence of ligand bound to the extracellular face of the protein. The tyrosine kinase pathway is an example, and the overall pathway is responsible for the activity of various growth factors, including insulin.

Another mechanism is used by very lipid-soluble ligands that cross cell membranes easily and act on some intracellular receptor. For example, glucocorticosteroids ultimately act in the nucleus and, through interaction with heat-shock protein (hsp90), eventually alter transcription of specific genes.

The third involves transmembrane ion channels, the "open" or "closed" states of which are controlled by ligand binding to the channel. This process applies to some of the important neurotransmitters, especially those in the brain (GABA, the main inhibitory neurotransmitter) and such amino acids as glycine, which exert "excitatory" actions. The nicotinic receptor for ACh fits in this category too.

30. The answer is c. (*Craig, p 382; Katzung, pp 68–70, 996–998.*) These are "pregnancy classifications." Drugs in Category A have been evaluated in controlled clinical studies in all trimesters, in humans, and they are deemed safe enough to pose only a remote risk of fetal harm. With categories B, C, and D, there is increasing evidence, whether from animal or human studies (or both), of risks and of the general risk-benefit ratio. Drugs in Category D have demonstrable risk, but may be used when, for example, the purpose is to manage a life-threatening condition and no safer alternatives are available. Notice of these pregnancy classification must be included in the package insert's Warning section, when necessary. Classification X means proven fetal harm, and the fetal risks from administering the drug usually far exceed the potential benefits to the mother.

31. The answer is d. (*Brunton, pp 131–135; Craig, pp 785–787; Katzung, pp 65–73.*) One of the most controversial (if not mind-boggling) aspects of marketing herbals, nutritional supplements, and other "nutriceuticals," is that manufacturers and sellers have to provide no prior or scientific proof of safety or efficacy to the FDA—something that must be provided, and with abundant and scientifically sound data, before the FDA will approve a drug for sale by prescription. Herbals, for example, came under the umbrella of the Dietary Supplement Health and Education Act (DSHEA) of 1994.

Such products, you may have noted, come with labels that state "serving size," rather than dose, as if we are going to be ingesting some carrots instead of a potentially active and dangerous drug.

Sellers of such products as herbals cannot make explicit claims that their products will prevent, diagnose, treat, or cure any disease. DHSEA allows a seller of a nutritional supplement to say such obtuse things as "boosts your memory," or "improves urinary tract health," but they cannot state "helps prevent or treat Alzheimer's disease" or "reduces urinary frequency and nocturia if you have benign prostatic hypertrophy." In fact, DSHEA simply requires that the label on the product states, in essence, that the FDA hasn't evaluated any of the claims the manufacturer has made, plainly or implicitly, on the label.

Moreover, while a drug company must provide and pay for the obligatory preclinical and clinical studies before a prescription drug gets the OK, if there is a reason or attempt to pull a nutriceutical from the market the FDA must do the work and pay the costs to prove that the product is unsafe or ineffective.

OTC drugs needn't be preapproved by the FDA as prescription drugs (answer a). While such prior approval is the trend, if not the norm (e.g., consider many antihistamines for allergy or insomnia; or drugs that inhibit gastric acid secretion being marketed for "heartburn" or "acid indigestion"), consider aspirin. It's been available OTC for decades and for its common uses (pain, fever, inflammation) it has never gotten an FDA blessing. Indeed, some say that if aspirin was being considered for approval as a prescription drug today, it would not be approved because of the risks of serious adverse responses (e.g., bleeding tendencies from antiplatelet effects; bronchospasm in many asthmatics) and drug-drug interactions. Nonetheless, we have many OTC drugs nowadays that first got approval for sale by prescription only . . . antihistamines, inhibitors of gastric acid secretion (noted above), and others. Approval for OTC sale was petitioned by the manufacturer, and then approved only after reviews by and recommendations from FDA expert advisory panels.

Answer c is incorrect. Once a drug gets approval for sale and use as a prescription drug, and for a given indication (or more, depending on data submitted and approved), the physician can prescribe that drug for any (reasonable) purpose for which he or she thinks is appropriate, safe, and effective. Physicians and scientists learn or hypothesize about new uses for a drug, conduct clinical studies, and overall can legally prescribe drugs for the off-label or unlabeled uses.

Phase III testing of drugs is conducted in usually no more than 5000 patients with a disease for which the drug is to be marketed. The main goal is to assess effectiveness for the stated use; and for overall safety. These are rather tightly controlled studies. The number of subjects, and the conditions in which the drug is given, are quite different from what happens in the "real world"—including Phase IV, which is the postmarketing surveillance phase of drug approval, where tens or hundreds of thousands of patients may get the drug in largely uncontrolled circumstances. Many drugs have come (been FDA-approved) and gone (pulled from the market because of adverse reactions or interactions, including those leading to death) because of what we've learned *after* the drug was approved by the FDA.

The Peripheral Nervous Systems: Autonomic and Somatic

Adrenergic agonists
Adrenergic antagonists
Cholinergic agonists
Cholinergic antagonists

Ganglionic blockers
Monoamine oxidase inhibitors
Skeletal muscle relaxants
Skeletal neuromuscular blockers

Questions

DIRECTIONS: Each item contains a question or incomplete statement that is followed by several responses. Select the **one best** response to each question.

Questions 32–37

[Note: The first seven questions in this chapter are based on a schematic diagram of the peripheral nervous system. I think this approach is the most appropriate, efficient, and briefest way to help you assess, or clarify, some essential "high yield" aspects of autonomic anatomy, (neuro)physiology, and pharmacology based on a few main "rules" and key exceptions to them. I hope this approach will be beneficial.]

The diagram shows, in schematized fashion, the main efferent pathways in the peripheral nervous systems—the autonomic (parasympathetic and sympathetic; PNS, SNS, respectively) and somatic nervous systems—"from the CNS/spinal cord (at the far left, not labeled) out" to peripheral target (effectors).

Those nerves are:

a. Preganglionic parasympathetic
b. Postganglionic parasympathetic
c. Preganglionic sympathetic
d. Postganglionic sympathetic to structures other than sweat glands
e. "Preganglionic" (functional equivalence) sympathetic to the adrenal (suprarenal) medulla
f. Preganglionic sympathetic, sweat gland innervation
g. Postganglionic sympathetic to sweat glands
h. Motor nerve, somatic nervous system

Schematic of Efferent Pathways in the Peripheral Nervous Systems

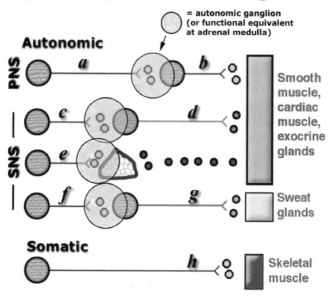

32. Anatomic, neurochemical, and pharmacologic studies of *nerves a, c, e, f,* and *h* indicate that they share one common property that is important to your understanding of peripheral nervous system pharmacology. Which of the following statements best summarizes what that property is?

a. Are cholinergic, activate postsynaptic nicotinic receptors
b. Are adrenergic, but receptor type on target cell depends on what/where the cell is
c. Cannot release their neurotransmitter(s) in the presence of atropine
d. Have the ability to directly activate all the adrenergic and all the cholinergic receptors
e. Recycle their neurotransmitter after each action potential, rather than synthesizing new transmitter *de novo*

33. Similar multidisciplinary assessments of *nerve d*, a "typical" postganglionic sympathetic nerve, indicate that it is quite different from all the other nerves shown in the schematic of the peripheral nervous systems. Which of the following statements accurately describes that difference?

a. Atropine selectively blocks activation of receptors by the neurotransmitter released from *nerve d*
b. It causes bronchodilation (airway smooth muscle relaxation) when it is activated
c. It is adrenergic (or noradrenergic if you wish to use that term instead)
d. The primary neurotransmitter synthesized by *nerve d* is epinephrine
e. When *nerve d* is physiologically activated by an action potential, actions of its released neurotransmitter are terminated mainly by hydrolysis in the synaptic cleft

34. Reuptake (into the nerve) is the main physiologic process for terminating the postsynaptic activity of a peripheral nervous system neurotransmitter. To which nerve does this process apply?

a. a
b. b
c. c
d. d
e. e
f. f
g. g
h. h

35. *Nerve d*, the typical postganglionic sympathetic nerve, is activated by a normally generated action potential. On which of the following receptor types does the neurotransmitter it releases act?

a. α_1 Adrenergic
b. α_2 Adrenergic
c. β_1 Adrenergic
d. β_2 Adrenergic
e. Muscarinic
f. Nicotinic
g. It depends on the target tissue (effector) type

36. Your studies also reveal that something is unique about *nerve g*, the postganglionic fibers that innervate sweat glands. Which of the following descriptive phrases best identifies that difference?

a. Cocaine blocks release of its neurotransmitter
b. Is adrenergic
c. Is cholinergic, but anatomically and functionally part of the SNS
d. Its neurotransmitter acts on nicotinic receptors
e. Uses epinephrine as its neurotransmitter

37. *Nerve g*, the postganglionic nerve innervating sweat glands, is activated by a normally generated action potential. On which of the following receptor types does the neurotransmitter it releases act?

a. α_1 Adrenergic
b. α_2 Adrenergic
c. Muscarinic
d. Nicotinic
e. β_1 Adrenergic
f. β_2 Adrenergic

38. Assume that all the efferent pathways in the schematic are tonically active (a quite reasonable assumption), even if at low levels. We add tubocurarine or pancuronium to the system, and as expected it blocks neurotransmitter activation of certain structures. Which of the following nerves innervates those structures and normally activates them in the absence of these or similar drugs?

a. a
b. b
c. c
d. d
e. e
f. f
g. g
h. h

Questions 39–45

The figure shows some of the main elements of norepinephrine (NE) synthesis, release, actions, and other steps in adrenergic neurotransmission. You do not need the diagram to answer this series of questions, but I do not think that showing it gives you an unfair advantage—just a little memory jolt and the "big picture"—that may aid your answering or reviewing. Note that the effector (target) cell on the far right will have either an α-adrenergic receptor *or* a β-adrenergic receptor, depending on what the effector cell is.

Adrenergic Neuroeffector Junction

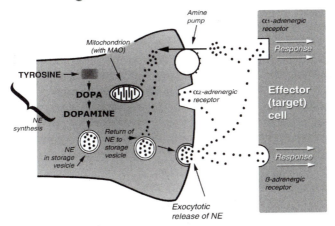

39. Mitochondria in the terminus of adrenergic nerve endings contain an abundance of monoamine oxidase (MAO). Which of the following best summarizes the biological role of that enzyme at that site?

a. Drives storage vesicles that contain NE to the nerve "ending" so that exocytotic release can occur in response to an action potential
b. Metabolically degrades NE that is free (not stored in vesicles) in the nerve terminal
c. Metabolizes dopamine to NE
d. Provides metabolic energy for nonexocytotic release of NE in response to amphetamines and other catecholamine-releasing drugs
e. Synthesizes ATP that is required to transport free intraneuronal NE into the storage granules/vesicles

40. Ultrastructural studies, combined with suitable histochemical techniques, show that the bulk of NE in the normal resting adrenergic neuron is stored in membrane-bound vesicles or granules. We administer a drug that, over time, depletes this supply of neurotransmitter and decreases the responses to sympathetic nerve activation. *In vitro* studies with chromaffin cells (dispersed cells from the suprarenal medulla) reveal that the drug acts by inhibiting uptake of the NE into the vesicles; it has no direct effect on catecholamine synthesis. Which of the following drugs fits this description best?

a. Pargyline
b. Prazosin
c. Propranolol
d. Reserpine
e. Tyramine

41. A substance abuser self-administers cocaine and experiences a variety of significant changes in cardiovascular function, in addition to the CNS-stimulating effects for which the drug is used. Which of the following is the most likely mechanism by which the cocaine causes its main peripheral and CNS effects?

a. Activation of α_2-adrenergic receptors leading to increased NE release
b. Blockage of NE reuptake via the amine pump
c. Direct activation postsynaptic α- and β-adrenergic receptors, leading to sympathomimetic (adrenomimetic) responses
d. Inhibition of MAO, leading to increased intraneuronal NE levels
e. Prevention of NE exocytosis

42. We administer a drug that is a selective agonist at the presynaptic α-receptors (α_2) in the peripheral sympathetic nervous system. It has no effect on α_1 receptors, β receptors, or any other ligand receptors that are important in peripheral nervous system function. Which of the following is the only response that is likely to occur?

a. Activation of NE exocytosis
b. Activation of the amine pump, stimulation of NE reuptake
c. Inhibition of dopamine β-hydroxylase, the enzyme that converts intraneuronal dopamine to NE
d. Inhibition of NE release in response to an action potential
e. Stimulation of intraneuronal MAO

43. We administer a therapeutic dose of a drug that selectively and competitively blocks the postsynaptic α-adrenergic ($α_1$) receptors. It has no effects on presynaptic α-adrenergic receptors ($α_2$) or β-adrenergic receptors found anywhere in the periphery, whether as an agonist or antagonist. Which of the following is the most likely drug?

a. Ephedrine
b. Labetalol
c. Phentolamine
d. Phenylephrine
e. Prazosin

44. Oxybutynin is indicated for the treatment of overactive bladder, reducing the symptoms of "urge incontinence," urinary urgency, and frequent urination. It prevents physiologic activation of the bladder's detrusor and simultaneously prevents relaxation of the sphincter. Side effects include constipation, dry mouth, blurred vision, photophobia, urinary retention, and slight increase in heart rate. The manufacturer also advises: "Heat stroke and fever due to decreased sweating in hot temperatures have been reported." Oxybutynin has no direct effect on blood vessels that might change blood pressure. Based on this information, which of the following prototype drugs is most like oxybutynin?

a. Atropine
b. β-Adrenergic blockers (e.g., propranolol)
c. Isoproterenol
d. Neostigmine
e. Phentolamine

45. A morbidly obese person visits the local bariatric (weight loss) clinic seeking a pill that will help shed weight. The physician prescribes dextroamphetamine. In addition to causing its expected centrally mediated anorexigenic (appetite-suppressant) effects it causes a host of peripheral adrenergic effects that, for some patients, can prove fatal. Which of the following best summarizes the main mechanism by which dextroamphetamine, or amphetamines in general, cause their peripheral autonomic effects?

a. Activates MAO
b. Blocks NE reuptake via the amine pump/transporter
c. Displaces, releases, intraneuronal NE
d. Enhances NE synthesis, leading to massive neurotransmitter overproduction
e. Stabilizes the adrenergic nerve ending by directly activating $α_2$ receptors

46. We administer a pharmacologic dose of epinephrine and observe (among other responses) a direct increase of cardiac rate, contractility, and electrical impulse conduction rates. Which of the following adrenergic receptors was responsible for these direct cardiac effects?

a. α_1
b. α_2
c. β_1
d. β_2
e. β_{3a}

47. A patient receives echothiophate during eye surgery. Which of the following enzymes is affected by this autonomic drug?

a. Tyrosine hydroxylase—stimulated
b. Acetylcholinesterase (AChE)—inhibited
c. Catechol-O-methyltransferase (COMT)—inhibited
d. Monoamine oxidase (MAO)—stimulated
e. DOPA decarboxylase—stimulated

48. We want to prescribe scopolamine, as a transdermal drug delivery system (skin patch), for a patient who will be leaving for an expensive cruise and is very susceptible to motion sickness. Which of the following comorbidities would weigh against prescribing the drug because it is most likely to pose adverse effects—or be truly contraindicated?

a. Angle-closure (narrow-angle) glaucoma
b. Bradycardia
c. History shellfish allergies
d. Resting blood pressure of 112/70
e. Hypothyroidism, mild
f. Parkinson's disease (early onset, not currently treated)

49. We have a patient with essential hypertension, and unusually high circulating catecholamine levels. Our goal is to block both α- and β-adrenergic receptors using just one drug. Which of the following is capable of doing that?

a. Labetalol
b. Metoprolol
c. Nadolol
d. Pindolol
e. Timolol

50. A man who has been "surfing the Web" in search of an aphrodisiac or some other agent to enhance "sexual prowess and performance" discovers yohimbine. He consumes the drug in excess and develops symptoms of toxicity that require your intervention. You consult your preferred drug reference and learn that yohimbine is a selective α_2-adrenergic antagonist. Which of the following should you expect as a response to this drug?

a. Bradycardia
b. Bronchoconstriction
c. Excessive secretions by exocrine glands (salivary, lacrimal, etc.)
d. Hypertension
e. Reduced cardiac output from reduced left ventricular contractility

51. A patient with Alzheimer's disease is taking an acetylcholinesterase inhibitor specifically approved for that indication, primarily because it is quite lipophilic and so enters the CNS well. Which of the following drugs is the patient most likely receiving?

a. Tacrine
b. Edrophonium
c. Neostigmine
d. Pyridostigmine
e. Ambenonium

52. A child overdoses on a drug that affects both the autonomic and somatic nervous systems. As blood level of the drug rises he experiences hypertension and tachycardia, accompanied by skeletal muscle tremor. Further elevations of the drug cause all the expected signs and symptoms of autonomic ganglionic blockade, plus weakness and eventual paralysis of skeletal muscle. Which of the following drugs did the child most likely ingest?

a. Bethanechol
b. Nicotine
c. Pilocarpine
d. Scopolamine
e. Tubocurarine

53. Review of a patient's chart reveals that two years ago she was treated with ritodrine. Which of the following was the most likely condition or reason for which this drug was given?

a. Parkinson's disease
b. Bronchial asthma
c. Depression
d. Hypertension
e. Premature labor

54. A patient receives bethanechol after abdominal surgery. Her heart rate falls slightly and she experiences some wheezing. Which of the following best accounts for or explains these cardiac and pulmonary responses?

a. Expected side effects
b. Idiosyncrasy
c. Parasympathetic ganglionic activation
d. Reflex (baroreceptor) suppression of cardiac rate
e. Undiagnosed asthma

55. A 35-year-old man who weighs 150 pounds and is 5 feet 10 inches tall is transported to the emergency department in severe distress. He complains of episodes of severe, throbbing headaches, profuse diaphoresis, and palpitations. Eighteen months ago his physician told him he is healthy except for what is assumed to be Stage 2 essential hypertension, but he refused medication and has not seen a health care provider for the last year and a half. He denies use of any drugs, whether prescription or over-the-counter, legal or otherwise.

Assessment now reveals that he is tachycardic and has an irregular pulse (sinus tachycardia, with occasional premature ventricular beats, are noted on his EKG). Heart rate at rest is approximately 130 beats/min, sometimes more. His resting blood pressure is approximately 200/140 mm Hg. These cardiovascular findings are shown in the figure.

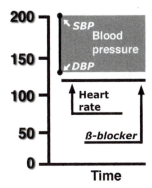

The first year house officer who is caring for this patient knows that all the orally effective β-adrenergic blockers are approved for use to treat essential hypertension, and concludes that prompt lowering of blood pressure is essential for this patient. Therefore, he orders intravenous administration of propranolol (at the arrow, in the figure), and a large dose of the drug since the symptoms seem severe.

Unknown to the MD is the fact that the patient's signs and symptoms are due to a pheochromocytoma (epinephrine-secreting tumor of the adrenal/suprarenal medulla).

Which of the following statements best describes the most likely ultimate outcome of administering this β blocker (or any other β blocker that lacks α-blocking activity), supplemented with no other medication, to this patient with an undiagnosed pheochromocytoma?

a. Heart failure, cardiogenic shock, death
b. Long-lasting normalization of heart rate, contractility, and blood pressure
c. Normalization of blood pressures but persistence of tachycardia
d. Restoration of normal sinus rate and rhythm, but no change of blood pressure from predrug levels.
e. Sudden and significant rise of systolic blood pressure and heart rate

56. The house officer considers prescribing nadolol for a 53-year-old patient. Which of the following preexisting conditions (comorbidities) would most likely contraindicate safe use of this drug?

a. Angina pectoris, chronic-stable (effort-induced)
b. Asthma
c. Essential hypertension
d. Heart failure, mild
e. Sinus tachychardia

57. A variety of ophthalmic drugs, working by several main mechanisms of action, are useful for managing chronic open-angle glaucoma. Which of the following reduces intraocular pressure by decreasing the formation of aqueous humor, rather than by changing the size of the pupil(s)?

a. Timolol
b. Echothiophate
c. Isoflurophate
d. Neostigmine
e. Pilocarpine

58. We give an "effective dose" of atropine to a person who was poisoned with an AChE inhibitor. Which of the following structures will continue to be overactivated by the excess ACh after the atropine is given?

a. Airway smooth muscle
b. SA node of the heart
c. Salivary and lacrimal glands
d. Skeletal muscle
e. Vascular smooth muscle

59. Guanadrel is an antihypertensive drug: it reduces arteriolar constriction, and in doing so lowers blood pressure, by reducing the amount of norepinephrine in peripheral adrenergic nerves. Lowered blood pressure is not accompanied by reflex tachycardia, and in fact a reduction of heart rate from predrug levels is the more common outcome. The main ocular effect of guanadrel is miosis. The widespread abolition of sympathetic influences throughout the body often causes diarrhea and urinary frequency. Based on this description, to which of the following drugs is guanadrel most similar in terms of its ultimate qualitative autonomic effects, but not specifically in terms of mechanism of action?

a. Acetylcholine
b. Atropine
c. Epinephrine
d. Isoproterenol
e. Norepinephrine
f. Propranolol
g. Reserpine

60. A patient with chronic obstructive pulmonary disease (COPD, e.g., emphysema) is receiving an orally inhaled muscarinic receptor-blocking drug to maintain bronchodilation. Which of the following drug is this patient most likely taking?

a. Albuterol
b. Diphenhydramine
c. Ipratropium
d. Pancuronium
e. Pilocarpine

61. We have a 48-year-old female patient with a history of myasthenia gravis. She has been treated with an oral acetylcholinesterase inhibitor for several years, and has done well till now. She presents with muscle weakness and other signs and symptoms that could reflect either a cholinergic crisis (excess dosages of her maintenance drug) or a myasthenic crisis (insufficient treatment). We will use a rapidly acting parenteral acetylcholinesterase inhibitor (AChE) to help make the differential diagnosis. Which of the following drugs would be most appropriate for this use?

a. Edrophonium
b. Malathion
c. Physostigmine
d. Pralidoxime
e. Pyridostigmine

62. It is common to include small amounts of epinephrine (EPI) in solutions of local anesthetics that will be administered by infiltration (injection around sensory nerve endings), as when a skin laceration needs suturing. Which of the following is the most likely reason for, or outcome of, including the EPI?

a. To antagonize the otherwise intense and common vasoconstrictor and hypertensive effects of the anesthetic
b. To counteract cardiac depression caused by the anesthetic
c. To prevent anaphylaxis in patients who are allergic to the anesthetic
d. To reduce the risk of toxicity caused by systemic absorption of the anesthetic
e. To shorten the duration of anesthetic action

63. A patient presents with an anaphylactic reaction following a bee sting. Which of the following is the drug of choice for treating the multiple cardiovascular and pulmonary problems that, if not promptly corrected, could lead to the patient's death?

a. Atropine
b. Diphenhydramine
c. Epinephrine
d. Isoproterenol
e. Norepinephrine

64. Phentolamine and prazosin are, basically, members of the same drug class. Which of the following properties or characteristics applies to *both* drugs?

a. Are competitive antagonists at α-adrenergic receptors
b. Profoundly inhibit gastric acid secretion
c. Cause a high incidence of bronchoconstriction in asthmatics
d. Cause bradycardia
e. Are used chronically for the treatment of primary hypotension

65. Left ventricular contractile force improves when dobutamine is given to a 60-year-old man with low cardiac output due to reductions of both heart rate and stroke volume. By which of the following adrenergic receptor-mediated actions is dobutamine causing these effects?

a. α-Adrenergic agonist
b. α-Adrenergic antagonist
c. β_1-Adrenergic agonist
d. β_1-Adrenergic antagonist
e. Mixed α and β agonist
f. Mixed α and β antagonist

66. It's fair to say that epinephrine, norepinephrine, and acetylcholine play the most important roles as agonists for the various receptors under control of the peripheral nervous systems. However, dopamine also plays a small but important role, particularly when administered IV at *low doses*. Which of the following functions in the periphery are affected by this catecholamine?

a. Bronchodilation via relaxation of airway smooth muscles
b. Direct activation of pressure receptors (e.g., baroreceptors) in response to blood pressure changes triggered by other agonists
c. Direct activation of the juxtaglomerular apparatus, release of aldosterone
d. Inhibition of epinephrine release from chromaffin cells (e.g., cells of the adrenal/suprarenal medulla)
e. Regulation of renal blood flow via control of renal arterial tone

67. We observe a rise of arterial pulse pressure during slow IV infusion of a drug to a normal subject. Which of the following drugs most likely caused this response?

a. Albuterol
b. Amphetamine
c. Epinephrine
d. Metoprolol
e. Phenylephrine

68. We are using novel *in vitro* methods to follow the fate and postsynaptic actions of norepinephrine, released upon an action potential generated in an adrenergic nerve. An action potential is generated and the postsynaptic effector briefly responds. Milliseconds later, the response is over. Which of the following processes mainly accounted for the brevity of the response, and termination of the released NE's actions?

a. Metabolism by enzyme(s) located near the postsynaptic receptor(s) and/or in the synaptic cleft
b. Reuptake into the nerve ending
c. Metabolism by catechol-O-methyltransferase (COMT)
d. Degradation by mitochondrial monoamine oxidase (MAO)
e. Conversion to a "false neurotransmitter" in the nerve ending

69. We are contemplating administration of a nonselective β-adrenergic blocker to a patient. In which of the following conditions is this considered generally acceptable, appropriate, and safe?

a. Angina, vasospastic ("variant"; Prinzmetal's)
b. Asthma
c. Bradycardia
d. Diabetes mellitus, insulin-dependent and poorly controlled
e. Heart block (second degree or greater)
f. Hyperthyroidism, symptomatic and acute
g. Severe congestive heart failure

70. A patient presents in the emergency department in great distress and with the following signs and symptoms:

bizarre behavior, delirium
facial flushing
clear lungs, no wheezing, rales, etc.
high heart rate
absence of bowel sounds
distended abdomen, full bladder
hot, dry skin
absence of lacrimal, salivary secretions
very high fever
dilated pupils that do not respond to light

Which of the following drugs has most likely caused these signs and symptoms?

a. AChE inhibitors
b. α-Adrenergic blockers
c. Antimuscarinics
d. β-Adrenergic blockers
e. Parasympathomimetics (muscarinic agonists)
f. Peripherally acting (neuronal) catecholamine depletors

71. Acebutolol and pindolol are classified as β blockers with intrinsic sympathomimetic activity (ISA). In a practical sense, what does this mean?

a. Are partial agonists (mixed agonist/antagonists)
b. Cause norepinephrine and epinephrine release
c. Induce catecholamine synthesis
d. Potentiate the actions of norepinephrine on α-adrenergic receptors
e. Useful when cardiac positive inotropic and chronotropic effects are wanted

72. A 10-year-old boy is diagnosed with Attention Deficit/Attention Deficit-Hyperactivity disorder (ADD/ADHD). Which of the following drugs is most likely to prove effective for relieving the boy's main symptoms?

a. Dobutamine
b. Methylphenidate
c. Pancuronium
d. Prazosin
e. Scopolamine
f. Terbutaline

73. During surgery we administer hexamethonium to an anesthetized patient. Which of the following effects should you expect in response to this drug?

a. Bradycardia mediated by activation of the baroreceptor reflex
b. Increased GI tract motility, possible spontaneous defecation
c. Increased salivary secretions
d. Miosis
e. Vasodilation

74. A patient with chronic open-angle glaucoma is treated with a topical ophthalmic β blocker. Which of the following is the most likely mechanism by which this drug lowers intraocular pressure?

a. Contracting the circular pupillary constrictor muscle
b. Contracting the iris dilator muscles
c. Decreasing aqueous humor synthesis/secretion
d. Dilating the uveoscleral veins
e. Directly opening the trabecular meshwork

75. A 65-year-old man is losing his vision. Retinal examination reveals optic nerve cupping. Visual field tests show peripheral vision loss, and tonometry shows that his intraocular pressure is increased. Following drug treatment he has improved visual acuity and near-normal intraocular pressure. Which of the following drugs was most likely given?

a. Baclofen
b. Homatropine
c. Phenylephrine
d. Scopolamine
e. Timolol

76. To facilitate or ease learning about the autonomic nervous system (or most other things), it's sometimes helpful to identify a generally applicable "rule" and then learn the one or two main exceptions to it. So, sympathetic innervation of which of the following structures is the exception to the general rule that "all postganglionic sympathetic nerves are adrenergic?"

a. Arterioles in the skin
b. Arterioles in the viscera
c. Radial muscle in the iris of the eye
d. Sinoatrial node of the heart
e. Sweat glands

77. A patient with a history of asthma experiences significant bronchoconstriction and urticaria, and drug-induced histamine release is a main contributor to these responses. Which of the following drugs is most likely to have caused these problems—not because it has any bronchoconstrictor or histamine agonist effects in its own right, but because it quite effectively releases histamine from mast cells?

a. Atropine
b. Neostigmine
c. Pancuronium
d. Propranolol
e. *d*-Tubocurarine

78. A patient receives a single injection of succinylcholine to facilitate preoperative intubation. The dose is correct for the vast majority of patients, and normally effects of this drug abate spontaneously over a couple of minutes. This gentleman remains apneic for an extraordinarily long time. A genetically based aberrant cholinesterase is eventually determined to be the cause. Which of the following would we administer if we were concerned about this unusually lengthy drug response?

a. Atropine
b. Bethanechol
c. Neostigmine
d. Nothing
e. Physostigmine
f. Tubocurarine

79. We administer an "effective" dose of a drug and observe the following responses:

Stimulates the heart
Dilates some blood vessels but constricts none
Dilates the bronchi
Raises blood glucose levels
Neither dilates nor constricts the pupil of the eye

Which of the following drugs most likely caused these responses?

a. Atropine
b. Epinephrine
c. Isoproterenol
d. Norepinephrine
e. Phenylephrine

80. "First-generation" (older) histamine H_1 blockers such as diphenhydramine, phenothiazine antipsychotic drugs (e.g., chlorpromazine), and tricyclic antidepressants (e.g., imipramine) have pharmacologic actions, side effects, toxicities, and contraindications that are very similar to those of which of the following?

a. Atropine
b. Bethanechol
c. Isoproterenol
d. Neostigmine
e. Propranolol

81. Physostigmine is the antidote for poisoning with antimuscarinic drugs (e.g., atropine). Another AChE inhibitor, neostigmine, is not suitable. That is because neostigmine cannot overcome the adverse effects of the antimuscarinic drug in or on which of the following?

a. Central nervous system (e.g., the brain)
b. Exocrine glands
c. Heart
d. Skeletal muscle
e. Smooth muscle

82. A patient presents with food poisoning that is attributed to botulism (Botulinus toxin poisoning). Which of the following is a correct characteristic, finding, or mechanism associated with this toxin?

a. Complete failure of all cholinergic neurotransmission
b. Favorable response to administration of pralidoxime
c. Impairment of parasympathetic, but not sympathetic, nervous system activation
d. Massive overstimulation of all structures having muscarinic cholinergic receptors
e. Selective paralysis of skeletal muscle

83. In between your M1 and M2 years you are volunteering in a hospital in a very poor part of the world. Their drug selection is limited. A patient presents with acute cardiac failure, for which your preferred drug is dobutamine, given intravenously. However, there is none available. Which of the following other drugs, or combination of drugs, would be a suitable alternative, giving the pharmacologic equivalent of what you want the dobutamine to do? (All these drugs are available in parenteral formulations.)

a. Dopamine (at a very high dose)
b. Ephedrine
c. Ephedrine plus propranolol
d. Norepinephrine plus phentolamine
e. Phenylephrine plus atropine

84. In general, structures that are affected by sympathetic activation respond to both sympathetic neural activation and to the hormonal component, epinephrine released from the adrenal medulla. Which of the following structures/functions is unique in that it responds to epinephrine, but not norepinephrine, and has no direct neural control?

a. Airway (tracheal, bronchiolar) smooth muscle: relaxation
b. Atrioventricular node: increased automaticity and conduction velocity
c. Coronary arteries: constriction
d. Iris of the eye: dilation (mydriasis)
e. Renal juxtaglomerular apparatus: renin release

85. The figure below shows several responses measured in a subject (healthy; receiving no other drugs) at rest (before) and after receiving a dose of an unknown drug. Note: The blood pressures shown can be considered mean blood pressures; the fall caused by the unknown was mainly due to a fall of diastolic pressure.

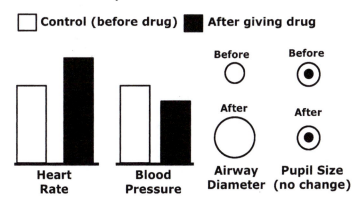

Which of the following drugs most likely caused the observed responses?

a. Atropine
b. Isoproterenol
c. Neostigmine
d. Phenylephrine
e. Propranolol

86. A patient received a single dose of succinylcholine for preoperative intubation. Skeletal muscle paralysis during a 3-hr surgery is maintained by a long-acting nondepolarizing type (i.e., curare-like) neuromuscular blocker. Surgery is over and the plan is to reverse the skeletal muscle paralysis. Which drug is administered first to block unwanted effects of the reversing agent on smooth muscles and glands, and then which drug is used to actually reverse the skeletal muscle paralysis?

a. Atropine to control smooth muscle, cardiac, and gland responses, then neostigmine to reverse skeletal muscle paralysis
b. β Blocker first to control cardiac responses, physostigmine for reversal
c. Belladonna alkaloids to block smooth muscle, cardiac, and gland responses, then pralidoxime to restore skeletal muscle function
d. Epinephrine first to control smooth muscle and glands, acetylcholine to reactivate skeletal muscle
e. Physostigmine to control smooth muscle and exocrine gland responses, followed by pancuronium for reversal of skeletal muscle paralysis

87. You are doing a summer research project that addresses biochemical mechanisms involved in the etiology of pheochromocytomas (most commonly a tumor of the catecholamine-secreting cells of the adrenal/suprarenal medulla). You want to assess activity of the *rate-limiting enzymatic step* in catecholamine synthesis, and drug effects thereupon. On which of the following enzymes should you focus your studies?

a. Catechol-*O*-methyltransferase (COMT)
b. Dopamine decarboxylase
c. Dopamine β-hydroxylase
d. Monoamine oxidase (MAO)
e. Phenylethanolamine N-methyltrasnferase
f. Tyrosine hydroxylase

88. Adrenergic nerves to the heart are activated, leading to a reflex increase of heart rate and cardiac contractility, in response to a sudden and significant fall of blood pressure. Those sympathetic nerves release norepinephrine (NE). Which of the following is the main physiologic mechanism by which the actions of the released NE are terminated?

a. Diffusion away from postsynaptic receptors
b. Hydrolysis by nonspecific deaminases
c. Metabolic inactivation by MAO
d. Metabolic inactivation by catechol-*O*-methyltransferase
e. Reuptake into the adrenergic nerve from which the NE was released

89. A 59-year-old man has a history of emphysema from 20 years of cigarette smoking; hypercholesterolemia that is being managed with atorvastatin; and Stage 2 essential hypertension for which he is taking metolazone. He presents in clinic today with his main new complaints: nocturia, urinary frequency, and an inability to urinate forcefully and empty his bladder. Following a complete workup, the MD arrives at a diagnosis of benign prostatic hypertrophy (BPH). We start daily therapy with tamsulosin. Which of the following is the most likely side effect the patient may experience from the tamsulosin, and about which he should be forewarned?

a. Bradycardia
b. Increased risk of statin-induced skeletal muscle pathology
c. Orthostatic hypotension
d. Photophobia and other painful responses to bright lights
e. Wheezing or other exacerbations of the emphysema

90. A patient walks out of the ophthalmologist's office and into bright sunlight after a comprehensive eye exam, for which he received a drug, applied topically. The drug has not only dilated his pupils but also impaired his ability to focus his eyes up close. The drug this patient received was most likely classified as, or worked most similar to, which of the following prototypes?

a. Acetylcholine
b. Epinephrine
c. Homatropine
d. Isoproterenol
e. Pilocarpine
f. Propranolol

91. We've received approval from the Institutional Review Board to study the *in vitro* (tissue bath) responsiveness of isolated human arteriolar segments (obtained during surgery) to a variety of pharmacologic and other interventions. The tissue samples are 1-cm-long "cylinders" of otherwise normal (but now denervated) arterioles obtained from the lower legs of patients undergoing amputation surgery for cancer.

Our set-up allows us to perfuse the vessels with a solution that will keep the tissue functionally and structurally intact for many hours; to monitor and change perfusion pressure (mm Hg; analogous to blood pressure in the intact organism) and perfusate flow (mL/min); and to assess the effects of various vasoactive drugs on the system.

We add to the perfusate a concentration of ACh identical to the serum concentration of ACh that causes "expected responses" in an intact human.

Under this experimental setup, adding ACh causes a rise of perfusion pressure and a decrease of flow, both of which basically reflect vasoconstriction.

Which of the following is the best explanation for these findings?

a. ACh released norepinephrine from the endothelium, which caused vasoconstriction
b. Atropine was added to the tissue bath before adding the ACh
c. Botulinum toxin was added to the bath before adding the ACh
d. The vascular endothelium has been damaged or removed (denuded)
e. This response is precisely what we'd expect with injection of ACh into the intact human

92. A 33-year-old woman becomes poisoned after receiving an injection of illicitly prepared and overly concentrated botulinum toxin. Which of the following is the main neurochemical mechanism by which this *Clostridium* toxin causes its effects?

a. Directly activates all muscarinic and nicotinic receptors
b. Inhibits ACh release from all cholinergic nerves
c. Prevents neuronal norepinephrine reuptake
d. Releases norepinephrine via a nonexocytotic process
e. Selectively and competitively blocks nicotinic receptors

93. A patient takes a massive overdose of diphenhydramine, suffering not only significant CNS depression but also numerous and serious peripheral autonomic side effects. Which of the following is the main mechanism by which diphenhydramine exerts its untoward peripheral autonomic actions?

a. Activation of both β_1 and β_2 adrenoceptors
b. Blockade of α-adrenergic receptors
c. Competitive antagonism of ACh actions on muscarinic receptors
d. Massive, direct overactivation of ganglionic nicotinic receptors
e. Sudden release of epinephrine from the adrenal medulla (suprarenal medulla)

94. A patient with a recent drug poisoning is transported to the emergency department. The physician orders (correctly, in this case) administration of pralidoxime as part of the comprehensive emergency treatment plan. Which one of the following best describes who the patient was?

a. A 13-year-old boy who took an overdose of methylphenidate for his ADD/ADHD
b. A 43-year-old who took an overdose of neostigmine, prescribed for her myasthenia gravis, in a suicide attempt
c. A 6-year-old who got into the family medicine cabinet and took 10 "adult doses" of her dad's prazosin
d. A farm/field worker accidentally doused with insecticide from an overflying crop-duster plane
e. An asthma patient who accidentally gave himself an intravenous injection of epinephrine in an attempt to self-treat a developing anaphylactic reaction

95. To facilitate a certain eye exam we want to cause mydriasis, but not alter normal control of accommodation. All of the following drugs are available as topical ophthalmic formulations. Which of the following would achieve our goals the best?

a. Atropine
b. Epinephrine
c. Homatropine
d. Isoproterenol
e. Pilocarpine
f. Timolol

96. A 26-year-old woman has rhinorrhea, excessive lacrimation, and ocular congestion from a bout with the common cold. Diphenhydramine provides symptomatic relief. Which of the following is the most likely mechanism by which this drug gave symptom relief in the presence of this rhinovirus?

a. α-Adrenergic activation (agonist)
b. β-Adrenergic blockade
c. Calcium channel blockade
d. Histamine (H$_1$) receptor blockade
e. Muscarinic receptor blockade

97. You have treated dozens of patients with acute hypotension from various causes, including overdoses of antihypertensive drugs, all of which can cause hypotension. Your usual approach to restoring blood pressure, and one that has worked well every time before, is to inject x mg of phenylephrine intravenously.

Today a patient with severe drug-induced hypotension presents in the emergency department. He has been taking this drug for many months. He is not volume-depleted, nor hemorrhaging.

You give the phenylephrine at the same dose and by the same route as you always have. It causes no change of blood pressure. Which of the following drugs did the patient most likely take an overdose of?

a. Atenolol
b. Bethanechol
c. Prazosin
d. Propranolol
e. Reserpine

98. This is a strange day for you in the emergency department. Now you have to treat another normovolemic patient with acute drug-induced hypotension, and give the usually correct and effective dose of phenylephrine. This time the drug causes a vasopressor response that is far greater than you've ever encountered: systolic pressure rises dramatically, if not dangerously.

Which of the following drugs did the patient most likely take an overdose of?

a. Atenolol
b. Bethanechol
c. Prazosin
d. Propranolol
e. Reserpine

99. A 43-year-old woman with diagnosed myasthenia gravis presents with profound skeletal muscle weakness. We are unsure whether she is experiencing a cholinergic crisis or a myasthenic crisis, so we administer a usually appropriate dose of parenteral edrophonium. Assume the patient was actually experiencing a cholinergic crisis. Which of the following is the most likely response to the drug?

a. Hypertensive crisis from peripheral vascular constriction
b. Myocardial ischemia, and angina, from drug-induced tachycardia and coronary vasoconstriction
c. Premature ventricular contractions from increased ventricular automaticity
d. Prompt improvement of skeletal muscle tone and function
e. Ventilatory distress or failure

The Peripheral Nervous Systems: Autonomic and Somatic

Answers

32. The answer is a. (*Brunton, pp 137–142; Craig, pp 83–88; Katzung, pp 75–83.*) Here's the simple rule. In the peripheral nervous systems—that is, both branches of the autonomic nervous system, and the somatic nervous system—"the first nerve out of the CNS is always cholinergic and the ACh released from those nerves always activates the nicotinic subtype of cholinergic receptor."

33. The answer is c. (*Brunton, pp 137–142; Craig, pp 83–88; Katzung, pp 75–83.*) Another rule: "all the efferents in the peripheral nervous systems are cholinergic except postganglionic sympathetics going to structures other than sweat glands." Count up all the nerves in our schematic of the peripheral nervous systems. There are eight. Seven of them—all except the majority of postganglionic sympathetics (*nerve d*)—are cholinergic (synthesize and release ACh as their neurotransmitter). The main postganglionic sympathetic fibers (except those innervating sweat glands) synthesize and release NE (not epinephrine; answer d) as their neurotransmitter, and so are adrenergic (or noradrenergic) nerves. What else can we call *nerve d*? A postganglionic sympathetic nerve to certain smooth muscles, to cardiac muscle, and certain exocrine glands except sweat glands. (Be sure to see the explanation for Question 36.)

Atropine (a) is incorrect. That drug selectively and competitively blocks the effects of ACh (and other muscarinic agonists) on muscarinic receptors. In the diagram, those receptors are found on structures innervated by nerves b and g.

Answer b is incorrect. NE, *nerve d*'s neurotransmitter, is an effective agonist for α-adrenergic receptors (α_1 and α_2) and for β_1s. Bronchodilation caused by sympathetic activation requires activation of β_2 receptors; NE cannot do that . . . but EPI, released from the adrenal (suprarenal) medulla, certainly can. And once NE has been released from its neurons and activates its postsynaptic receptors, its actions are promptly terminated by reuptake (via an "amine pump" that can be blocked by cocaine or tricyclic antidepressants). Hydrolysis in the synaptic cleft (e) is the mechanism by which the action of ACh, released from cholinergic nerves, is terminated.

34. The answer is d. (*Brunton, pp 146–150; Craig, pp 89–92; Katzung, pp 75–76.*) The actions of norepinephrine (NE), released from adrenergic nerves, are terminated by neuronal reuptake. (Don't forget that this reuptake process is inhibited by cocaine and tricyclic antidepressants, and the outcome is increased and more prolonged adrenergic effects of NE.) All the other nerves shown in the diagram are cholinergic; the actions of the ACh they release are terminated promptly by hydrolysis (via acetylcholinesterase).

35. The answer is g. (*Brunton, pp 139–141; Craig, p 93; Katzung, pp 76, 84–86.*) The neurotransmitter released from *nerve d*, the postganglionic sympathetic fibers (to structures other than most sweat glands), is norepinephrine. NE can activate α-adrenergic receptors (both α_1 and α_2), and β_1 receptors (not β_2). Of course, different structures have different subtypes of adrenergic receptors: such structures as arterioles and the iris dilator muscle have α_1 receptors; β_1s are found in the heart, while β_2 receptors (not activated by NE) are found on various smooth muscles in the GI and urinary tracts and airways. So, the only correct response to the question "which receptors are activated?" really depends on which structure is being innervated. This is precisely why you need to memorize where the various receptors and their subtypes are located, as well as key agonists and antagonists for those receptors and the responses most likely to occur when those receptors are activated or blocked.

36. The answer is c. (*Brunton, pp 138–140, 140f, 144t; Craig, pp 83–84; Katzung, pp 75–76, 84–86.*) The postganglionic sympathetic fibers innervating sweat glands are cholinergic. That is the *exception* to the rule that "*all postganglionic sympathetic fibers are adrenergic.*" How do we know it's cholinergic? A variety of biochemical and histochemical methods can prove that ACh is the neurotransmitter. They also show that there is abundant acetylcholinesterase (AChE), which hydrolyzes ACh, at the synaptic cleft. Pharmacologically we can prevent release of neurotransmitter from *nerve g* with botulinum toxin, which affects only cholinergic nerves; and we can prevent the response of the sweat glands innervated by *nerve g* with atropine, the prototype muscarinic (cholinergic) receptor antagonist—a drug that has no effects on nicotinic (or other) receptors (e.g., answer d). Likewise, nicotinic receptor blockers (or nicotine itself) have no effect at this site—another reason why answer d is incorrect. And how we do know it's part of the SNS? Sweat glands are activated (secretions are increased) when the rest of the SNS is activated; and if we trace the origins of the preganglionic nerves that activate the postganglionic ones, they emanate from the same regions of the spinal cord from which all other sympathetic preganglionic fibers arise—the thoracic and lumbar regions of the cord.

Cocaine (a) is incorrect. It, and tricyclic antidepressants (e.g., amitriptyline, imipramine), block neuronal reuptake of NE. That is, its site of action is at the neuroeffector junction of postganglionic sympathetic neurons (*nerve d*)—all of them except those that innervate sweat glands, of course.

37. The answer is c. (*Brunton, pp 138–141, 150–153; Craig, pp 84, 92–93, 121–123; Katzung, pp 75–76, 86–87.*) The nerve is cholinergic, so the neurotransmitter it acts on, postsynaptically, must be either nicotinic or muscarinic. Nicotinic receptors are found on cell bodies of all postganglionic nerves (in both SNS and PNS), on the adrenal medulla, and on skeletal muscle (somatic nervous system)—at the "first synapses out of the CNS." Cholinergic receptors at all other sites are muscarinic, "defined" by the fact that those receptors are competitively blocked by atropine. Be sure to see the explanation for Question 36.

38. The answer is h. (*Brunton, pp 220–225; Craig, pp 338–340, 342–344; Katzung, pp 75–76.*) Pancuronium and tubocurarine (as well as metocurine and several related drugs) are nondepolarizing skeletal neuromuscular blockers (quite differently, mechanistically, from succinylcholine, a depolarizing blocker). They specifically and competitively block activation of nicotinic receptors on skeletal muscle by ACh, thereby preventing depolarization of skeletal muscle; and have no effect on muscarinic receptors or any of the adrenergic receptor subtypes. (Remember something about the natives of the Amazon obtaining a poisonous substance from the skin of certain species of frogs, putting it on the tips of their darts, and using that to kill their dinner with a blowgun? That was curare . . . *d*-tubocurarine, or the prototype nondepolarizing skeletal neuromuscular blocker, as we've come to know it.)

39. The answer is b. (*Brunton, pp 158–164; Craig, pp 89–92; Katzung, pp 81–82, 90.*) While mitochondria in virtually all cells in which they are found are important for oxidative phosphorylation and ATP synthesis, we asked about the MAO that is rich in adrenergic neurons. There MAO will degrade NE that is free (i.e., not safely stored away) in the storage vesicles. If that intravesicular uptake is inhibited, NE stores will be depleted.

40. The answer is d. (*Brunton, pp 158–164, 171t, 172t; Craig, pp 89–92; Katzung, pp 81–82, 90.*) Reserpine blocks intraneuronal storage of NE, thereby exposing the free NE to degradation by intraneuronal MAO. Reserpine also blocks vesicular uptake of dopamine, for example, in parts of the CNS. This is important because the final synthesis of NE from its precursor occurs in the vesicles; if dopamine entry is blocked, NE synthesis is thereby inhibited (or dopaminergic nerves don't accumulate their neurotransmitter).

Pargyline (a) is a MAO inhibitor. Note that unlike reserpine, MAO inhibitors do not inhibit intraneuronal storage of NE. Rather, they metabolically inactivate NE (or, at other sites, other monoamines). Prazosin (b) and propranolol (c) are adrenergic receptor blockers (α_1- and β-, respectively) and have no direct effect on NE storage. Tyramine (e) is an indirect-acting sympathomimetic that displaces and releases neuronal NE *via* a process that does not involve exocytosis.

41. The answer is b. (*Brunton, pp 158–162, 171t, 239, 377, 620; Craig, pp 89–92, 94, 407; Katzung, pp 81, 90.*) Cocaine and tricyclic antidepressants such as imipramine are classic examples of drugs that inhibit NE reuptake by the "amine pump," which is the main process by which released NE reenters the neuron and its receptor-mediated effects are terminated physiologically. In the presence of cocaine or a tricyclic, released NE lingers and accumulates in the synapse (neuroeffector junction), and so pertinent adrenergic responses appear heightened or more intense, and prolonged.

Provided an adrenergic nerve is present (as it is in the diagram), the effects of cocaine or a tricyclic antidepressant are not affected by or dependent on whether the effector (target) is smooth muscle, cardiac muscle, or an exocrine gland of any sort.

There is no direct functional link between the amine pump and such processes as NE release (exocytotically or otherwise) or activation of presynaptic (α_2-) adrenergic receptors.

42. The answer is d. (*Brunton, pp 167–170, 172t; Craig, pp 90–94; Katzung, pp 81–90, 125, 134, 165–167.*) The adrenergic neuronal α_2 (presynaptic) receptor, like all other adrenergic receptors, are G-protein-coupled. When the α_2 receptor is activated by a suitable agonist, it signals the neuron to stop further NE release. NE itself is one such agonist; its activation of the presynaptic α_2 receptor (which occurs concomitant with activation of postsynaptic [α_1 or β_1] adrenergic receptors) provides a physiologic "feedback" signal that halts further NE release. That is, released NE regulates the release of more NE from the very neuron from which the neurotransmitter came.

Although activation of both the presynaptic α_2 receptors and NE reuptake by the amine pump/transporter occur simultaneously, there is no direct functional or biochemical linkage between the two. That is, activating (or blocking) the α_2 receptor will not directly affect NE reuptake, nor will drugs that affect the amine pump necessarily have any effect on the α_2 receptors and the function they serve.

Note: Clonidine, which you typically (and correctly) think of as a centrally acting antihypertensive drug, acts as an α_2 agonist in the periphery. Its as "turning off" of NE release, then, can contribute to reduced vasoconstriction (and other adrenergic processes mediated by NE), which in turn helps lower blood pressure. However, clonidine is a very lipophilic drug. When it is given in usual doses, by the usual route (oral), the drug enters the CNS well, and rather promptly, and it acts there (in the cardiovascular control center of the brain's medulla) to inhibit sympathetic outflow. It is that central effect that accounts for the drug's main antihypertensive mechanism.

43. The answer is e. (*Brunton, pp 144–145, 172t, 269–270, 246–247; Craig, pp 111–113, 231; Katzung, p 172.*) Prazosin selectively blocks α_1 adrenergic receptors and, unlike many other α blockers (phentolamine, phenoxybenzamine) has virtually no presynaptic (α_2) effects.

None of the other drugs fit the bill: ephedrine (a) exerts sympathomimetic (adrenomimetic) effects in part by releasing intraneuronal NE, and in part by directly but weakly acting as an agonist on all the adrenergic receptors. It has no antagonist activity with respect to any adrenergic (or cholinergic) receptors. (Related drugs are pseudoephedrine and phenylpropanolamine, and the lesser-known drug metaraminol.) Labetalol (b) blocks both α- and β-adrenergic receptors and is an agonist for neither. (A mechanistically related and important drug is carvedilol.) Phentolamine (c) nonselectively blocks both α_1 and α_2 receptors, has no β-blocking activity, and is an agonist for none of the adrenergic receptors. Phenylephrine (d) is a strong agonist for all the α-adrenergic receptors, has no α agonist activity, and exerts no effects of any type on β receptors.

44. The answer is a. (*Brunton, pp 166t, 189–195, 197; Craig, pp 134–139; Katzung, pp 116, 116t.*) You may never have learned about oxybutynin (although you've probably seen an ad for its brand-name product on TV). But it makes no difference to answering this rather easy question. The description of this unusual drug is, in reality, also an excellent description of many of the properties of atropine, the prototype muscarinic receptor blocking drug.

You should also be able to eliminate incorrect answers by a simple process of elimination. For example, do β blockers (b) cause the visual, urinary tract, sweat gland, or cardiovascular responses we noted? Not at all., nor do isoproterenol (c; β_1/β_2 agonist), neostigmine (d; cholinesterase inhibitor, which produces precisely the opposite responses that oxybutynin does), or phentolamine (e; nonselective α blocker).

45. The answer is c. (*Brunton, pp 161–163, 171t–172t, 257–259; Craig, pp 105–106, 349–351; Katzung, pp 81–90.*) Amphetamines (dextroamphetamine, methamphetamine, amphetamine, and several related drugs) can be classified as indirect-acting sympathomimetics (adrenomimetics). They are taken into the adrenergic nerve ending by the amine pump, displace NE from its storage vesicles (via processes that are not dependent on an action potential) and cause the stored neurotransmitter to be released into the synaptic space. At that point, all the expected effects of NE on its receptors and effectors occur. These drugs have no direct effects, whether as an agonist or antagonist, on the adrenergic receptors. Their actions are wholly dependent on intraneuronal NE stores.

46. The answer is c. (*Brunton, pp 243–246; Craig, pp 100–102; Katzung, pp 129–130.*) The inotropic (contractility), chronotropic (rate), and dromotropic (conduction velocity-related) effects of epinephrine on the heart are mediated through activation of β_1-adrenergic receptors. These receptor sites mediate an epinephrine-induced increased firing rate of the SA node (spontaneous, or Phase 4, depolarization), increased conduction velocity through the AV node and the His-Purkinje system, and increased contractility and conduction velocity of atrial and ventricular muscle. Epinephrine activation of α adrenoceptors does not affect cardiac function in any physiologically or therapeutically important way—except for the crucial role of α adrenoceptors as mediators of coronary artery vasoconstriction (clearly a vascular smooth muscle, not cardiac muscle, phenomenon). The β_2-adrenergic receptors play virtually no direct role in cardiac stimulation. They are more important in the relaxation of tracheobronchial smooth muscle, dilation of arterioles that serve skeletal muscles, increased secretion of insulin by the pancreas, and to a lesser degree relaxation of the detrusor of the urinary bladder. (Lipolysis in fat cells and melatonin secretion by the pineal gland appear to involve stimulation of β_3-adrenergic receptors. However, we do not have any clinically useful drugs that selectively activate or block the β_3 receptors, and so you might want to question how much you learn about the β_3s.)

47. The answer is b. (*Brunton, pp 205, 207t, 1720t, 1723; Craig, pp 126–130; Katzung, pp 101–104.*) Echothiophate is a long-acting ("irreversible," which basically means "very long acting" in terms of the duration of clinical effects) acetylcholinesterase inhibitor. It is used topically on the eye for the treatment of various types of glaucoma. Maximum reduction of intraocular pressure occurs within 24 h, and the effect may persist for several days. The drug is water-soluble, which affords a practical advantage over the lipid-soluble isoflurophate (another cholinesterase inhibitor used to treat glaucoma). (Had we listed a drug with a generic name ending in the suffix "-stigmine," you no doubt would have answered correctly and immediately. However, echothiophate is one of those cholinesterase inhibitors that is not a stigmine. If you're unfamiliar with the drug—this one or anyone as you work your way through the questions—by all means look it up!)

Tyrosine hydroxylase (a) is involved in the biosynthesis of catecholamines. COMT (c) is involved in extraneuronal metabolism of catecholamines, while MAO (d) is the major intraneuronal enzyme that degrades NE in adrenergic nerves. Forms of MAO are also found in, and important in, the liver and parts of the CNS. DOPA decarboxylase (e) catalyzes the metabolism of DOPA (dihydroxyphenylalanine) to dopamine as part of the catecholamine biosynthetic pathway.

48. The answer is a. (*Brunton, pp 192, 196, 1711, 1722; Craig, pp 138–139; Katzung, p 118.*) With any antimuscarinic drug—and scopolamine certainly is one—narrow-angle glaucoma (which accounts for only about 10% of all glaucomas) is the biggest concern. The drug might provoke significant rises of intraocular pressure as it further reduces aqueous humor drainage, causing not only pain but vision problems that might be severe or permanent. Bradycardia is not a concern; if anything, the scopolamine would increase heart rate a bit. Should the patient eat some bad shellfish, the incidence or severity diarrhea might be reduced or prevented altogether by the scopolamine, due to its effects on longitudinal muscles in the gut (inhibited) and on sphincters (activated). A resting blood pressure of 112/70 (or thereabouts) is not at all uncommon or worrisome, and not likely to be changed at all by the drug. Hypothyroidism typically is associated with slight bradycardia; again, no envisaged problem with scopolamine. And if our patient had mild Parkinson's disease, we might actually, eventually, see a little improvement with this drug. Recall, one strategy to manage parkinsonism—basically a central imbalance between dopamine and ACh, is to block the muscarinic receptors (with such drugs as benztropine or trihexyphenidyl; see CNS chapter).

49. The answer is a. (*Brunton, pp 283t, 285; Craig, pp 113, 116–117; Katzung, p 142.*) Labetalol is a competitive antagonist at both α- and β-adrenergic (both β_1 and β_2) receptors. (This "trick" might help you remember that labetalol blocks both main types of adrenergic receptors: take the first two letters of the generic name and reverse them—*la* tranposes to al, as in alpha—and then add the next four letters—*beta.* You'll simply have to memorize the name of another important α/β blocker, carvedilol.) Note, too, that the generic names of all the drugs listed end in *-olol*—a great tip-off that a drug has β-blocking activity. (Can you think of a major drug's generic name that ends in *-olol* and is not a β blocker? There isn't any. Might this help your learning?)

    Labetalol's α-blocking actions are weak compared with its actions at the β receptors. This relative difference is somewhat concentration-dependent: at relatively low serum levels, as might be achieved with typical oral doses, it is about three times more potent as a β blocker than as an α blocker (do not commit this to memory!). With higher serum concentrations, such as those often achieved with parenteral (e.g., IV) dosing, the intensity of β blockade increases considerably with little increase in α-blocking efficacy (another ultimately important point, but not priority knowledge now!). One of labetalol's main uses is for managing essential hypertension (all the orally administered β blockers are indicated for essential hypertension, and most are indicated for chronic-stable angina). Given parenterally (IV), it is often a first-choice agent for managing urgent hypertensive crises when more efficacious (and potentially more dangerous) IV drugs aren't indicated or cannot be given safely.

Metoprolol (and atenolol and acebutolol, not listed) have a preferential effect on β_1 receptors ("cardioselectivity") vs. β_2, and have no α-blocking actions. Nadolol and timolol are nonselective β blockers. (One property to remember for nadolol is its relatively long half-life; for timolol you might want to recall that a topical ophthalmic dosage form is often used for chronic open-angle glaucoma.) Pindolol is a nonselective β blocker and also exerts strong intrinsic sympathomimetic activity (ISA; that is, partial agonist-antagonist activity).

50. The answer is d. (*Brunton, pp 166t, 174, 264, 264f, 271; Craig, pp 94, 787t; Katzung, pp 81, 84, 146, 189.*) Whether you memorize that yohimbine is a selective α_2 antagonist is up to you, but you should know what the main effects of a selective α_2 antagonist are. That, of course, depends on knowing what α_2 receptors—at least in the peripheral autonomic nervous system—do in the physiological sense. Recall that the preponderance of physiologically important α_2 receptors are located on adrenergic nerve terminals (or nerve "endings"). When stimulated by a suitable agonist, the response is a turning-off of further NE release. Because NE is the neurotransmitter released from adrenergic nerves and it is an excellent α agonist, the presynaptic α_2 receptors upon which NE acts serve as the main physiologic mechanism for regulating neurotransmitter release.

So, when we block those receptors with yohimbine, we enhance the apparent overall activity of the sympathetic nervous system on its effectors by interfering with NE's ability to turn off its own release. Of the responses listed, only hypertension (owing to the vasoconstrictor effects of NE on postsynaptic α-adrenergic receptors) occurs as a result of yohimbine (or of NE excess). The other main effects you should anticipate would be cardiac stimulation (rate, contractility, electrical impulse conduction rates; all β_1-mediated effects) and, probably of less clinical consequence, mydriasis (α).

In terms of the aphrodisiac effects, the drug probably increases arousal via an action in the CNS, but the mechanism isn't known for sure; and it increases the vigor of ejaculation, which is predominantly an α-mediated effect. (Recall that erection primarily involves muscarinic-cholinergic vascular effects, mediated by enhanced production of endothelium-derived relaxing factor . . . i.e., nitric oxide.)

51. The answer is a. (*Brunton, pp 204, 211, 214, 538–540; Craig, pp 128, 130, 371; Katzung, pp 105, 1010–1011.*) Patients with Alzheimer's disease present with progressive impairment of memory and cognitive functions such as a lack of attention, disturbed language function, and an inability to complete common tasks. Although the exact defect in the central nervous system (CNS) has not been elucidated, evidence suggests that a reduction in cholinergic nerve function or receptor activation plays an important role in the etiology. At the very least, increasing central cholinergic receptor activation seems to reduce symptom severity.

Tacrine has been found to be somewhat effective in patients with mild-to-moderate symptoms of this disease for improvement of cognitive functions. The drug is primarily a reversible cholinesterase inhibitor that increases the concentration of functional ACh in the brain. However, the pharmacology of tacrine is complex; the drug also acts as a muscarinic receptor modulator in that it has partial agonistic activity, as well as weak antagonistic activity on muscarinic receptors in the CNS. In addition, tacrine appears to enhance the release of ACh from cholinergic nerves, and it may alter the concentrations of other neurotransmitters such as dopamine and NE.

Of all the reversible cholinesterase inhibitors, only tacrine and physostigmine cross the blood-brain barrier in sufficient amounts to make these compounds useful for disorders involving the CNS. Physostigmine has been tried as a therapy for Alzheimer's disease; however, it is more commonly used to antagonize the effects of toxic concentrations of drugs with antimuscarinic properties, including atropine, antihistamines, phenothiazines, and tricyclic antidepressants. Neostigmine, pyridostigmine, and ambenonium are used mainly in the treatment of myasthenia gravis; edrophonium is useful for the diagnosis of this disease because of its fast onset and short duration.

52. The answer is b. (*Brunton, pp 152–154, 231–233; Craig, pp 85, 92, 142–144; Katzung, pp 97, 106.*) Nicotine initially stimulates and then blocks nicotinic-muscular (NM) (skeletal muscle) and nicotinic-neural (NN) (autonomic ganglia) cholinergic receptors. Initial ganglionic stimulation leads to vasoconstriction and hypertension. Bradycardia may or may not occur; parasympathetic ganglionic activation is likely to increase the predominant parasympathetic (bradycardic) tone on heart rate, but sympathetic activation may cause the opposite effect. Initial stimulation of skeletal muscle nicotinic receptors would account for the tremor. As nicotine's blood levels rise we get autonomic ganglionic blockade (depolarization of postganglionic cells), leading to hypotension and bradycardia. Blockade at the skeletal neuromuscular junction leads to muscle weakness and respiratory depression caused by interference with the function of the diaphragm and intercostals. Bethanechol (a) and pilocarpine (c) are cholinomimetics that exert their primary effects as direct agonists on muscarinic receptors for ACh, not on nicotinic receptors such as those responsible for skeletal muscle activation. Scopolamine (d) is a muscarinic blocker with virtually no effects on skeletal muscle (nicotinic responses). Tubocurarine (e) is a competitive nicotinic receptor antagonist, acting almost exclusively on skeletal muscle. It is not at all likely to cause direct autonomic effects, whether by blocking muscarinic receptors or by other likely mechanisms.

53. The answer is e. (*Brunton, pp 251–254; Craig, p 720; Katzung, pp 135, 138.*) Ritodrine is a selective β_2-adrenergic agonist that relaxes uterine smooth muscle. It also has the other effects attributable to β-adrenergic receptor agonists, such as bronchodilation, cardiac stimulation, enhanced renin secretion, and hyperglycemia. Yes, it is classified the same as, for example, albuterol, salmeterol, or terbutaline, and several other drugs typically used as adrenergic bronchodilators. But ridodrine is approved for use as a tocolytic (uterine-relaxing) drug. Will it, or can it, cause bronchodilation? Absolutely! And when blood levels become sufficiently high the selective activation of β_2 receptors is lost, and the drug behaves like isoproterenol, the prototype β_1/β_2 agonist. This loss of β_2 adrenergic agonist selectivity is a property of all the drugs classified, rather inappropriately, as "selective" β_2 agonists or selective adrenergic bronchodilators.

54. The answer is a. (*Brunton, pp 186–189; Craig, pp 93, 123–126; Katzung, pp 98–100.*) These are expected side effects from bethanechol, a muscarinic agonist (parasympathomimetic drug). They occur even though the effects of the drug—the ones for which it is given—are "predominately" on the bladder musculature. These effects are common and dose- (and patient-) dependent, and not at all idiosyncratic reactions. Bethanechol has no sympathetic (or parasympathetic) ganglionic blocking actions. If the patient had undiagnosed asthma (and the presence of asthma would contraindicate use of the drug), the pulmonary response would be much more significant than "some wheezing." Potentially fatal bronchospasm could occur because the airway smooth muscles of asthmatic individuals are exquisitely (hyper)sensitive to muscarinic agonists, with even small doses of those drugs capable of causing a lethal outcome.

55. The answer is a. (*Brunton, pp 164, 269–270, 855, 857; Craig, p 231; Katzung, pp 146–147.*) The figure approximates what is likely to happen following administration of a β blocker to a patient with a pheochromocytoma.

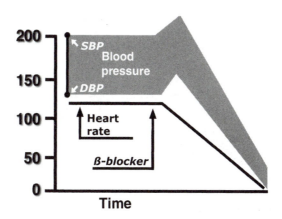

To answer this question correctly you must integrate your basic knowledge of both autonomic pharmacology and cardiovascular physiology. With a pheochromocytoma we have what might be described as "massive" amounts of catecholamines—mainly epinephrine—being released from the tumor into the bloodstream. Germane to our problem, then, is excessive stimulation of cardiac rate, contractility, impulse conduction, and automaticity (β_1); intense vasoconstriction (α); and vasodilation in some vascular beds (β_2).

Nonetheless, while the patient we've described is not at all healthy, he is still alive before we give the β blocker. But what happens after we give the β blocker is critical. The β blocker does nothing to block the α-mediated vasoconstriction, so in terms of only vascular effects BP will remain very high. If you wish to opine that blocking β_2-mediated vasodilation will raise BP a bit, that's fine; we've shown that in the figure. (Remember: Usually effective doses of a β blocker will either lower BP [most common response], or not affect it at all, in patients with essential hypertension. If pressure rises in response to a β blocker, *suspect pheochromocytoma*.)

Nonetheless, there will not be a sudden and significant rise or normalization of BP and/or cardiac function (b, c, d). Likewise, heart rate will not rise significantly (e); it can't: the β_1 receptors necessary for that to occur are blocked.

Next you must recall that the inotropic state of the heart (i.e., of the left ventricle, LV) is critical. This is critical because LV peak systolic pressure must exceed aortic pressure in order to establish the LV-aortic pressure gradient to expel blood into the aorta, and propel blood throughout the circulation. If aortic diastolic pressure exceeds LV peak systolic pressure, blood will not flow out of the heart. But until we give the β blocker, the heart can maintain (for a while) its function thanks to catecholamine-mediated stimulation.

But when we give just a β blocker to the pheochromocytoma patient we have done little if anything to lower the already high aortic pressure, and simultaneously have inhibited cardiac contractiilty, rate, and other key parameters. The function of the heart as a pump is suppressed. It now faces a very high aortic pressure, and ultimately it fails. Cardiac output falls, the patient develops cardiogenic shock, and is then likely to die.

This is why, when treating hypertension associated with a pheochromocytoma, we give an α blocker first. Blood pressure will fall. We then deal with the excessive cardiac stimulation (which may be intensified, *via* the baroreceptor reflex, in response to a sudden and significant BP fall) by giving a suitable β blocker immediately thereafter.

56. The answer is b. (*Brunton, pp 272–278, 287–288; Craig, pp 115–117; Katzung, pp 148–154, 157.*) You probably learned that nadolol is a β blocker, and perhaps that it's a nonselective (β_1/β_2) blocker with a rather long duration of action and half-life. If not, you should have been able to recognize that since the generic name ends in "-olol" it is, indeed, some kind of β blocker. You should also know that asthma is one of the main contraindications for β blocker administration. β-Adrenergic blockade results in an increase in airway resistance (by antagonism of bronchodilation mediated by epinephrine) that can be fatal in some asthmatic patients. Nadolol, and all the other orally effective β blockers, are approved for treating chronic-stable angina (a) and essential hypertension (c). They are critical elements in contemporary therapy of heart failure (d; except when it is severe and cardiac output is profoundly depressed); and have beneficial effects to control heart rate in such conditions as sinus tachycardia (e).

57. The answer is a. (*Brunton, pp 186–188, 207–208, 212, 1720–1722; Craig, p 115; Katzung, p 156.*) When applied topically to the eye, both the direct-acting cholinomimetic agents (e.g., pilocarpine) and those that act by inhibition of AChE (e.g., echothiophate, isoflurophate, and physostigmine) cause miosis by contracting the sphincter muscle of the iris and reducing intraocular pressure by contracting the ciliary muscle, allowing better drainage of aqueous humor. In patients with glaucoma, this latter effect permits greater drainage of the aqueous humor through the trabecular meshwork in the canal of Schlemm and a reduction in resistance to outflow of the aqueous humor. Certain β-adrenergic blocking agents (e.g., timolol and levobunolol), applied to the eye(s), are also very useful in treating chronic wide-angle glaucoma. These drugs appear to act by decreasing the secretion (or formation) of aqueous humor by antagonizing the effect of circulating catecholamines on β-adrenergic receptors in the ciliary epithelium. Echothiophate (b), isoflurophate (c), and neostigmine (e) are acetylcholinesterase inhibitors and all constrict the pupil. Pilocarpine (d) is muscarinic receptor agonist; it, too, causes miosis.

58. The answer is d. (*Brunton, pp 209–211; Craig, pp 126–129, 131, 134–137; Katzung, pp 102–103, 116–117.*) In "cholinesterase poisioning" we are dealing with overstimulation (from accumulated ACh) of both peripheral muscarinic and nicotinic receptors. Recall that atropine is a specific muscarinic receptor blocker, and the muscarinic receptors are the ones found on such structures as smooth muscle, cardiac nodal tissue, and exocrine glands. In contrast, the cholinergic receptor on skeletal muscle is nicotinic, so skeletal muscle isn't affected by atropine. If one receives a lethal dose of a cholinesterase inhibitor, he or she may be a little more comfortable (less defecation, urination, respiratory tract mucus hypersecretion and bronchoconstriction, and all that) after the atropine is given, but they are still likely to die from skeletal muscle (nicotinic) overstimulation and then fatigue and paralysis (of which paralysis of the diaphragm and intercostals muscles are the most lethal consequences).

59. The answer is g. (*Brunton, pp 161–162, 171t, 173–174, 855–856; Craig, pp 94, 234–235; Katzung, pp 90, 167–170.*) The qualitative effects of guanadrel are very similar to those of reserpine. Both drugs cause what has been described as a "chemical sympathectomy," markedly reducing sympathetic (adrenergic) influences on usual target structures and thereby exposing opposing parasympathetic influences. For example, in the presence of either drug miosis, diarrhea, and urination; arterioles dilate and blood pressure falls (because there's little/no norepinephrine to be released, because it's been depleted from the nerve endings); and heart rate does not increase reflexly because it can't (again, no norepinephrine to be released to stimulate the heart). Indeed, heart rate falls markedly. Reserpine causes its effects mainly by interfering with intraneuronal storage of NE, exposing the neurotransmitter to metabolic inactivation by MAO and ultimately depleting the NE. Guanadrel releases NE directly, and gradually, eventually leading to a state of intraneuronal NE depletion with signs and symptoms very similar to those caused by reserpine.

60. The answer is c. (*Brunton, pp 189–190, 194–196; Craig, pp 138, 461, 464; Katzung, pp 115, 327–328.*) Ipratropium, a quaternary antimuscarinic drug, is FDA-approved for use as an inhaled bronchodilator for COPD. (It is used, but not FDA-approved for, some cases of asthma.) Its action involves blockade/antagonism of ACh-mediated bronchoconstrition, and it is often used adjunctively with albuterol or other β_2 agonists.

Albuterol certainly is an inhaled bronchodilator for asthma or COPD, but it works, of course, as a β_2-adrenergic agonist. Diphenhydramine has bronchodilator activity (by blocking both histamine H_1 and muscarinic receptors), but it is not given by inhalation; moreover, for ambulatory patients with asthma the mucus-thickening effects of muscarinic receptor blockade can do more harm than good. Pancuronium is a curare-like skeletal neuromuscular blocker (nicotinic/skeletal muscle competitive antagonist of ACh). Pilocarpine is a muscarinic agonist, used mainly for causing miosis in patients with angle-closure glaucoma. It will cause bronchoconstriction—an effect that may be harmful for patients with COPD and certainly would be harmful for asthmatics. A wide variety of clinical conditions are treated with antimuscarinic drugs. Dicyclomine hydrochloride and methscopolamine bromide are used to reduce GI motility, although side effects—dryness of the mouth, loss of visual accommodation, and difficulty in urination—may limit their acceptance by patients. Cyclopentolate hydrochloride is used in ophthalmology for its mydriatic and cycloplegic properties during refraction of the eye. Trihexyphenidyl hydrochloride is one of the important antimuscarinic compounds used in the treatment of parkinsonism. For bronchodilation in patients with bronchial asthma and other bronchospastic diseases, ipratropium bromide is used by inhalation. Systemic adverse reactions are low because the actions are largely confined to the mouth and airways.

61. The answer is a. (*Brunton, pp 203–204, 211–213, 1724; Craig, pp 126–130, 347; Katzung, pp 101–104.*) Although several of the listed drugs inhibit the activity of AChE, only edrophonium is used in the diagnosis of myasthenia gravis. The drug has a more rapid onset of action (1 to 3 min following intravenous administration) and a shorter duration of action (approximately 5 to 10 min) than pyridostigmine. This fast acting/short duration profile is precisely what we want in this situation. We can quickly get our diagnostic answer, yet not have to deal too long with adverse responses (such as ventilatory paralysis) if the patient was experiencing a cholinergic crisis (excessive doses of their oral cholinesterase inhibitor); and we've now worsened the situation by inhibiting the metabolic inactivation of ACh even more with our diagnostic medication. (The short duration and the need for parenteral administration preclude use of edrophonium as a practical drug for long-term treatment of myasthenia gravis.)

Malathion (b) is used topically to treat head lice and is never used internally (intentionally). Pyridostigmine (e) is used orally for maintenance therapy of myasthenia gravis. Physostigmine (c) is indicated for treatment of glaucoma (given topically), and is also a valuable parenteral drug for treating toxicity of anticholinergic drugs such as atropine. They are all cholinesterase inhibitors. Pralidoxime (d) is a "cholinesterase reactivator" and is used adjunctively (with atropine) in the treatment of poisonings caused by "irreversible" cholinesterase inhibitors, such as the "nerve gases" used as bioweapons and some commercial insecticides.

62. The answer is d. (*Brunton, pp 247, 375; Craig, pp 334–335; Katzung, p 137.*) There are several reasons for and outcomes of adding a vasoconstrictor (usually epinephrine) to some local anesthetics, including those given by infiltration. The vasoconstrictor confines the local anesthetic to the desired site of action (site of administration) by reducing local blood flow and the rate of anesthetic entry into the bloodstream. It is the bloodstream (or, more precisely, it is the presence of anesthetic in the systemic distribution system) that delivers the drug to sites where signs and symptoms of toxicity occur. Slow down anesthetic absorption rates and the drug will enter the circulation slowly enough that it can be metabolized (inactivated) fast enough to prevent accumulation to toxic levels. That is, we reduce the risk of systemic toxicity with added vasoconstrictor.

Another outcome of including a vasoconstrictor is to prolong (and certainly not shorten) the duration of local anesthetic effect. That occurs also because reduced local blood flow keeps the anesthetic in the vicinity of sensory nerves longer (since the anesthetic is not being removed as quickly by blood flow).

More on this issue will be presented in the CNS questions. But for now: Local anesthetics (except cocaine) can cause vasodilation (not vasoconstriction; a), but unless the local anesthetic dosages are quite high (toxic), the vasodilation is not intense; hypotension is uncommon with usual dosages. Likewise, cardiac depression can occur, but again that is a manifestation of overdose. We don't routinely include epinephrine in a local anesthetic to combat or prevent these cardiac-depressant problems (b), and the amount of epinephrine found in these preparations is far too low to do anything meaningful to remedy these adverse responses should they occur. Likewise, the amounts of vasoconstrictor are far too low to prevent (or treat) anesthetic-induced anaphylaxis (c)—a reaction that requires only a few molecules of antigen to occur.

So what the vasoconstrictor does is essentially cause a pharmacologic tourniquet, reducing regional blood flow that otherwise would quickly "wash away" the anesthetic. This essentially confines the anesthetic to the desired site longer (not shorter; e) than otherwise, and decreases the potential systemic reactions (d). Some local anesthetics cause vasodilation, which allows more compound to escape the tissue and enter the blood. Procaine is an ester-type local anethetics with a short duration of action due to rather rapid biotransformation in the plasma by cholinesterases. The duration of action of the drug during infiltration anesthesia is greatly increased by the addition of epinephrine, which reduces the vasodilation caused by procaine.

Finally, in plastic surgery and many other types of surgery the direct vasoconstricor effects of EPI not only antagonize the local vasodilator effects of a local anesthetic, but also cause direct vasoconstriction in the region, and thereby limit blood loss further.

63. The answer is c. (*Brunton, pp 244–247, 262, 640; Craig, p 104; Katzung, p 138.*) Epinephrine is the drug of choice to relieve the symptoms of an acute, systemic, immediate hypersensitivity reaction to an allergen (anaphylactic shock). Subcutaneous administration of a 1:1000 solution of epinephrine rapidly relieves itching and urticaria, but more importantly may save the life of the patient when laryngeal edema and bronchospasm threaten suffocation; and severe hypotension, and cardiac arrhythmias become life-endangering too. Norepinephrine, isoproterenol, and atropine are ineffective therapies. Angioedema is responsive to antihistamines (e.g., diphenhydramine), but epinephrine is necessary in the event of a severe reaction.

64. The answer is a. (*Brunton, pp 263–270; Craig, pp 111–113; Katzung, pp 142–146.*) Both phentolamine and prazosin competitively block the postsynaptic (α_1-) adrenergic receptors. Phentolamine, but not prazosin, also blocks α_2 (presynaptic) receptors.

Phentolamine, a parenteral drug, is used for acute hypertension, whether drug-induced or due to such pathologic processes as pheochromocytoma. The drug triggers significant reflex tachycardia, which poses major clinical problems. For that reason, and others, phenylephrine is being used less and less. When adrenergic blockade is indicated for rapid control of hypertension due to causes other than overdoses with a pure α agonist (e.g., phenylephrine), the combined α/β blocker labetalol is almost always used instead.

Prazosin, as you certainly know, is a selective α_1-adrenergic receptor blocker that, at therapeutic doses, has little activity at α_2-adrenergic receptors and clinically insignificant direct vasodilating activity. This oral drug is usually selected as a second-line agent for managing essential hypertension or as an adjunct to managing pheochromocytoma long-term. Since prazosin has no appreciable α_2-blocking effects, it does not interfere with the ability of norepinephrine to suppress its own neuronal release. This is one of the reasons why reflex tachycardia is more severe and common with phentolamine than with prazosin.

65. The answer is e. (*Brunton, pp 250–251, 890; Craig, p 105; Katzung, pp 133, 136, 208–209.*) Dobutamine raises LV developed pressure by acting as a β_1-selective agonist, and that is the mechanism by which it causes its positive inotropic effect (and, to a lesser degree, positive chronotropy).

To be precise, the drug is a racemic mixture: the (+) isomer, which is a potent β_1 agonist that also has some α_1-antagonist effects; the (−) isomer is an efficacious and potent α_1 agonist. So, there are probably several ways that we might classify the drug.

Nonetheless, when the drug is used for acute heart failure the intent of its use—and, indeed the main mechanism by which it does what we want—is to activate β_1 receptors. The positive inotropic and chronotropic effects raise myocardial oxygen demand, which may be problematic for patients with ischemic heart disease. On occasion, the drug may cause significant increase of blood pressure, mainly through α-mediated vasoconstriction. That is a dose-dependent phenomenon; the cardiac stimulant effects persist after the dose is dropped. Dobutamine is used clinically as a β_1-selective agonist. It is useful in CHF because of its ability to increase cardiac output while causing a decrease in ventricular filling pressure. It may not benefit patients with ischemic heart disease because it tends to increase heart rate and myocardial oxygen demand.

66. The answer is e. (*Brunton, pp 248–250; Craig, pp 47t, 103–104, 157; Katzung, pp 133, 136–137.*) Infusing low doses of dopamine activates D_1 receptors, raises vascular smooth muscle cAMP levels, and causes vasodilation in the kidneys and mesentery. (Clinicians often refer to these as "renal doses" because, in such conditions as low cardiac output, the drug is given to increase renal blood flow and urine output.) The outcome of the increased renal blood flow is increased glomerular filtration and sodium excretion. A similar D_1/cAMP-mediated effect also occurs in the renal tubules (particularly the proximal tubules and the medullary region of the thick ascending limb in the loop of Henle); this inhibits a Na^+-K^+-ATPase, which further increases renal sodium loss (by inhibiting sodium reabsorption).

67. The answer is c. (*Brunton, pp 243–245; Craig, pp 100–102; Katzung, pp 129–131.*) Recall that pulse pressure is the difference between systolic and diastolic pressures. Epinephrine's β_1 activity directly increases left ventricular pressure development, which leads to an increase in peak systolic arterial pressure. Its peripheral vasoconstricting effect (in most vascular beds), mediated by agonist activity, increases systolic pressure further. However, the drug also causes dilation in some other peripheral vascular beds (e.g., large arterioles in the extremities). This occurs via β_2 activation and tends to lower diastolic pressure (under the conditions we described). So, pulse pressure is increased by the epinephrine.

68. The answer is b. (*Brunton, pp 163–164; Craig, pp 90–92; Katzung, pp 81–83.*) Norepinephrine (and other monoamine neurotransmitters such as dopamine) is removed from its receptors by an "amine pump" located in the neuronal membrane. Recall that this reuptake process can be blocked by (among other drugs) cocaine and tricyclic antidepressants. (You might ask "what about 'stimulation' of presynaptic α_2 receptors?" Well, that answer might work, but it wasn't one of the choices here. Moreover, presynaptic α_2 receptor activation only inhibits release of additional NE; it does not stop the effects of NE that has already been released.)

Monoamine oxidase (MAO), and to a lesser degree catechol-*O*-methyl transferase (COMT), are enzymes responsible for metabolic degradation of NE (the former intraneuronally as far as monoaminergic nerves go, the other extraneuronally). However, they are not important in terminating the immediate actions of released NE, which is a process dependent mainly on neuronal reuptake following each action potential and which is not affected by MAO or COMT inhibitors.

69. The answer is f. (*Brunton, pp 290, 1522–1523, 1530; Craig, pp 113–117; Katzung, pp 154–156.*) The tachycardia associated with symptomatic, untreated hyperthyroidism reflects to a great degree thyroid hormone-related hyperreactivity of β-adrenergic receptors to catecholamines. The untoward and potentially dangerous cardiac response can be managed, symptomatically, with a β blocker. Of the conditions listed, this is the only indication for propranolol or virtually any other β blocker; and the only one that is not likely to worsen some aspect of the current clinical presentation.

Recall from your studies of cardiovascular pharmacology that β blockers (particularly such ones as labetalol and carvedilol, which also have α-blocking activity) now play important roles in managing heart failure, so long as the degree of failure is not "severe" (i.e., so long as cardiac output/ejection fraction, heart rate, or A-V nodal conduction velocity, are not so low that reducing them further could be life-threatening).

Recall, too, that even very small doses of a β blocker (even a topical β blocker that might be used for glaucoma, and even the so-called selective $β_1$ blockers such as atenolol or metoprolol) can prove lethal for some asthmatics.

β-Blockers may pose significant problems for patients with severe, poorly controlled diabetes mellitus. They can, for example, prevent tachycardia that is one signal to the patient that blood glucose levels are too low, and they can delay the recovery of blood glucose levels following an episode of hypoglycemia. However, for many patients with mild and well-controlled diabetes (especially Type 2), in such conditions as mild-to-moderate heart failure (and others) the judicious use of a β blocker probably provides more benefit than harm.

Bradycardia or heart (A-V nodal) block can be worsened by any β blocker. Administration of any β blocker to a patient with second or third degree (complete) heart block can have devastating consequences.

Finally (see the cardiovascular chapter for more), remember that β blockers may be safe and effective for chronic-stable angina, but they may worsen and be contraindicated in patients with vasospastic (variant, or Prinzmetal's) angina because they may block β-mediated coronary vasodilation and leave α-mediated constrictor (spasm-favoring) effects unopposed.

70. The answer is c. (*Brunton, p 198; Craig, p 138; Katzung, pp 116–117.*) These are among the classic signs and symptoms of atropine (antimuscarinic) poisoning. Although you may have not learned this this way, put a Lewis Carroll/*Alice in Wonderland* spin on the main findings. Maybe that will help your memory. The antimuscarinic drug-poisoning syndrome has the patient:

red as a beet (characteristic facial flushing; a so-called "atropine flush");
dry as a bone (no exocrine gland secretions, no fecal or urinary output because bowel and bladder motility are inhibited);
hot as a furnace (profound fever; a CNS "problem" compounded by a lack of body heat loss normally afforded by sweating);
blind as a bat (paralysis of accommodation and dilated pupils do not respond to even very bright light);
mad as a hatter (CNS problems, including delirium).

You may never see true atropine poisoning. As you know, that prototype antimuscarinic is not used clinically that much, except in some particular specialties. However, you should realize that many common groups of drugs (see Question 80), some of which are available over-the-counter, exert strong antimuscarinic effects. The signs and symptoms of "atropine poisoning" are an important component of their overdose syndromes.

71. The answer is a. (*Brunton, pp 23–25, 272, 274t, 276, 282t; Craig, pp 113–114; Katzung, pp 150, 153–154.*) The β blockers with intrinsic sympathomimetic activity (ISA) are partial agonists—they act simultaneously as both β agonists and competitive β blockers. How can that be? At usual doses, and in the presence of low (e.g., resting) sympathetic tone, they act as weak agonists for β-adrenergic receptors. Under these conditions, then, they may actually but slightly increase such β-mediated responses as heart rate. However, while these drugs are occupying the β-adrenergic receptors, they simultaneously block (antagonize) the effects of more efficacious ("stronger") β agonists, for example, epinephrine and norepinephrine, or such exogenous agents (drugs) as isoproterenol. Thus, although they weakly increase resting heart rate, when catecholamine levels are high (as with stress, or exercise), such β-mediated responses as acceleration of heart rate and contractility are less intense than they would be had these drugs with ISA not been present. See Question 22 (in the General Principles chapter) for more information, because it was based on the effects of a β blocker with ISA/partial agonist activity.

72. The answer is b. (*Brunton, pp 257–259, 263; Craig, pp 94, 106, 349–351; Katzung, pp 134, 139.*) Methylphenidate is similar to amphetamine and acts as a CNS stimulant, with more pronounced effects on mental than on motor activities. It does so by releasing neuronal norepinephrine and dopamine via a nonexocytotic (not dependent on action potentials) mechanism. It is used to treat narcolepsy and attention-deficit hyperactivity disorders. Dobutamine (a) is a β_1-adrenergic agonist. Pancuronium (c) is a nondepolarizing skeletal neuromuscular blocker (nicotinic receptor competitive antagonist). Prazosin (d) is a competitive and selective α_1-adrenergic blocker. Scopolamine (e) is an antimuscarinic (atropine-like) drug with greater efficacy for causing sedation and antimotion sickness effects. Terbutaline (f) is an agonist predominantly selective for β_2-adrenergic receptors at "low" doses, but it can exert nonselective (isoproterenol-like) β_1- and β_2-agonist effects at high doses, including doses that may commonly be given therapeutically.

73. The answer is e. (*Brunton, pp 142–145, 233–235; Craig, pp 141–142, 145–146; Katzung, pp 118–120.*) Answering this question requires knowledge of two things: how hexamethonium is classified (what it does); and which branch of the autonomic nervous system, parasympathetic or sympathetic, exerts "predominant resting tone" over various structures and their functions. Hexamethonium can be considered the prototypic autonomic ganglionic blocking drug, and so by blocking neurotransmission across all autonomic ganglia (and activation of the adrenal/suprarenal medulla) we essentially denervate distal structures by a pharmacologic means. (If you have not specifically learned or read about hexamethonium, perhaps you know about other ganglionic blocking drugs such as trimethaphan or mecamylamine. It's OK to consider them equivalent for the purpose of answering this question.) Now, we observe how things change.

For the structures and functions listed (and several others that weren't), it is the parasympathetic nervous system that exerts the predominant resting tone. In contrast, control of vascular smooth muscle tone (and, therefore, of blood pressure) is primarily regulated by the sympathetic nervous system. Block all ganglionic transmission and vasodilation will occur as predominant SNS influences on the vessels are removed. As far as the other structures go—all of which, we said, have predominant PNS tone at rest—we would observe a rise of heart rate; decrease of bladder and gut tone (e.g., reduced tone of the bladder detrusor and longitudinal muscles of the gut); contraction of sphincters in the GI and urinary tracts; mydriasis; and reduced salivary secretions (xerostomia). Sweat gland secretions, which are mainly under sympathetic-cholinergic influences, would decrease too.

Finally, realize that in the presence of an autonomic ganglionic blocking drug no autonomic reflexes (e.g., baroreceptor reflexes; pupillary constriction in response to bright light) can occur. Although the afferent pathways that are important in eliciting those reflexes are unimpaired, responses such as changes in heart rate or pupil size depend on intact efferent pathways, and ganglionic blockade interrupts them.

74. The answer is c. (*Brunton, pp 143t, 278, 279t, 282t–283t, 1709–1711, 1720–1722; Craig, pp 113–115; Katzung, pp 151–152.*) The secretion of aqueous humor occurs in response to activating β_2-adrenergic receptors located on ciliary epithelia. β-Adrenergic antagonists decrease secretory activity and lower intraocular pressure. Muscarinic agents induce contraction in the circular pupillary constrictor muscles. Ciliary muscle contraction facilitates opening of the trabecular meshwork, leading to better outflow of aqueous humor. α-Adrenergic agonists cause contraction of the radially oriented pupillary dilator muscles.

75. The answer is e. (*Brunton, pp 264f, 274t, 278, 1709–1710, 1720–1722; Craig, pp 113–114; Katzung, p 152.*) Timolol is a nonselective β-adrenergic blocker, and one of a handful available in a topical ophthalmic formulation that is used for chronic open-angle glaucoma, which our patient most likely has. The drug presumably works by inhibiting synthesis of aqueous humor. (Recall that drugs with either β-agonist or -antagonist activity have no effect on pupil size.)

Baclofen (a) is a centrally acting (spinal cord or higher centers) antispasmodic that is used for controlling skeletal muscle spasticity of various etiologies. It suppresses hyperreflexia probably by virtue of its GABA-mimetic actions (recall that GABA is the main inhibitory neurotransmitter in many parts of the CNS, including the spinal cord). Homatropine (b) and scopolamine (d) are atropine-like (antimuscarinic) drugs; in ophthalmology they are used mainly for diagnostic purposes to cause both mydriasis and cycloplegia (paralysis of accommodation). The mydriatic effect would have no benefits in open-angle glaucoma and could increase intraocular pressure further (by virtue of reducing aqueous humor outflow from the anterior chamber of the eye) in patients with angle-closure (narrow-angle) glaucoma. Phenylephrine (c) is the prototypic α-adrenergic agonist. Topical ophthlalmic preparations are used to cause mydriasis or conjunctival decongestion, and they do not lower intraocular pressure; oral and some topical preparations are used for mucous membrane decongestion; and parenteral formulations are generally used to raise blood pressure in hypotensive states such as those which are drug-induced (as opposed to being caused by excessive fluid/blood loss).

76. The answer is e. (*Brunton, pp 140–144, 194; Craig, pp 84, 93; Katzung, pp 86t, 91.*) By way of review of a point made (and question asked; Question 36) earlier: sympathetic innervation of sweat glands involves postganglionic sympathetic nerves that are cholinergic, not adrenergic. We know that the neurotransmitter is ACh, and more specifically that they are muscarinic, because sweat gland activation can be competitively blocked by atropine or other drugs with antimuscarinic activity. We know that this innervation is part of the sympathetic nervous system because (1) sweating occurs as part of the sympathetic "fight or flight" response to stress and (2) anatomically, the preganglionic cell bodies and the ganglia in the efferent pathway located at sites consistent with the rest of the sympathetic nerves (i.e., thoracic and lumbar origins, paravertebral ganglia).

77. The answer is e. (*Brunton, pp 154–158, 172t, 220–226; Craig, p 343; Katzung, pp 438–439.*) Tubocurarine, arguably the prototypic nondepolarizing skeletal neuromuscular blocker (competitive antagonist of the effects of ACh on skeletal muscle nicotinic receptors), differs from most of the other nondepolarizing neuromuscular blockers (including pancuronium; c) because it triggers histamine release. It exerts a "direct" degranulating effect on mast cells, not one involving activation of mast cell antibodies. This histamine-releasing effect is not clinically significant for patients who do not have asthma, but for many who do the bronchoconstriction can be intense and problematic (even though the patient is intubated). In the absence of (released) histamine, curare and the other neuromuscular blockers would have no effect on airway smooth muscle activity, since these drugs block only nicotinic receptors on skeletal muscle. Tubocurarine is not an agonist for histamine—or other—receptors.

Atropine (a) causes bronchodilation by blocking muscarinic receptors on airway smooth muscle cells. Propranolol (d) can provoke severe and sometimes fatal airway smooth muscle contraction in asthmatics, but that is due to blockade of epinephrine's agonist (bronchodilator) actions on β_2 receptors. The same outcome can be caused by neostigmine (b), but that occurs because the drug inhibits metabolic inactivation (by AChE) of acetylcholine—another bronchoconstrictor agonist to which the airways of asthmatics are exquisitely sensitive.

78. The answer is d. (*Brunton, pp 223, 227–228; Craig, p 342; Katzung, p 433.*) While this may seem like a trick question, the point is that even with markedly deficient cholinesterase activity, the succinylcholine eventually will be metabolized and its effects will disappear. All that needs to be done is to maintain adequate mechanical ventilatory support.

Succinylcholine exerts its effects by activating nicotinic receptors on skeletal muscle (powerfully but normally briefly, owing to prompt metabolism) and depolarizing the myocytes. Atropine will not work. It blocks only muscarinic receptors. Bethanechol is a muscarinic agonist. Although it may have some nicotinic activating actions at extraordinarily high doses, that effect would add to, not resolve, the effects of the succinylcholine.

Some texts note that under some conditions succinylcholine can cause what is termed Phase II block: a type of neuromuscular blockade that is curare-like (i.e., nondepolarizing). Because nondepolarizing blockade can be (and is, clinically) reversed with acetylcholinesterase inhibitors (mainly neostigmine; physostigmine would work but is not used because of its CNS effects), the implication is that we could administer a cholinesterase inhibitor here and reverse the paralysis. However, this so-called Phase II block is a manifestation of excessive (toxic) doses of succinylcholine and is not likely to apply here. Regardless, the approach is to give nothing and to ventilate the patient as long as needed, as noted.

79. The answer is c. (*Brunton, pp 143t–144t, 250; Craig, pp 93, 102; Katzung, pp 128–131.*) Piece things together. Some tip-offs to help arrive at the correct answer: no effect on the size of the pupil, so rule out any drug that has effects on the "parasympathetic" side, whether as an agonist or antagonist (here, atropine), and rule out any drug with α effects. (As noted above, no β receptors control the size of the pupil of the eye.)

Does isoproterenol fit all the other criteria/properties? Yes. And none of the other choices have all the stated properties, only some of them.

80. The answer is a. (*Brunton, pp 191–194, 198; Craig, p 138; Katzung, pp 109–115.*) These drugs all possess antimuscarinic (atropine-like) actions that often are sufficiently strong to cause all the side effects and adverse responses associated with atropine itself. Likewise, it is prudent to assume they share all the contraindications and precautions associated with atropine and that managing severe overdoses of those drugs or drug groups will resemble (and need to be treated) in quite the same way as those of the prototype antimuscarinic. That would include the potential need to administer physostigmine, the acetylcholinesterase inhibitor that plays an important role in managing atropine poisoning.

Note that of all the drugs with atropine-like actions, diphenhydramine (and, to a somewhat lesser extent the other first generation antihistamines) are available over-the-counter. Although you may do your best to avoid prescribing drugs with atropine-like actions for patients who should not receive them, atropine-like problems can arise in patients who self-prescribe these nonprescription medications.

Clearly, the effects of bethanechol (muscarinic agonist) and neostigmine (acetylcholinesterase inhibitor) are the opposite of those you'd expect to see with atropine (muscarinic receptor blocker). You might argue that isoproterenol (β_1 and β_2 agonist) causes some effects (e.g., tachycardia) that you would expect with atropine. True. However, despite any similarities in appearance, the mechanism is quite different, the spectrum of all effects caused by the drug is different, and certainly most contraindications and toxic manifestations are very different. Propranolol (prototype nonselective β blocker) is radically different from atropine in nearly every important way.

81. The answer is a. (*Brunton, pp 198, 211–214; Craig, pp 126–131; Katzung, pp 101–104.*) Physostigmine is basically the only clinically useful AChE inhibitor that gets into the brain, a major target of atropine/antimuscarinic poisoning. That is because it lacks the quaternary structure (it is charged at virtually all pH values likely to be found in a living person) that nearly all the other common alternatives possess, and lacking that structure it can cross the blood-brain barrier.

Alternatives such as neostigmine, pyridostigmine, and others will combat peripheral effects of atropine poisoning, just as physostigmine will. Unfortunately, some of the CNS manifestations (e.g., severe fever, leading to seizures) contribute greatly to the morbidity and mortality associated with high dose of antimuscarinics, and the quaternary agents simply will not combat them in the CNS.

You won't encounter too many patients overdosed on atropine itself, but you'll see many people suffering toxicity from older antihistamines (e.g., diphenhydramine), older (tricyclic or tetracyclic) antidepressants (e.g., imipramine), some of the centrally acting antimuscarinics that are used for parkinsonism (e.g., benztropine and trihexyphenidyl), scopolamine (used for motion sickness), and most of the phenothiazine antipsychotics (e.g., chlorpromazine). Owing to the often strong antimuscarinic side effects of these drugs, treating overdoses of any of them probably will involve managing what amounts to "atropine poisoning"—and many other problems too.

(You may not know this, and perhaps it will have some meaning or help jog your memory: the trade name for physostigmine is Antilirium. Recall that one of the hallmark CNS signs of atropine/antimuscarinic poisoning is delirium. Hence, Antilirium.)

82. The answer is a. (*Brunton, pp 24, 151–152, 171, 224–225, 229; Craig, pp 67t, 94t, 340–341; Katzung, p 90.*) Botulinus (botulinum) toxin prevents release of acetylcholine (from storage vesicles) by virtually all cholinergic nerves in the autonomic and somatic nervous systems. (Take a look at the schematic of the peripheral nervous systems on Page 40 to refresh your memory about where these sites are.) Thus, there is no activation (let alone "massive overstimulation," d) of any cholinergic receptors, whether nicotinic or muscarinic.

Noteworthy findings, then, include an inability to activate all postganglionic neurons (sympathetic and parasympathetic), no physiologic release of epinephrine from the adrenal/suprarenal medulla, and flaccid skeletal muscle paralysis due to failure of ACh release from motor nerves. The cause of death is ventilatory failure because the intercostals muscles and diaphragm are paralyzed—but of course that's not the only problem.

Pralidoxime (b) is a cholinesterase reactivator, an antidote for poisonings with "irreversible" cholinesterase inhibitors such as soman, sarin ("nerve gases"), and many organophosphorus insecticides. Because no ACh is being released in botulinus poisoning, "reactivation" of the enzyme that normally metabolizes the neurotransmitter is irrelevant (and ineffective).

83. The answer is d. (*Brunton, pp 238, 240t–241t, 250–251; Craig, pp 101–102, 112t; Katzung, pp 136–137, 212–213.*) Dobutamine behaves, for all practical purposes, as a selective β_1 agonist. Norepinephrine is a β_1 agonist that also activates α-adrenergic receptors effectively. However, when it is administered with phentolamine (prototype α blocker) its spectrum of activity is, qualitatively, identical to that of dobutamine.

High doses of dopamine (a) cause positive inotropic and chronotropic effects, but also release neuronal norepinephrine and probably activate α-adrenergic receptors directly (causing unwanted vasoconstriction). These vasoconstrictor effects would negate vasodilator effects due to stimulation of dopamine D_1 receptors found in some arterioles and of D_2 receptors found on some ganglia, and in the cardiovascular control center of the CNS.

Ephedrine (b) weakly activates all adrenergic receptors and also leads to norepinephrine release. Overall, its effects are quite similar to those produced by norepinephrine itself. Regardless, if one administers ephedrine with propranolol (c), the prototypic nonselective (β_1 and β_2) beta blocker, ephedrine's remaining actions amount to selective α-adrenergic activation (i.e., phenylephrine-like)—not at all like dobutamine, and not at all what we want in this situation.

Phenylephrine (α agonist) plus atropine (muscarinic antagonist) (e) causes effects that in no way resemble those of dobutamine or the norepinephrine-phentolamine combination. From a cardiovascular perspective, this combination would give us a rise of blood pressure due to peripheral vasoconstriction. The vasoconstriction would elicit a baroreceptor reflex tantamount to withdrawing sympathetic tone and increasing opposing parasympathetic tone. However, the presence of atropine would blunt parasympathetic-mediated cardiac slowing. The overall and combined effect on heart rate of reduced sympathetic tone to the SA node, and concomitant blockade of ACh–mediated cardiac slowing (also an effect on the SA node) can vary. However, it would be reasonable to predict a slight increase of rate over predrug rates. Nonetheless, there would not be a positive inotropic response, which is what would occur with either dobutamine or a norepinephrine-phentolamine combination.

84. The answer is a. (*Brunton, pp 143t, 243–246; Craig, pp 93, 103; Katzung, p 130.*) With only one major exception (sweat glands), the neurotransmitter released by postganglionic sympathetic nerves (adrenergic nerves) to activate their targets is norepinephrine (NE). Of course, NE is a "good" agonist for only α- and β₁-adrenergic receptors. In contrast, epinephrine (from the adrenal medulla) is a good agonist for both classes of adrenergic receptors and their main subtypes, including β_2. Of the responses listed in the question, only airway smooth muscle relaxation is a process that involves (depends on) activation of β_2-adrenergic receptors. There is no innervation of these muscles, and so no NE to be released. Even if NE were injected, its lack of β_2 agonist activity would render it ineffective as a bronchodilator.

85. The answer is b. (*Brunton, pp 143t–145t, 234t; Craig, p 93; Katzung, pp 86, 129–131.*) To me, the tip-off that helps get to the correct answer, isoproterenol, is to focus (no pun intended) on the fact that the unknown drug did not change the size of the pupil of the eye. Of all the main autonomic receptor types, adrenergic and cholinergic, only the β receptors play no role in regulating the size of the pupil. That narrows things down to isoproterenol or propranolol. Propranolol might lower BP (particularly in a hypertensive patient), but it would not raise heart rate or dilate the bronchi. Only isoproterenol fits the bill.

And the other answers? Atropine might raise heart rate, it is not likely to lower BP, it will dilate the airways, but it would also cause mydriasis. Neostigmine would slow heart rate, maybe lower BP (probably not), and constrict the airways and pupils. Phenylephrine would raise BP, and if the BP rise is sufficiently high and quick, reflexly lower heart rate. It would do nothing to airway diameter, but would cause mydriasis.

86. The answer is a. (*Brunton, pp 227–228; Craig, p 137; Katzung, pp 440–441.*) Skeletal muscle paralysis from curare-like drugs involves competitive blockade of skeletal muscle nicotinic receptors. We reverse that by administering an ACh esterase inhibitor (e.g., neostigmine). Of course, the increased peripheral ACh levels will not only overcome skeletal muscle blockade, but also exert expected muscarinic-activating effects of various smooth muscles (e.g., the airways), the heart, and exocrine glands. We prevent those unwanted "parasympathomimetic" effects by giving atropine (antimuscarinic) right before giving the cholinesterase inhibitor. None of the other approaches are rational or used for "reversal."

87. The answer is f. (*Brunton, pp 158–164; Craig, pp 90–92; Katzung, p 82f.*) The hydroxylation of dietary tyrosine by tyrosine hydroxylase is generally considered to be the rate-limiting step in the synthesis of all the catecholamines:

dopamine (DA), epinephrine (EPI), and norepinephrine (NE). Catechol-*O*-methyltransferase (a) metabolically inactivates of many catecholamines (endogenous or given as drugs) extraneuronally; Dopamine decarboxylase (b) is actually one of several L-amino acid decarboxylases, and in the nervous systems it catalyzes the conversion of DOPA (dihydroxyphenylalanine) to dopamine. Dopamine β-hydroxylase (c) converts dopamine to norepinephrine. Monoamine oxidase (MAO; d) is a main intracellular (mitochondrial) enzyme involved in the degradation of catecholamines and many other pharmacologically active monoamines. Phenylethanolamine N-methyltransferase (e), in the presence of sufficient amounts of S-adenosylmethionine, converts NE to EPI (e.g., in the adrenal/suprarenal medulla), and follows the synthesis of dopamine that is the metabolic precursor of both NE and EPI.

88. The answer is e. (*Brunton, pp 163–164; Craig, pp 90–92; Katzung, pp 79–82.*) In short, the answer is "reuptake." A norepinephrine transporter plays the main role in terminating the activity of neuronally (physiologically) released NE. This transporter is blocked by cocaine and tricyclic antidepressants (e.g., imipramine). Diffusion of released NE from the synaptic space, leading to metabolism by such enzymes as COMT (d), is overall a minor process in terms of the physiologic inactivation of the effects of NE. Metabolic inactivation by MAO (c) requires reuptake of the catecholamines into the neuron, since the MAO that degrades catecholamines is located intraneuronally (and intramitochondrially).

89. The answer is c. (*Brunton, pp 263–270; Craig, pp 111–113; Katzung, pp 144–146, 148.*) Tamsulosin is a selective α_1-adrenergic blocker, and presumably its affinity is greater for α receptors on smooth muscles in the prostate (hence, its use for BPH, due to relaxation of smooth muscles there) than for those in the peripheral vasculature. Nonetheless, its pharmacologic profile is most similar to that of prazosin, which can be considered the prototypic α_1-selective adrenergic blocker that is mainly used to treat hypertension because it competitively blocks vasoconstriction caused by α agonists such as epinephrine and norepinephrine. (Remember: drugs with a generic name that ends in "-osin" or "-zosin" are selective α_1-adrenergic blockers: for example, tamsulosin, prazosin, terazosin, doxazosin.)

So, of the answers listed above, orthostatic hypotension is the most likely side effect. Among the many classes of adrenergic drugs, bradycardia would most likely be caused by a β blocker (or lesser prescribed drugs such as reserpine, a catecholamine depletor), or a muscarinic agonist or cholinesterase inhibitor, and certainly not by a drug that has no direct cardiac effects and is more likely to elicit reflex cardiac stimulation secondary to reduced blood pressure. There are no known interactions between α blockers and atorvastatin or related drugs. Photophobia is an unlikely problem: it is usually caused by drugs that cause mydriasis (e.g., α-adrenergic agonists or antimuscarinics), and if anything tamsulosin is likely to prevent the mydriasis that is a common cause of photophobia. Exacerbations of emphysema, whether due to bronchoconstriction or other causes, is unlikely too. From an autonomic perspective, epinephrine is the main bronchodilator substance (via β_2 activation), ACh is the main autonomic bronchoconstrictor (via muscarinic activation). Tamsulosin affects neither.

90. The answer is c. (*Brunton, pp 186–188, 1712, 1720–1722; Craig, pp 134–138; Katzung, pp 111–115.*) There are a couple of ways you could (should?) have arrived at this answer, even if you did not learn specifically about homatropine being a shorter-acting, semisynthetic derivative of atropine, the prototypic antimuscarinic drug.

First off, consider major autonomic innervation of the eye. The sympathetic nervous system, via α-adrenergic receptors, controls mainly the size of the pupil of the eye; there is very little influence on the ciliary muscle or other structures that control accommodation. (β-Adrenergic influences play no role in controlling pupil size or tone of the ciliary muscle.) The parasympathetic branch of the ANS, and its influences on muscarinic receptors, can alter both pupil size and accommodation—precisely what we have here. So, we can rule out any "sympathetic" drug, agonist or antagonist, as a correct answer. Thus, we reject epinephrine (b), an α and β agonist that would cause mydriasis; isoproterenol (d), the β_1/β_2 agonist; and propranolol (f), the β_1/β_2 blocker, that affect neither pupil size nor accommodation.

We reject ACh (A); this muscarinic agonist would cause miosis and facilitates accommodation. The same applies to pilocarpine (e). This leaves us with homatropine (c). So you could arrive at this correct answer either by the process of elimination, or by making an educated guess (correctly, of course) that *hom*atropine is an atropine-like (antimuscarinic) drug.

91. The answer is d. (*Brunton, pp 30, 177, 184–187, 395–396; Craig, pp 123–124; Katzung, pp 98–100.*) ACh, *in vivo* or *in vitro*, causes its vasodilator response *via* an action on the endothelium, where the muscarinic receptors are located. The vasodilator response ultimately depends on endothelial cell formation of nitric oxide (NO), which in the case of ACh is a process that emanates from and involves endothelial cell integrity. When the endothelium is damaged or removed (d; the most likely case described here), the direct effect of ACh on vascular smooth muscle is contraction (constriction of arterioles). Atropine, the prototype muscarinic antagonist, will prevent ACh-mediated vasodilation of intact arterioles (b), with intact endothelium, by blocking the interaction between ACh and endothelial cell muscarinic recptors, but it will not cause vasoconstriction when the endothelium is intact (it is important here to distinguish between preventing vasodilation and causing vasoconstriction). Botulinum toxin (c) prevents ACh release from cholinergic nerves, but in our experimental setup that is irrelevant because the *in vitro* preparation is devoid of innervation, and ACh is added directly to the tissue bath. Moreover, even if the smooth muscle preparation were innervated, botulinum toxin would not convert the usual vasodilator response to ACh into a vasoconstrictor one.

92. The answer is b. (*Brunton, pp 151–152, 171, 224, 229; Craig, pp 66–67, 341–342; Katzung, p 90t.*) The toxin inhibits release of ACh from all cholinergic nerves. It has no agonist (a) activity on any cholinergic receptors, nor an ability to block nicotinic (e) or muscarinic receptors. The toxin has no direct effects on adrenergic nerves (other than preventing their physiologic activation by ACh, normally released by preganglionic sympathetic nerves. Thus, NE reuptake is not affected (c; recall that cocaine and tricyclic antidepressants do inhibit NE reuptake) nor is NE released (d) as occurs with, say, amphetamines.

93. The answer is c. (*Brunton, pp 197–198, 634t, 637–640, 642, 1002; Craig, pp 138t, 370, 453–455; Katzung, pp 114, 264–266.*) The peripheral autonomic actions of diphenhydramine (an ethanolamine-type "first generation" histamine H-1 antagonist) are very similar to those of atropine, the prototypic competitive muscarinic receptor antagonist. These effects are seen with both therapeutic doses (e.g., dry mouth, blurred vision, and occasionally urinary retention or constipation) and toxicity. In life-threatening cases physostigmine, the "antidote for atropine poisoning" may be a valuable adjunct. Diphenhydramine, and other H_1 blockers, have no direct effects (either as agonist or antagonist) on adrenergic receptors; and no nicotinic receptor-activating activity, whether in autonomic ganglia or at the adrenal medulla (suprarenal gland).

94. The answer is d. (*Brunton, pp 210–211; Craig, pp 66–67, 127–128; Katzung, pp 103, 117, 989t.*) Pralidoxime is classified as a "cholinesterase reactivator" and is used specifically, and adjunctively, for managing poisoning with the long-acting ("irreversible") organophosphate cholinesterase inhibitors that are found in some insecticides; and "nerve gases" such as soman, sarin, and VX. Pralidoxime, an oxime, has very high affinity for phosphorus in the organophosphates. If given early enough in the poisoning it will prevent or reverse the binding of the organophosphate to, and long-term inhibition of, the active binding site on the cholinesterase. The need for early pralidoxime administration is critical: if it is delayed too long the enzyme will "age," yielding a largely permanent and irreversible enzyme configuration.

Methylphenidate (a) is an indirect-acting (norepinephrine-releasing or amphetamine-like) sympathomimetic; pralidoxime has no effect on its actions, nor on the actions of epinephrine (b) or prazosin (e), a selective α_1-adrenergic blocker. Although neostigmine (d) is a cholinesterase inhibitor it is not an organophosphate (it is a carbamate), and it is spontaneously and relatively quickly hydrolyzed leading to loss of cholinesterase-inhibitory activity. Thus, use of pralidoxime for excesses of neostigmine (or other carbamate) doses would be both ineffective (mechanistically) and unnecessary.

95. The answer is b. (*Brunton, pp 143t, 1720–1722; Craig, pp 92–94; Katzung, pp 86t, 91f, 131, 138.*) Start off with a fundamental review of autonomic innervation of the eye insofar as control of pupil size, and effects on the ciliary muscle (which affects accommodation . . . the ability of the lens of the eye to thicken so we can see close-up). The sympathetic nervous system, via α-adrenergic receptor activation, has the ability to cause mydriasis. Activate those receptors and the pupil dilates; or block the opposing parasympathetic influences (via muscarinic receptor blockade) and the same thing happens, since there's a relatively comparable influence of both branches of the autonomic nervous system on pupil size. However, there is little resting influence of the sympathetic nervous system (or adrenergic receptors) on the tone of the ciliary muscle. That is mainly a parasympathetic-dependent phenomenon that indirectly affects the shape of the lens of their eyes and, so, the point of sharp focus. And, for all practical purposes, β receptor activation has no influence on pupil size or accommodation.

Now, classify the drugs by their sites and mechanisms of action.

Eliminate atropine (a) as a possible answer choice. By blocking all ocular effects of normal parasympathetic innervation (muscarinic blockade), it will both dilate the pupil and impair accommodation. The same applies to homatropine (c), a drug that is, for all practical purposes, atropine-like. Pilocarpine (e), a muscarinic agonist, will *constrict* the pupil of the eye and impair cholinergic mechanisms involved in focusing of the lens. Isoproterenol (d) activates all β-adrenergic receptors, timolol (f) blocks them all, and as we said, β receptors are not relevant in terms of pupil size or accommodation. This leaves us with epinephrine: it has both α-adrenergic and β-adrenergic activating activity, and no cholinergic/muscarinic activity. It will dilate the pupil and not significantly affect accommodation.

96. The answer is e. (*Brunton, pp 631–632, 640–641; Craig, pp 138t, 453–455; Katzung, pp 109, 266.*) You may have chosen d (histamine H_1 receptor blocker) as your answer to this question. However, although diphenhydramine is an "antihistamine," histamine plays a minor role in the symptoms of rhinovirus infections (in contrast with a much more important role in, say, seasonal allergies). As a result, blocking the effects of histamine on its receptors does not cause profound symptom relief in this situation. The drying up of nasal secretions afforded by diphenhydramine (an ethanolamine-type H_1 blocker and the prototype of the first generation agents) in this instance is due to the drug's rather intense muscarinic receptor-blocking (atropine-like) actions.

97. The answer is c. (*Brunton, pp 254, 260, 263–267, 269–271; Craig, pp 105, 111–113; Katzung, pp 122–124, 130–131, 142–145.*) Phenylephrine raises blood pressure by activating α-adrenergic receptors on vascular smooth-muscle cells. Prazosin competitively blocks those receptors, and when present at sufficiently high doses (as might occur with an acute, severe overdose) may eliminate the vasopressor response to even higher than usual doses of phenylephrine. β Blockers (atenolol, propranolol) have no α-blocking activity and so won't reduce the vasopressor response to phenylephrine. Nor will bethanechol, which causes vasodilation by activating muscarinic receptors for ACh. And reserpine? See the answer to Question 98.

98. The answer is e. (*Craig, pp 94, 97; Brunton, pp 161–162, 171t, 173–174, 856; Katzung, p 89.*) Reserpine treatment of sufficient duration depletes neuronal norepinephrine. This accounts for the lowered blood pressure with therapeutic doses or frank hypotension with overdoses. One consequence of this, long-term, is development of adrenergic receptor supersensitivity because the receptors just aren't being activated as they should. And a consequence of that, in turn, will be heightened (and sometimes extreme) responses to a given dose of adrenergic agonists that can activate adrenergic receptors (α- or β-) directly, including the phenylephrine you administered. (That is, the dose-response curve for direct-acting adrenergic agonists is "shifted to the left" after long-term reserpine treatment.)

99. The answer is e. (*Brunton, pp 205–207, 212–214; Craig, pp 126–130, 347; Katzung, pp 101–104.*) Edrophonium is fast- and short-acting parenteral acetylcholinesterase inhibitor—one of the relatively few members of that therapeutic class with a generic name that doesn't end in "-stigmine."

The question states that we are dealing with a patient experiencing a cholinergic crisis. That means, of course, that she has received either relatively or absolutely excessive doses of the oral cholinesterase inhibitor (e.g., pyridostigmine, neostigmine, several others) used to manage her myasthenia gravis. Because of the dosage excess, and the excess ACh accumulating at the skeletal neuromuscular junctions (owing to reduced metabolic inactivation of the neurotransmitter), her skeletal muscles are weakened and fatigued from what amounts to overstimulation of nicotinic receptors by the ACh. This skeletal muscle hypofunction involves not only muscles in the extremities, but also the diaphragm and intercostals that must function normally for adequate ventilation. So, when we give a cholinesterase inhibitor to patients like the one described above, who is already experiencing excessive cholinergic effects, further (over)activation of the diaphragm and intercostals may be sufficient to cause ventilatory distress or total ventilatory failure. This is the main reason why the "edrophonium test" is so dangerous should the underlying problem actually be the cholinergic crisis, and why edrophonium is preferred to other ACh esterase inhibitors because it has a very short duration of action (highly desirable should adverse effects occur).

Edrophonium is not at all likely to trigger a hypertensive crisis (a). It and other drugs in its class, or direct muscarinic agonists (e.g., bethanechol) for that matter, have no vasoconstrictor activity (when vascular endothelial cells are intact). Cholinesterase inhibitors are far more likely to lower heart rate (*via* indirect muscarinic receptor activation secondary to inhibited ACh hydrolysis at the SA node) than stimulate it (b); and just as the drug causes no peripheral vasoconstriction, it causes no coronary vasoconstriction. Ventricular automaticity is likely to decrease further, not increase (c), in response to increased muscarinic activation. Edrophonium will not improve skeletal muscle tone and function (d) if the problem is a cholinergic crisis; that is the expected response, however, if the patient has a myasthenic crisis (reflecting inadequate dosages of the cholinesterase inhibitor used for maintenance therapy).

Note: For many patients with myasthenia gravis, and who are being treated with an oral cholinesterase inhibitor, you should be able to differentiate between a myasthenic and a cholinergic crisis without resorting to the "edrophonium test." You simply need to assess your patient carefully, and apply some basic autonomic pharmacology knowledge. In either crisis, the main common features are skeletal muscle fatigability, weakness, or paralysis due to inadequate (myasthenic crisis) or excessive (cholinergic crisis) activation of nicotinic receptors on skeletal muscle.

With a myasthenic crisis the primary problems are *confined to skeletal muscle* function (and secondary consequences of that, such as inadequate ventilation).

Things usually present quite differently, however, if the underlying problem is a cholinergic crisis. Remember that cholinesterase inhibitors do not act only at skeletal neuromuscular junctions. They also act at all cholinergic synapses in the peripheral nervous systems: at all the postganglionic parasympathetic nerve "endings" and at the synapses between postganglionic sympathetic fibers and sweat glands—inhibiting ACh metabolism there, and leading to signs and symptoms of muscarinic activation in addition to nicotinic/skeletal muscle effects.

Thus, in patients who are experiencing a cholinergic crisis many or most of the signs and symptoms typically associated with parasympathetic (muscarinic) activation will occur, and they will be useful to you in making the differential diagnosis if you look and listen carefully: miosis and excessive lacrimation, salivation, bradycardia (and possibly A-V block determined by an EKG), wheezing or other manifestations of bronchoconstriction and/or increased airway mucus secretions; gut and bladder hypermotility (e.g., defecation, urinary frequency or incontinence, increased bowel sounds), and diaphoresis. See some of these in addition to skeletal muscle dysfunction and you should be thinking cholinergic crisis and placing myasthenic crisis further down on your list of possible diagnoses.

The Central Nervous System

Antidepressants and other mood-stabilizing drugs
Antiepileptics
Antiparkinson's
Antipsychotics
Anxiolytics
Central nervous systems
Stimulants and anorexigenic agents

Ethanol and related alcohols
General anesthetics and anesthesia adjuncts
Opioid analgesics and antagonists
Psychotomimetics
Sedatives, hypnotics

Questions

DIRECTIONS: Each item contains a question or incomplete statement that is followed by several responses. Select the **one best** response to each question.

100. A 42-year-old woman develops akathisias, parkinsonian-like dyskinesias, galactorrhea, and amenorrhea, during drug therapy. Which of the following drug-receptor-based mechanisms, occurring in the central nervous system, most likely caused these responses?

a. Blockade of α-adrenergic receptors
b. Blockade of dopamine receptors
c. Blockade of muscarinic receptors
d. Supersensitivity of dopamine receptors
e. Stimulation of nicotinic receptors

101. A patient on the trauma-burn unit receives a drug to ease the pain of debridement and dressing changes. The patient experiences good, prompt analgesia, but despite the absence of pain sensation during the procedure her heart rate and blood pressure rise considerably, consistent with the concept that the sympathetic nervous system was activated by the pain and not affected by the analgesic drug. As the effects of the drug develop, the patient's skeletal muscle tone progressively increases. The patient appears awake at times because the eyes periodically open. As drug effects wear off, the patient hallucinates and behaves in a very agitated fashion. Which of the following drug was most likely given?

a. Fentanyl
b. Ketamine
c. Midazolam
d. Succinylcholine
e. Thiopental

102. A patient who has been treated with levodopa is switched to a regimen with a proprietary product that contains both levodopa and carbidopa. Which of the following is the main action of carbidopa that provides the rationale for using it in this combined approach?

a. Blocks ACh release in the CNS, thereby facilitating levodopa's ability to restore a dopamine-ACh balance
b. Helps activate dietary vitamin B_6, a deficiency of which occurs during levodopa therapy
c. Increases permeability of the blood-brain barrier to levodopa, giving levodopa better access to the CNS
d. Inhibits metabolic conversion of levodopa to dopamine outside the CNS
e. Reduces levodopa-induced hypotension by blocking vascular dopamine receptors

103. The attending with whom you are working in the emergency department quizzes you on your basic knowledge of local anesthetics and their uses. She asks you to identify the drug that is suitable for topical administration (e.g., to mucous membranes), but cannot be given parenterally because of its physicochemical properties, which render it very poorly soluble. Which of the following drugs is the best answer to her question?

a. Benzocaine
b. Bupivacaine
c. Etidocaine
d. Mepivacaine
e. Procaine

104. A physician considers placing a patient on long-term (months, years) phenobarbital for control of a relatively common medical condition. For most of these indications, newer and arguably more efficacious drugs are available and preferred. For which of the following, however, is it still considered reasonable and appropriate to use this barbiturate?

a. Alcohol withdrawal signs/symptoms
b. Anxiety management
c. Certain epilepsies
d. Endogenous depression (adjunct to SSRIs)
e. Sleep disorders such as insomnia

105. One reason for the declining use of tricyclic antidepressants such as imipramine, and the growing use of newer classes, is the prevalence of common tricyclic-induced side effects or adverse responses. Which of the following best describes the side effects or adverse responses that are most likely to occur with the administration of a tricyclic?

a. Anticholinergic (antimuscarinic) effects
b. Arrhythmias
c. Hepatotoxicity
d. Nephrotoxicity
e. Seizures

106. A 17-year-old male was diagnosed with epilepsy after developing repeated episodes of generalized tonic-clonic sezures following a motor vehicle accident in which he received a closed head injury. After treating acute seizures with the proper injectable drugs, he is started on a regimen of oral phenytoin, the daily dose titrated upwards until symptom control and a therapeutic plasma concentration were reached. The elimination half-life of the drug during initial treatment was measured to be 24 h, a value that is quite typical for otherwise healthy adults taking no other drugs.

Today he presents in the neurology clinic with nystagmus, ataxia, diplopia, cognitive impairment, and other signs and symptoms consistent with phenytoin toxicity. A blood sample, drawn at noon, has a plasma phenytoin concentration of 30 mcg/mL. That value is 50% higher than typical peak therapeutic serum concentrations and twice the usual minimum effective blood level. These values are summarized in the figure.

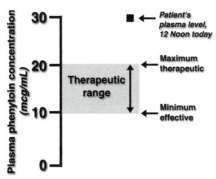

We will withhold further doses of phenytoin until plasma levels fall into the therapeutic range, and the patient is largely free of signs and symptoms of phenytoin toxicity. However, which of the following statements correctly summarizes what we should do, or expect to occur, next?

a. Administer flumazenil, which will quickly reverse signs and symptoms of phenytoin toxicity but may cause seizures to recur

b. Elimination of phenytoin from the plasma will follow zero-order kinetics for several days

c. Give an amphetamine or other CNS stimulant to reverse generalized CNS depression due to the phenytoin excess

d. Give phenobarbital to induce the P450 system, thereby hastening phenytoin's metabolic elimination

e. Plasma phenytoin concentrations will fall to 15 mcg/mL, in the middle of the therapeutic range, by noon the next day (24 h later, per the usual half-life)

107. We have a patient with Parkinson's disease. Signs and symptoms can be classified as "moderate" now but progressive and not responding well to current drug therapy. The physician decides to empirically assess an antiparkinson drug that is a selective inhibitor of monoamine oxidase type B (MAO-B). Which of the following drugs would that be?

a. Bromocriptine
b. Carbidopa
c. Phenelzine
d. Selegiline
e. Tranylcypromine

108. Meperidine is similar to morphine in many ways. However, with very high blood levels or with true overdoses, meperidine can cause significant adverse responses that simply aren't seen with morphine or most other opioid analgesics. Which of the following best identifies that rather unique effect of meperidine?

a. Constipation leading to paralytic ileus
b. Heightened response to pain (paradoxical hyperalgesia)
c. Intense biliary tract spasm
d. Psychosis-like state, possibly seizures
e. Respiratory depression, apnea, ventilatory arrest

109. Chlorpromazine and haloperidol can be considered prototypes of two relatively old but still used antipsychotic drugs—the phenothiazines and the butyrophenones—respectively. While many of the actions and side effects of these drugs are qualitatively similar, they are different quantitatively: that is, in terms of incidence and severity. Which of the following effects or side effects typically occur more frequently, and could be said to be more severe, with haloperidol?

a. Extrapyramidal reactions
b. Intense atropine-like side effects
c. Lethal blood dyscrasias
d. Orthostatic hypotension
e. Urinary retention necessitating bladder catheterization

110. A patient is transported to the emergency department. A friend who accompanies the patient to the ED says "he was experimenting with (PCP phencyclidine)." Which of the following best describes the actions of phencyclidine?

a. Causes its peripheral and central effects via antimuscarinic properties
b. Causes significant withdrawal symptoms
c. Has hallucinogenic properties
d. Has strong opioid receptor-activating activity
e. Overdoses should be treated with flumazenil

111. After a few weeks on a drug, a patient reports profound thirst and the production of copious volumes of clear (dilute) urine each day. Which of the following drugs is most likely responsible for the signs and symptoms?

a. Diazepam
b. Fluoxetine
c. Haloperidol
d. Lithium
e. Phenytoin

112. A 12-year-old boy has been treated with methylphenidate for the last 3 years. His younger sister finds the bottle of pills and consumes enough to cause significant toxicity. Which of the following findings would you most likely expect?

a. Hypertension, tachycardia, seizures
b. Hypotension, bronchospasm
c. Drowsiness, obtunded reflexes, diarrhea
d. Miosis, bradycardia, profuse salivation, sweating
e. Hypothermia, skeletal muscle weakness or paralysis, pupils that are not responsive to light

113. Two inhaled general anesthetics, A and B, have the following MAC values:

A. MAC = 2%
B. MAC = 100%

Based on this information alone, which of the following statements is true?

a. Drug A has a longer duration of action than Drug B
b. Drug A is more soluble in the blood than Drug B
c. Drug B causes greater analgesia and skeletal muscle relaxation than Drug A
d. The concentration of drug in inspired air that is needed to cause adequate surgical anesthesia is higher for Drug B than for Drug A
e. The time to onset of adequate general anesthesia is 50 times longer for Drug B than for Drug A

114. A 31-year-old woman has been treated with fluoxetine for 5 months. She is diagnosed with another medical problem and receives one or more drugs that, otherwise, would be suitable and probably problem-free. She is rushed to the ED with unstable vital signs, muscle rigidity, myoclonus, CNS irritability and altered consciousness, and shivering. Which of the following add-on drugs most likely causes these responses?

a. Codeine for cough
b. Loratadine for seasonal allergies
c. Midazolam and fentanyl, used to ease discomfort from endoscopy
d. Sumatriptan for migraine
e. Zolpidem for short-term insomnia

115. A 72-year-old woman with a long history of anxiety that has been treated with diazepam decides to triple her daily dose because of increasing fearfulness about "environmental noises." Two days after her attempt at self-prescribing, she is found extremely lethargic and nonresponsive, with markedly obtunded reflexes and reaction to painful stimuli. Respirations are 8/min and shallow. Which of the following drugs should we give specifically to reverse these signs and symptoms?

a. Dextroamphetamine
b. Flumazenil
c. Naltrexone
d. Physostigmine
e. Pralidoxime

116. A patient who has been treated for Parkinson's disease for about a year presents with purplish, mottled changes to her skin. Which of the following drugs is the most likely cause?

a. Amantadine
b. Bromocriptine
c. Levodopa (alone)
d. Levodopa combined with carbidopa
e. Pramipexole

117. A young boy who has been treated for epilepsy for a year is referred to a periodontist for evaluation and probable treatment of massive overgrowth of his gingival tissues. Some teeth are almost completely covered with hyperplastic tissue. Which of the following drugs was the most likely cause of the oral pathology?

a. Carbamazepine
b. Lorazepam
c. Phenobarbital
d. Phenytoin
e. Valproic acid

118. A patient with undiagnosed coronary artery disease is given a medication. Shortly thereafter she develops intense tightness and "crushing discomfort" of her chest. An EKG reveals ST–segment changes indicative of acute myocardial ischemia. The patient suffered acute myocardial ischemia and angina pectoris as a result of the drug. Which of the following drugs most likely causes this reaction?

a. Clozapine
b. Pentazocine
c. Phenytoin
d. Sumatriptan
e. Zolpidem

119. A patient with status epilepticus has received an IV dose of lorazepam. At the institution at which you trained, phenytoin would be given next, but the attending orders fosphenytoin. Which of the following best describes the main advantage of the fosphenytoin over phenytoin itself?

a. Causes less vascular/venous irritation, can be injected at a faster rate
b. Directly stimulates ventilation (action in brain's medulla) that is compromised during status epilepticus
c. Has a mechanism of anticonvulsant action that is different from and more effective than plain phenytoin
d. Has such a long duration of action that oral anticonvulsant therapy is not needed once the status epilepticus has been stopped
e. Lacks intrinsic anticonvulsant activity but slows lorazepam clearance, thereby prolonging lorazepam's anticonvulsant action

120. Nitrous oxide is a common component in the technique of balanced anesthesia. It is used in conjunction with such other drugs as a halogenated hydrocarbon volatile liquid anesthetic, and usually included as 80% of the total inspired gas mixture. Which of the following best summarizes why nitrous oxide cannot be used alone for general anesthesia?

a. Almost total lack of analgesic activity, regardless of concentration
b. Inspired concentrations > 10% tend to profound cardiac negative inotropic effects
c. MAC (minimum alveolar concentration) is > 100%
d. Methemoglobinemia occurs even with low inspired concentrations
e. Such great solubility in blood that its effects take an extraordinarily long time to develop
f. Very high frequency of bronchospasm

121. A patient develops a severe and rapidly worsening adverse response to a drug. The physician orders prompt administration of antipyretics, IV hydration, and bromocriptine or dantrolene to manage symptoms and hopefully to prevent a fatal outcome. Which of the following drugs or drug groups most likely causes these adverse responses?

a. Benzodiazepines, especially those used as hypnotics
b. Chlorpromazine
c. Levodopa
d. Phenytoin
e. SSRIs

122. Ropinirole is a relatively new drug that recently was approved to treat what's commonly called restless legs syndrome (also known as Ekbom syndrome). The drug works as a dopamine receptor agonist in certain parts of the brain. Given this mechanism of action, which of the following other disorders is most likely another indication for this drug?

a. Daytime anxiety
b. Hypersomnia (excessive sleepiness)
c. Parkinson's disease
d. Schizophrenia
e. Status epilepticus
f. Treatment of severe pain

123. A 34-year-old man with mild anxiety and depression symptoms has heard about buspirone on television and asks whether it might be suitable for him. According to the latest diagnostic criteria, the drug would be appropriate, particularly for short-term symptom control. Which of the following best describes an important property of this drug?

a. Associated with a withdrawal syndrome that, if unsupervised, is frequently lethal
b. Has a significant potential for abuse
c. Is likely to potentiate the CNS depressant effects of alcohol, benzodiazepines, and sedative antihistamines (e.g., diphenhydramine), so such interactants must be avoided at all cost
d. Requires almost daily dosage titrations in order to optimize the response
e. Seldom causes drowsiness

124. A patient in the neurology unit at your hospital develops status epilepticus. Which of the following is the best first IV drug to give?

a. Carbamazepine
b. Lorazepam
c. Phenobarbital
d. Phenytoin
e. Valproic acid

125. A patient has had a documented severe allergic reaction to ester-type local anesthetics. Which one of the following is also a member of the ester class, and so would be the most likely to provoke an allergic or anaphylactic reaction if this patient received it?

a. Bupivicaine
b. Lidocaine
c. Mepivacaine
d. Prilocaine
e. Tetracaine

126. A 66-year-old woman is diagnosed with Alzheimer's disease, with symptoms being described as mild-to-moderate. Which of the following pharmacologic approaches best summarizes a mechanism of action by which current drugs, used for early Alzheimer's and having actions mainly in the CNS, provide some slowing of the underlying brain pathology?

a. Activate a population of serotonin receptors
b. Block dopamine release or receptor activation
c. Inhibit acetylcholinesterase
d. Inhibit MAO
e. Dissolve cerebral vascular thrombi

127. Trihexyphenidyl is prescribed as an adjunct to other drugs being used to manage a patient with Parkinson's disease. Which of the following is the most likely purpose or action of this drug as part of the overall drug treatment plan?

a. To counteract sedation that is likely to be caused by the other medications
b. To help correct further the dopamine-ACh imbalance that accounts for parkinsonian signs and symptoms
c. To manage cutaneous allergic responses that are so common with "typical" antiparkinson drugs
d. To prevent the development of manic/hypomanic responses to other antiparkinson drugs
e. To reverse tardive dyskinesias if the parkinsonism was induced by an antipsychotic drug

128. In early 2006 the FDA granted approval to market a new prescription drug ("Drug X") that will be administered in the form of a dermal patch (apply the patch to intact skin, the drug is absorbed from there).

This new drug belongs to a very old class of drugs that, when given by its usual route—orally—can interact with foods such as cheese and processed meats (and certain breads, other foods, and alcoholic beverages) leading to an interaction that can elevate blood pressure (to severe and sometimes fatal levels). After more than a decade of testing, the FDA approved its use for adults. In its lowest dose, no dietary restrictions are required. "

Based on this information, how is this new drug, Drug X, most likely classified, and which of the following is its most likely clinical use?

a. Amphetamine-like agent for ADD/ADHD
b. Barbiturates used for daytime anxiety
c. Benzodiazepine for anxiety and sleep
d. MAO inhibitor for depression
e. Morphine-like analgesic for severe/chronic pain

129. The pediatrician writes a prescription for a combination (of several drugs) product that contains dextromethorphan, which is an isomer of a codeine analog. The patient is a 12-year-old boy. Which of the following is the most likely purpose for which the drug was prescribed?

a. Control mild-moderate pain after the lad broke his wrist playing soccer
b. Manage diarrhea caused by food-borne bacteria
c. Provide sedation because the child has ADD/ADHD
d. Suppress severe cough associated with a bout of influenza
e. Treat nocturnal bed-wetting

130. We administer a "usually effective" and otherwise therapeutic dose of thiopental to a patient. It is given by IV bolus injection. Within a matter of seconds the patient is asleep. We give no other drug. Which of the following is most likely to occur thereafter?

a. Significant and clinically useful analgesia will persist for an hour or so
b. Significant increase in cerebral oxygen consumption
c. The drug will be promptly metabolized by the hepatic P450 system
d. The patient develops acute seizures (e.g., status epilepticus)
e. The patient will awake in about 3–5 min

131. Many legal jurisdictions have imposed various restrictions on over-the-counter sale of products that contain pseudoephedrine, for example, various oral decongestant products. That is because pseudoephedrine can be rather easily used to synthesize which of the following highly psychoactive and abuse-prone drug?

a. Methamphetamine
b. Morphine
c. Oxycodone
d. Pentazocine
e. Phencyclidine ("PCP")

132. The anesthesiologist prepares to administer several drugs to a patient as part of normal pre- and intraoperative care. Which of the following lacks, as its normal spectrum of action, a direct ability either to suppress overall CNS function or the patient's level of consciousness, or to provide analgesia?

a. Clonidine
b. Droperidol
c. Pancuronium
d. Propofol
e. Thiopental

133. A 26-year-old woman with depression has been on antidepressant therapy for several months. Today she complains of missing her period and having galactorrhea, and your careful assessment suggests she has developed some dyskinesias not unlike those you would typically associate with a phenothiazine or butyrophenone (e.g., haloperidol) antipsychotic drug. Pregnancy tests are negative. Which of the following is most likely to have caused these findings?

a. Amoxapine
b. Citalopram
c. Fluoxetine
d. Sertraline
e. Tranylcypromine

134. A patient has been taking an oral monoamine oxidase inhibitor (MAOI), but that fact is unknown to the health team who is now taking care of her, for unrelated medical conditions, in the hospital. The patient receives a drug that leads to a fatal response characterized by profound fever, delirium, psychotic behavior, and status epilepticus. It was found to have occurred because of an interaction with the MAOI. Which of the following drugs, or class of drugs, was most likely administered by the attending health team?

a. A barbiturate
b. Diazepam
c. Meperidine
e. Morphine
e. Phenytoin

135. A young woman is taken to the emergency department by some of her friends. It seems they were out on "bar night" and someone slipped something into her alcoholic beverage, the first and only one she consumed that night. She is now extraordinarily drowsy and has little recall of what happened between the time she sipped her drink and now. Someone overheard another bar patron talking about "roofies." Being knowledgeable about your pharmacology you suspect her drink was spiked with rohypnol. Assuming your guess is correct, which of the following drugs is most likely to reverse the flunitrazepam's effects?

a. Diazepam
b. Flumazenil
c. Ketamine
d. Naltrexone
e. Triazolam

136. In deciding on pharmacotherapy for many patients you've diagnosed with depression, you've usually considered starting with an SSRI or, in some cases, a tricyclic. Today you assess a patient and suspect endogenous depression. While discussing treatment options they refer to a drug by name and ask you about it; they've seen many advertisements for it in magazines and on television. The drug (generic name) is bupropion. Which of the following statements best describes bupropion in terms of how it differs from either or both the SSRIs or tricyclics?

a. Higher incidence of CNS depression, drowsiness
b. Higher incidence of weight gain
c. Less drug-induced sexual dysfunction
d. Much more common and severe falls of resting blood pressure and orthostatic hypotension
e. More severe and more frequent peripheral anticholinergic (atropine-like) side effects
f. Stronger inhibition of monoamine oxidase

137. A 33-year-old woman patient treated with haloperidol is seen in the emergency department (ED). Her husband describes complaints of rapidly worsening fever, muscle stiffness, and tremor. Her level of consciousness is diminishing. Her temperature is 104°F, and her serum creatine kinase (CK) level is elevated. Which of the following is the best explanation for these findings?

a. Allergic response to her medication
b. Neuroleptic malignant syndrome (NMS)
c. Overdose
d. Parkinsonism
e. Tardive dyskinesia

138. A patient will receive bupivacaine, infused continuously via an epidural catheter, for prolonged analgesia during postoperative recovery. Which of the following is the greatest concern when using this drug, compared with what one might expect with otherwise equianalgesic doses of the overall local anesthetic prototype, lidocaine?

a. Arrhythmias
b. Greater paralysis of skeletal muscle (motor block) than sensory block
c. Higher risk of bronchospasm
d. Hypertension, hypertensive crisis
e. Nephrotoxicity

139. Nearly all the drugs used as primary therapy, or as adjuncts, for the treatment of Parkinson's disease or drug-induced parkinsonism exert their desired effects directly in the brain's striatum. Which of the following exerts its main effects in the gut, not in the brain?

a. Amantadine
b. Benztropine
c. Bromcriptine
d. Carbidopa
e. Selegiline

140. You have a patient with severe postoperative pain, who is not getting adequate analgesia from usually effective doses of morphine. The physician orders an immediate switch to pentazocine (at usually effective analgesic doses). Which of the following is the most likely outcome of stopping the morphine and immediately substituting the pentazocine?

a. Abrupt, added respiratory depression
b. Acute development of physical dependence
c. Coma
d. Seizures
e. Worsening of pain

141. Our chosen pharmacologic approach to managing a patient with mild and recently diagnosed parkinsonism will be to enhance specifically the activity of endogenous brain dopamine by inhibiting its metabolic inactivation. Which one of the following drugs works primarily by that mechanism?

a. Benztropine
b. Selegiline
c. Trihexyphenidyl
d. Bromocriptine
e. Chlorpromazine

142. Chlorpromazine has been prescribed for a patient with schizophrenia, and the patient has been taking the drug, at usually effective doses, for about 6 months. Today he comes to the hospital with other medical conditions that require surgery and the administration of other drugs, and we decide it is unwise to stop the chlorpromazine and run the risk of psychotic behavior while we perform other interventions. Which of the following other signs/symptoms that the patient may also have or acquire as the result of surgery and drug therapy is most likely to be affected beneficially by the continued use of chlorpromazine?

a. Epilepsy and the risk of seizures
b. Hypotension
c. Nausea and vomiting
d. Urinary retention caused by abdominal surgery
e. Xerostomia (dry mouth) caused by antimuscarinic drugs used to prevent intraoperative bradycardia

143. There are, rightfully, concerns about cocaine abuse, and too many deaths have occurred from smoking "crack" cocaine or injecting or nasally inhaling the drug. Which of the following statements best describes the main mechanism by which cocaine exerts its deleterious effects in the central nervous system or in the periphery?

a. Directly activates, as an agonist, both α- and β₁-adrenergic receptors
b. Enhances neuronally-mediated adrenergic-receptor activation by inhibiting neuronal-norepinephrine reuptake
c. Inhibits catecholamine inactivation by inhibiting MAO and catechol-O-methyltransferase
d. Produces bradycardia and vasodilation, leading to hypotension and acute heart failure, by blocking neuronal NE release
e. Stimulates autonomic nerve conduction effectively, leading to increased neuronal norepinephrine release

144. We administer a drug with a pharmacologic profile consistent with selective activation (as an agonist) of dopamine D_2 receptors. Which of the following is the most likely drug?

a. Bromocriptine
b. Chlorpromazine
c. Fluphenazine
d. Haloperidol
e. Promethazine

145. We perform a meta-analysis on the ability of various antipsychotic drugs to cause constipation, urinary retention, blurred vision, and dry mouth—all of which reflect significant blockade of muscarinic receptors in the peripheral nervous system. Which of the following drugs, or the main drug class to which it belongs, was most likely to cause these unwanted effects?

a. Chlorpromazine
b. Clozapine
c. Haloperidol
d. Olanzapine
e. Sertraline

146. A patient is on long-term methadone therapy as part of a holistic plan to curb the opioid addiction and abuse. Which of the following best describes a characteristic of this drug?

a. Causes pentazocine-like activation of κ receptors and blockade of μ receptors
b. Has greater oral bioavailability than morphine, especially when oral administration is started
c. Remarkably devoid of such typical opioid analgesic side effects as constipation and respiratory depression
d. Useful for maintenance therapy in opioid- (e.g., heroin-) dependent individuals, but lacks clinically useful analgesic effects
e. When abruptly stopped after long-term administration, causes a withdrawal syndrome that is more intense, but briefer, than that associated with morphine or heroin withdrawal

147. A 14-year-old girl is brought to the ED by her mother, who has observed that her daughter has abruptly experienced frequent impairments of consciousness associated with episodes of staring into space lasting approximately 30 s. Further neurologic evaluation indicates signs and symptoms consistent with absence seizures. With which of the following drugs should we start treatment?

a. Alprazolam
b. Diazepam
c. Ethosuximide
d. Midazolam
e. Phenytoin

148. A 43-year-old woman becomes hypertensive and suffers a fatal acute coronary syndrome shortly after starting therapy on a drug. Autopsy shows little in the way of coronary atherosclerosis, but EKG changes noted just before her death revealed significant myocardial ischemia in the myocardium served by the left anterior descending and circumflex coronary arteries. The cause of death is thought to involve coronary vasospasm. Which of the following drugs most likely precipitated this event?

a. Bromocriptine for Parkinson's disease
b. Ergotamine given to abort a migraine attack
c. Morphine for post-trauma analgesia
d. Phenoxybenzamine used for carcinoid syndrome
e. Phenytoin to manage generalized tonic-clonic seizures

149. A 20-year-old man with absence seizures is treated with ethosuximide. Which of the following is the principal mechanism of action of ethosuximide?

a. Calcium channel blockade
b. Increase in the frequency of the chloride channel opening
c. Increase in GABA
d. Increased potassium channel permeability
e. Sodium channel blockade

150. Promethazine, a phenothiazine derivative with substantial antiemetic, antitussive, and H_1 histamine receptor blocking activity, has a clinical profile quite similar to diphenhydramine. Recently the FDA mandated a "black box warning" for this widely used drug. The FDA now warns against use of the drug, in all doses and forms, for children aged 2 years or younger. Fatalities have occurred in these young patients, even in response to dosages that previously were considered therapeutic and safe. Which of the following is the most likely cause of death from promethazine in these patients?

a. Complete heart block followed by asystole
b. Hypertensive crisis, intracranial hemorrhage
c. Parkinsonian-like dyskinesias, including tardive dyskinesias
d. Severe and refractory diarrhea leading to fluid and electrolyte loss
e. Ventilatory depression, apnea, excessive CNS depression

151. A patient in the emergency department requires suturing of a deep 2-cm laceration. To reduce discomfort we first infiltrate the surrounding area with lidocaine. Which of the following functions or sensations is most likely to disappear first as the drug's effects build up, and the last to reappear as the drug's effects wear off?

a. Autonomic efferent function
b. Motor nerve activity
c. Pain
d. Pressure (deep or heavy pressure)
e. Temperature

152. A 55-year-old woman undergoes surgery. She receives several drugs for preanesthesia care, intubation, and intraoperative skeletal muscle paralysis; and a mixture of inhaled anesthetics to complete the balanced anesthesia. Toward the end of the procedure she develops hyperthermia, hypertension, hyperkalemia, tachycardia, muscle rigidity, and metabolic acidosis. Which of the following drugs is most likely to have participated in this reaction?

a. Fentanyl
b. Halothane
c. Ketamine
d. Midazolam
e. Propofol

153. A 30-year-old woman with partial seizures is treated with vigabatrin. Which of the following is the principal mechanism of action of vigabatrin?

a. Sodium channel blockade
b. Increase in frequency of chloride channel opening
c. Increase in GABA
d. Calcium channel blockade
e. Increased potassium channel permeability
f. NMDA receptor blockade

154. A patient with epilepsy is started on oral therapy with an appropriate anticonvulsant. Not long after treatment starts he manifests psychotic behaviors that were not present before antiepileptic drug therapy started. Of the following antiepileptic agents, which is associated with the highest risk of causing psychosis?

a. Ethosuximide
b. Phenobarbital
c. Phenytoin
d. Valproic acid
e. Vigabatrin

155. A 24-year-old woman has a history of epilepsy that is being treated with phenytoin. She is healthy otherwise. She becomes pregnant. Which of the following should we do throughout the remainder of her pregnancy?

a. Add valproic acid
b. Discontinue all anticonvulsant medication
c. Increase daily dietary iron intake
d. Prescribe daily folic acid supplements
e. Switch from the phenytoin to phenobarbital

156. A patient is transported to the emergency department by ambulance after repeated episodes of fainting. The cause was attributed to severe drug-induced orthostatic hypotension due to α-adrenergic blockade from one of the drug's main side effects. Which of the following drugs was the most likely cause of this problem?

a. Buspirone
b. Chlorpromazine
c. Diphenhydramine
d. Haloperidol
e. Zolpidem

157. A patient who is going to have an uncomfortable endoscopic procedure is pretreated with midazolam and fentanyl, both given IV. Both drugs cause generalized CNS depression and desired sedation. Which of the following is the main effect for which the midazolam was used as a supplement?

a. Causes amnesia of short duration
b. Causes analgesia to supplement the sedative effects of fentanyl
c. Counteracts the tachycardic effects of the fentanyl
d. Prevents fentanyl-induced rises of blood pressure
e. Prevents/blocks fentanyl-induced ventilatory depression

158. Clozapine, as an example of the "atypical antipsychotics," seldom is used as first-line (initial) therapy of schizophrenia. Compared with the older antipsychotics, it is associated with a much higher risk of a serious adverse response. Which of the following best summarizes what that greater risk is?

a. Agranulocytosis
b. Extrapyramidal side effects (parkinsonian)
c. Hypoglycemia
d. Hypotension, severe
e. Ventilatory depression or arrest

159. A woman has been taking a prescribed drug throughout her pregnancy. Starting about a month before her expected delivery date we start administering oral vitamin K supplements, and when the baby is born he/she is given an injection of vitamin K. The goal is to reduce the risks of excessive or abnormal bleeding, caused by drug-induced impairments of hepatic vitamin K-dependent clotting factors, in the newborn. For which of the following drugs are these precautions most likely to be needed?

a. Bupropion
b. Diazepam
c. Methadone
d. Naloxone
e. Phenytoin

160. A patient has frequent facial tics and spontaneous outbursts of foul language (coprolalia). Which of the following drugs would most likely be the best and probably most efficacious and safe initial treatment for this, assuming no specific contraindications to using it?

a. Clozapine
b. Haloperidol
c. Levodopa
d. Methylphenidate
e. Phenobarbital

161. When we administer carbidopa along with levodopa for Parkinson's disease, we increase the bioavailability of levodopa by inhibiting the formation of dopamine in the gut. However, the carbidopa-induced inhibition of dopa decarboxylase favors the peripheral metabolism of levodopa to another metabolite (3-O-methyldopa) that competes with levodopa for transport across the blood-brain barrier. This is catalyzed by catechol-O-methyltransferase (COMT). Which of the following drugs inhibits COMT, and so can increase the central bioavailability and effects of levodopa?

a. Donepezil
b. Entacapone
c. Selegiline
d. Tacrine
e. Trihexyphenidyl

162. A patient has a long history of excessive alcohol consumption. He was arrested for drunk driving and was referred to a physician for therapy. The MD prescribed a drug to stifle further alcohol ingestion, to be used along with other interventions. The patient was instructed not to consume any alcohol, not to use alcohol-containing mouthwashes, or even apply alcohol-based toiletries, because alcohol may cause a disturbing, if not dangerous interaction with his medication. The patient ignored the advice and decided to have a cocktail. Within minutes he develops flushing, a throbbing headache, nausea, and vomiting. Which of the following medications was he most likely taking?

a. Naltrexone
b. Diazepam
c. Disulfiram
d. Phenobarbital
e. Tranylcypromine

163. We start a patient with endogenous depression on a drug that selectively inhibits neuronal serotonin (5-HT) reuptake and has minimal effect on the reuptake of norepinephrine or dopamine. Which of the following drugs best fits this description?

a. Amitriptyline
b. Bupropion
c. Fluoxetine
d. Imipramine
e. Venlafaxine

164. A 29-year-old man uses secobarbital and alcohol to satisfy his addiction to barbiturates and other CNS depressants. During the past week he has been incarcerated and is not able to obtain the drugs. He is brought to the medical ward because of the onset of severe anxiety, increased sensitivity to light, dizziness, and generalized tremors due to drug withdrawal. On physical examination, he is hyperreflexic. Which of the following agents is the best choice to diminish his withdrawal symptoms?

a. Buspirone
b. Chloral hydrate
c. Chlorpromazine
d. Lorazepam
e. Trazodone

165. A 50-year-old man has been consuming large amounts of ethanol on an almost daily basis for many years. One day, unable to find any ethanol, he ingests a large amount of methanol (wood alcohol) that he had bought for his camp lantern. Which of the following drugs should we administer to best treat the poisoning and the signs and symptoms that occurred?

a. Diazepam
b. Ethanol
c. Flumazenil
d. Phenobarbital
e. Phenytoin

166. Many news reports in the spring and summer of 2006 have told of a large number of deaths of opioid abusers who had purchased and self-administered illicit drugs that contained lethal amounts of fentanyl. One patient who received this fentanyl-laced drug presents in your emergency department, barely alive. Which of the following drugs should you administer first, with the best hope that it can promptly reverse the lethal effects of the fentanyl?

a. Diazepam
b. Flumazenil
c. Naloxone
d. Naltrexone
e. Phenytoin

167. A 10-year-old boy has nocturnal enuresis. His parents take him to a clinic that specializes in management of this condition. The physician writes an order for a low dose of imipramine. After a couple of weeks on the drug, the episodes of bed-wetting decrease dramatically. Which of the following best accounts for the beneficial effects of the drug in this patient?

a. Alleviates depression signs and symptoms by increasing neuronal catecholamine reuptake
b. Blocks muscarinic receptors in the bladder musculature
c. Causes sedation such that the boy sleeps through the night without voiding
d. Reduces renal blood flow, glomerular filtration, and urine output
e. Releases antidiuretic hormone (ADH)

168. A patient is transported to your emergency department because of a seizure. A review of his history reveals that he has been treated by different physicians for different medical conditions, and there has been no dialog between the two doctors in terms of what they've prescribed. One physician has prescribed a drug for short-term management of depression. Another has prescribed the very same drug to help the patient quit smoking cigarettes. Which of the following was most likely prescribed by both doctors, and was the most likely cause of the seizures?

a. Bupropion
b. Chlordiazepoxide
c. Fluoxetine
d. Imipramine
e. Lithium

169. About one year ago you diagnosed schizophrenia signs and symptoms in a 23-year-old otherwise healthy man. As a result of intensive psychotherapy, careful titration of chlorpromazine dosages, and remarkably good compliance on the patient's part, he is well enough to return to work. Several months later, at a scheduled visit, you observe numerous signs and symptoms of drug-induced parkinsonism, and the patient reports rather distressing symptoms of akathisias. However, he states no recurrences of schizophrenia manifestations. Which of the following approaches is most likely to alleviate the motor and subjective parkinsonian responses, and poses the lowest risk of causing schizophrenia signs and symptoms to reappear?

a. Add a catechol-*O*-methyltransferase inhibitor (e.g., tolcapone)
b. Add a centrally acting cholinesterase inhibitor (e.g., donepezil or tacrine)
c. Add benztropine
d. Add levodopa or levodopa plus carbidopa
e. Switch from chlorpromazine to haloperidol

170. Isoflurane and halothane are good examples of volatile liquid general anesthetics. Which of the following statements best compares or contrasts their actions?

a. Halothane and isoflurane typically raise blood pressure, via direct vasoconstrictor effects
b. Halothane is associated with a higher risk of renal and hepatic toxicity, especially in patients who have been anesthetized with this drug before
c. Isoflurane prolongs the QT interval (ventricular repolarization), and is associated with a much higher risk of causing potentially fatal ventricular tachyarrhythmias, than halothane
d. Isoflurane sensitizes the myocardium to the arrhythmogenic effects of catecholamines much more than halothane does
e. Use of isoflurane for balanced anesthesia requires adjunctive use of nitrous oxide and neuromuscular blockers, use of halothane does not

171. We have a patient with Parkinson's disease, and administer a drug that acts in the CNS as an agonist for dopamine receptors. It has no direct effects on dopamine synthesis, neuronal reuptake, or metabolic inactivation. Which of the following drugs best fits this description?

a. Amantadine
b. Apomorphine
c. Belladonna
d. Bromocriptine
e. Selegiline

172. A patient develops profound fever, skeletal muscle rigidity, and autonomic and systemic electrolyte imbalances as part of a severe adverse response to a psychoactive drug. The working diagnosis is neuroleptic malignant syndrome. In addition to administering dantrolene in an attempt to restore some semblance of normal skeletal muscle function, which of the following other drugs is most likely to be given to help provide additional symptom relief?

a. Benztropine
b. Bromocriptine
c. Diazepam
d. Flumazenil
e. Naloxone
f. Propranolol

The Central Nervous System

Answers

100. The answer is b. (*Brunton, pp 477–481; Craig, pp 364–366, 399–402; Katzung, pp 472–475.*) Unwanted extrapyramidal side effects produced by antipsychotic drugs (e.g., chlorpromazine, as the exemplar of the phenothiazines; and, more so, by haloperidol as the prototype of the butyrophenones) include Parkinson-like syndrome, akathisia, dystonias, galactorrhea, amenorrhea, and infertility. These side effects are due to the ability of these agents to block dopamine receptors. The phenothiazines also block muscarinic and α-adrenergic receptors, which are responsible for other effects in both the CNS and (especially) in the periphery. The incidence and severity of these autonomic side effects is much greater with low-potency antipsychotics (e.g., chlorpromazine and other phenothiazines) than with the high-potency butyrophenones (e.g., haloperidol).

101. The answer is b. (*Brunton, pp 351–353; Craig, pp 292t, 297; Katzung, pp 411–412, 415–416.*) The scenario describes most of the classic responses to ketamine, a "dissociative anesthetic": analgesia; an ostensibly light sleep-like state; a trance-like and cataplectic state (including increased muscle tone); and activation of most cardiovascular parameters (in patients with normal cardiovascular status to begin with). The various psychosis-like emergence reactions are the main disadvantages to using a drug that, otherwise, causes many of the desired elements of balanced anesthesia, usually without the need for complicated and expensive anesthesia administration devices or personnel. Ketamine undergoes significant metabolism in humans, with about 20% of the absorbed dose recovered as metabolites. The only other drug listed that provides adequate analgesia is fentanyl (a). Midazolam (c; benzodiazepine), succinylcholine (d; depolarizing neuromuscular blocker), and thiopental (e; thiobarbiturate) lack analgesic activity; moreover, if any cardiovascular or autonomic changes were to occur in response to any of those drugs, they would be better characterized as depression, not activation.

102. The answer is d. (*Brunton, pp 533–534; Craig, pp 366–369; Katzung, pp 448–451.*) When levodopa is administered orally, the vast majority of the administered dose (about 90%) is metabolized in the gut to dopamine by DOPA decarboxylase. However, dopamine cannot cross the blood-brain barrier, and so only a fraction of the parent drug gets into the CNS, to be metabolized and cause its desired effects there. Carbidopa inhibits DOPA decarboxylase in the periphery (it cannot cross the blood-brain barrier), reducing peripheral metabolism of levodopa to dopamine and "sparing" a bigger fraction of the dose so it can be metabolized in the nigrostriatum. By reducing peripheral conversion of levodopa to dopamine, the adjunctive use of carbidopa may also allow management of parkinsonian signs and symptoms with lower doses of levodopa. One additional benefit of that is a reduction in the number and severity of peripheral side effects of the levodopa (or, more precisely, its metabolite, dopamine). Adding carbidopa to a regimen involving levodopa only may also help (at least transiently) combat such problems as dopamine's "on-off" phenomenon and "end-of-dose" failure.

103. The answer is a. (*Brunton, pp 370–371, 379; Craig, pp 334–335; Katzung, p 419.*) Nearly all local anesthetics contain a lipophilic functional group, and most have a hydrophilic group (e.g., amine). Benzocaine does not contain the terminal hydrophilic group; thus, it is only slightly soluble in water and is extraordinarily slowly absorbed. It is, therefore, only useful as a topical anesthetic (e.g., on mucous membranes).

104. The answer is c. (*Brunton, pp 126, 416t, 418, 510–511, 522–523; Craig, pp 294–295, 381, 411–412; Katzung, pp 361–363.*) Phenobarbital's role in the primary management of all of the conditions given in the answer list in Question 104 has waned dramatically, and appropriately, as newer drugs have been developed. The only one in the list, for which phenobarbital is still considered reasonable for long-term therapy, is for managing certain epilepsies (mainly as an alternative to phenytoin). Benzodiazepines are almost always preferred, and used, for managing alcohol withdrawal and anxiety management. Benzodiazepines, or the benzodiazepine-like agents zaleplon or zolpidem, are almost always turned to for insomnia. Major reasons for selecting a benzodiazepine over a barbiturate include fewer drug-drug interactions (phenobarbital is a classic P450 inducer); a lower risk of dependence; withdrawal syndromes that are typically less severe or dangerous; lower risk of fatal ventilatory depression with oral overdoses (and the availability of flumazenil, the specific benzodiazepine antagonist, to treat them); and less narrowing between lethal and effective doses (better therapeutic index or margin of safety) as use continues.

Note that even though benzodiazepines may be preferred, treatment for such problems as anxiety and insomnia should be kept as short as possible. Phenobarbital (or other barbiturates) is not indicated for treating endogenous depression.

105. The answer is a. (*Brunton, pp 433–434, 447–448; Craig, pp 388t, 389–391; Katzung, pp 483, 486, 488–490, 493.*) The most common side effects associated with tricyclic antidepressants are their antimuscarinic effects, which may occur in over 50% of patients. Clinically, these effects may manifest as dry mouth, blurred vision, constipation, tachycardia, dizziness, and urinary retention. At therapeutic plasma concentrations these drugs usually do not cause changes in the EKG—but with severe overdoses lethal arrhythmias often do occur.

106. The correct answer is b. (*Brunton, pp 509–510, 1860t; Craig, pp 53, 377–378; Katzung, pp 380–382.*) The hepatic enzymes responsible for phenytoin metabolism (mainly CYP 2C9) become saturated at plasma drug concentrations above approximately 10–15 mcg/mL, which are clearly within the typical therapeutic range yet well below maximum or peak therapeutic levels. At daily dosages associated with or below those 10–15 mcg/mL values, dose increases give relatively proportional increases in plasma drug concentrations, and phenytoin elimination follows usual first-order kinetics (a constant fraction of drug is eliminated with the passing of each half-life). Once the metabolic capacity is exceeded (as it has in our patient, which may arise with intentional or inadvertent increases in the daily dose), small increases in dosage lead to disproportionately large increases of serum concentrations (and effects) because, in essence, "drug in greatly exceeds drug out": zero-order kinetics now describes the drug's elimination, such that a constant amount (not fraction) of drug is eliminated per unit time. Therefore, the first-order half-life does not apply; elimination is slower, and the plasma concentration will be much greater than 15 mcg/mL (half of 30 mcg/mL; ans. e) 24 h after the initial blood sample is taken.

The figure shows an *approximation* of the relationship between plasma phenytoin levels and daily doses (the placement of the curve can vary from patient to patient along the x-axis). From the rapid rise in the curve at dosages above about 300 mg/day you can deduce a significant reduction of clearance rates owing to slowed metabolism (since metabolism is the main pathway for phenytoin's elimination).

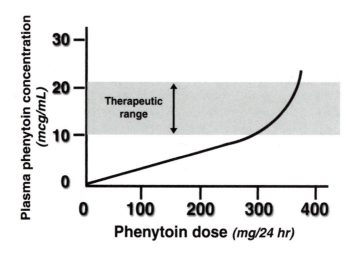

Answer (a) is incorrect; flumazenil is a benzodiazepine receptor antagonist (competitive blocker) that has no effects (beneficially or not; pharmacokinetic or otherwise) on the elimination or effects of phenytoin. It would be inappropriate—and dangerous—to give an amphetamine or any other CNS stimulant to counteract the excess CNS depression. Titrating upwards the dose of a CNS stimulant to combat CNS depression (whether caused by a drug or from another cause) is a risky endeavor, due to the chance of inducing seizures from excessive CNS stimulation, and the risks are far greater in a person with a history of seizure disorders.

Phenobarbital (d) is a classic example of a P450 inducer, and indeed it is metabolized mainly by CYP2C9, on which phenytoin's elimination is mainly dependent. In theory, giving phenobarbital might increase phenytoin's metabolism *via* P450 induction. In reality, the pharmacokinetic outcomes of a phenobarbital-phenytoin interaction are quite variable (and dependent on blood levels of each drug), but the more likely consequence is inhibited phenytoin elimination as the barbiturate competes with it for conversion by the same cytochromes. Regardless, adding phenobarbital is likely to add to the generalized CNS depression caused by the phenytoin, and complicate both the clinical picture and its management. Therefore, this approach, too, would be inappropriate.

107. The answer is d. (*Brunton, pp 174, 299, 443, 529–533, 535, 537; Craig, p 369; Katzung, pp 83, 453.*) Two of the important types of MAO are: (1) MAO-A, which metabolizes norepinephrine and serotonin and other biogenic amines, and is the predominant hepatic form of the enzyme; and (2) MAO-B, which metabolizes dopamine and other monoamines in the brain. Selegiline is a selective inhibitor of MAO-B. It therefore inhibits the breakdown of dopamine and prolongs the therapeutic effectiveness of levodopa (endogenous or that provided pharmacologically) in parkinsonism. The risks of serious drug interactions in patients taking nonselective MAO inhibitors (e.g., phenelzine, tranylcypromine), such as hypertensive crisis in response to mixed- and indirect-acting sympathomimetics (tyramine, pseudoephedrine, amphetamines) are much less (but still possible) with selegiline.

Bromocriptine (a) is a dopamine receptor agonist. Carbidopa (b) inhibits the peripheral metabolism of levodopa. Both are useful in the treatment of some cases of idiopathic (but not antipsychotic drug-induced) parkinsonism. Phenelzine (c) and tranylcypromine (e) are nonselective MAOIs. Combining them with L-dopa may lead to a potentially fatal hypertensive crisis, and thus they are not used in the therapy of parkinsonism. A similar interaction may occur with tyramine-rich foods and beverages; and with catecholamine-releasing sympathomimetics (ephedrine, pseudoephedrine, amphetamines, and amphetamine-like drugs). As a result of these common and potentially lethal interactions, nonselective MAO inhibitors are rarely used for anything.

108. The answer is d. (*Brunton, pp 568–571; Craig, pp 322–323; Katzung, p 511.*) High or frankly toxic serum levels of meperidine can cause seizures, hypertension, and a psychosis-like state, in addition to typical morphine-like effects (e.g., analgesia and ventilatory depression). It appears that administration of naloxone to combat excessive effects of meperidine may increase the risk of seizures; this is something we typically don't see when naloxone is administered to combat excessive effects of morphine and most other opioids.

The rather unique adverse effects attributed to meperidine are probably due to a major metabolite, normeperidine. A weak opioid analgesic, propoxyphene (structurally related to methadone), can produce toxic reactions similar to those of meperidine. One of its metabolites, norpropoxyphene, is thought to be the cause.

Meperidine, like other opioids, can cause constipation (a) through its actions on longitudinal muscles and sphincters in the GI tract. Hyperalgesia (b) does not occur. Biliary spasm (c) is much less likely to occur than with most other opioids (say, the prototype, morphine). Indeed, the risks of biliary tract/gall bladder problems are said to be less with meperidine than with most alternatives, and so can be considered a preferred opioid (for short-term) use for patients with moderate-severe pain and gall bladder disease. Because of the toxicity risk, however, meperidine should not be used for more than brief analgesic effects.

Respiratory depression, possibly leading to ventilatory arrest, is a property shared by all the opioid analgesics, but of course to varying degrees based on their efficacy and dose.

109. The answer is a. (*Brunton, pp 474, 477–481, 572t; Craig, pp 399–400; Katzung, pp 462–463, 466–467, 471.*) It is common to classify chlorpromazine and other phenothiazine antipsychotics as "low potency" agents, in comparison with haloperidol (butyrophenone class), which has been called a "high potency" antipsychotic. Potency, of course, usually refers to the dose needed to cause a stated effect of a certain intensity, and does not necessarily give us good insight into a particular drug's efficacy. Nonetheless, haloperidol is more potent than phenothiazines and is more selective for blocking dopamine D_2 receptors. But another implied and arguably more important meaning of using the "low potency—high potency" terminology is that chlorpromazine and other phenothiazines tend to cause a higher incidence of peripheral autonomic side effects (from α-adrenergic blockade and antimuscarinic effects) than haloperidol (as a representative high potency antipsychotic); and a lower incidence of extrapyramidal reactions, which can be severe and of sudden onset with haloperidol—a very rapidly acting drug, especially when given parenterally (as for acute psychosis).

110. The answer is c. (*Brunton, pp 332, 624–625; Craig, pp 417–418; Katzung, pp 523–525.*) Phencyclidine (PCP; angel dust) is an hallucinogen with an amphetamine-like mechanism of action. Thus, the problems that arise are due to blockade of neuronal reuptake of such monoamines as dopamine, norepinephrine, and serotonin. The drug does not have central or peripheral muscarinic receptor antagonist activity (d), nor opioid agonist actions (b). A withdrawal syndrome (a) has not been described for this drug in human subjects. In overdose, the treatment of choice for manifestations of drug-induced psychosis is the haloperidol, although rapidly acting and highly sedating benzodiazepines may be used instead. Flumazenil (e) is a selective benzodiazepine receptor antagonist with no use in phencyclidine toxicity.

111. The answer is d. (*Brunton, pp 429, 485–490; Craig, pp 393–395; Katzung, pp 477–478.*) Lithium treatment (for bipolar illness) frequently causes polyuria and (as a consequence of excessive renal fluid loss) polydipsia. The collecting ducts of the kidney lose the capacity to conserve water via antidiuretic hormone. This amounts to drug-induced diabetes insipidus. Such findings are not associated with diazepam (a; prototype benzodiazepine anxiolytic); fluoxetine (b; the prototypic SSRI antidepressant); haloperidol (c; butyrophenone antipsychotic); or phenytoin (e; hydantoin anticonvulsant).

112. The answer is a. (*Brunton, pp 259, 263; Craig, pp 106, 349–350, 407; Katzung, pp 521–523, 990.*) Methylphenidate, which is widely used to manage ADD–ADHD, has amphetamine-like sympathetic and CNS-stimulating effects. Indeed, amphetamine itself is used for treatment of ADD–ADHD.

Peripheral sympathetic (adrenergic) effects arise from the drugs' ability to release neuronal norepinephrine. Related findings would include increased vasoconstriction (greater α_1 receptor activation of vascular smooth muscle), and therefore increased blood pressure; and tachycardia (plus increased cardiac contractility and electrical impulse conduction rates, probably accompanied by tachyarrhythmias, from β_1 activation).

At toxic doses, the CNS effect of the drug is likely to cause seizures.

There is no mechanism by which direct effects of methylphenidate or amphetamine (whether at normal or toxic doses) would cause bronchospasm, bronchoconstriction, or even bronchodilation (because norepinephrine that is released has no ability to activate or block β_2 receptors on airway smooth muscle). Miosis (which occurs with either muscarinic activation or α blockade) would be the opposite of what you would predict in terms of ocular effects.

In terms of autonomic effects, skeletal muscle weakness or paralysis are findings you would expect from drugs that either blocked nicotinic cholinergic receptors (e.g., tubocurarine or another similar nondepolarizing neuromuscular blocker) or stimulated them in excessive and prolonged fashion (e.g., succinylcholine).

113. The answer is d. (*Brunton, p 344; Craig, pp 298–302; Katzung, pp 402–405.*) MAC (minimum alveolar concentration) is an expression of inhaled anesthetic "potency." It is defined as the minimum inspired concentration needed to abolish a specified painful response in 50% of treated patients. (Thus, it is much like the ED_{50}, measured in a population dose-response curve, for most other drugs.) Obviously, giving a drug at a dose that suppresses a response in only half the treated patients is not desirable, so inhaled anesthetics are typically given at a dose more than the MAC. (Recall, too, that MAC is not absolute: it can change depending on the use of other anesthesia adjuncts and such other factors as body temperature, ventilatory rate, presence of other diseases, etc.)

A drug's MAC gives us no useful information about onsets or durations of action. We cannot state correctly that Drug B (MAC = 100%) causes greater analgesia and/or skeletal muscle relaxation than another drug any more than we can say that a drug with an ED_{50} of 5 mg causes a greater response than one with ED_{50} = 1 mg. It all depends on the dose given, not the MAC or ED_{50}.

114. The answer is d. (*Brunton, pp 305–306, 441–442, 450, 446–447; Craig, pp 386–388; Katzung, pp 271, 493–494, 991.*) This patient has the serotonin syndrome. Serotonin is already present in increased amounts in synapses because of blockade of its reuptake by the SSRIs. When sumatriptan (or other triptans used for migraine therapy; they are 5-$HT_{1B/2D}$ agonists) is added, rapid accumulation of serotonin and/or the triptan in the brain can occur.

The risk of the serotonin syndrome in SSRI–treated patients is much higher when MAO inhibitors are used concomitantly. Nonetheless, such severe reactions from an SSRI–triptan interaction have been reported. In addition, do not forget that MAO inhibitors can also cause an acute and potentially fatal hypertensive crisis when coadministered with tricyclic/tetracyclic antidepressants (e.g., imipramine); such combined use should be avoided.

115. The answer is b. (*Brunton, pp 402–406, 413–414, 615; Craig, pp 296, 357; Katzung, pp 357–360, 364, 989.*) Flumazenil is a competitive antagonist of benzodiazepines at the GABA receptor. Repeated administration is necessary because of its short half-life relative to that of most benzodiazepines— especially diazepam, which forms many long-lasting active metabolites.

Dextroamphetamine (a) is a CNS stimulant that increases the patient's level of consciousness, but it is not indicated for this use. Naltrexone (c) specifically antagonizes the effects of opioid agonists on μ and k receptors and is used to diagnose or treat opioid overdoses; it has no benzodiazepine receptor-blocking activity. Physostigmine (d) is a lipophilic acetylcholinesterase inhibitor that may be a life-saving intervention for severe poisoning with many drugs (a key exception being tricyclic antidepressants) having significant antimuscarinic (atropine-like) actions. Pralidoxime (e) is a cholinesterase reactivator used in the adjunctive management of poisoning with such "irreversible" cholinesterase inhibitors as the organophosphate insecticides and many "nerve gases" (soman, sarin, VX).

116. The answer is a. (*Brunton, pp 538, 1256–1258; Craig, p 370; Katzung, p 454.*) This cutaneous response, called *livedo reticularis*, is characteristically associated with amantadine. Recall that this seldom-used antiparkinson drug probably works by releasing endogenous dopamine and blocking its neuronal reuptake. Livedo reticularis is not associated with levodopa (used alone or with carbidopa; c or d), nor with the dopamine agonists bromocriptine (d) or pramipexole (e; a newer and generally preferred drug for starting treatment of mild parkinsonian signs and symptoms). (You might also recall that amantadine is also used for prophylaxis of some strains of influenza virus infections.)

117. The answer is d. (*Brunton, pp 509–510; Craig, p 378; Katzung, p 383.*) For many years, phenytoin has been cited as a classic example of a drug that can cause gingival hyperplasia. (Among oral surgeons and dentists, it is often referred to as Dilantin hyperplasia, in recognition of phenytoin's common proprietary name.) The mechanism is unknown, but we suspect the drug alters collagen metabolism in the gingival tissues. Although phenytoin isn't the only drug associated with potential gingival hyperplasia (verapamil is another common one), it is the only one listed as a choice. Note that phenobarbital, which is often used as an alternative to phenytoin, does not cause gingival hyperplasia. It is precisely for that reason that phenobarbital is sometimes prescribed for children with responsive seizure disorders in lieu of phenytoin.

118. The answer is d. (*Brunton, pp 308, 447, 450, 570; Craig, pp 283–284; Katzung, pp 271, 493–494, 991.*) The serotonin receptor agonist actions of the "triptans," including the prototype, sumatriptan, can trigger intense vasoconstriction in various vascular beds. The cerebral vasoconstrictor effects of these drugs contribute importantly to the relief they afford in migraine headaches.

However, coronary vasospasm can occur also; it may be particularly intense and potentially life-threatening in patients with coronary vasospastic disease (i.e., variant or Prinzmetal's angina), for whom the triptans are contraindicated.

None of the other drugs listed have any significant coronary (or other) vasoconstrictor effects. Indeed, some such as phenytoin and zolpidem (a benzodiazepine-like hypnotic) may cause slight cardiovascular changes (e.g., afterload reduction) that would actually reduce the degree of myocardial ischemia and the risk of angina.

119. The answer is a. (*Brunton, pp 509–510; Craig, p 383; Katzung, pp 380, 397–398.*) Fosphenytoin is the prodrug form of phenytoin. It is its metabolite (the phenytoin itself) that is responsible for anticonvulsant effects, and so the mechanism of actions are identical. Using fosphenytoin does not: have a faster onset of action than phenytoin; eliminate the need for giving such drugs as lorazepam first, nor prolong lorazepam's half-life; eliminate (for most patients) the need for long-term seizure control with suitable oral agents; or stimulate ventilation. The main advantages of fosphenytoin are less vascular irritability, the ability to be injected faster, and greater physical compatibility with IV solutions that might be used to dilute or administer it (e.g., phenytoin must be diluted before injection, but it is physically incompatible with glucose-containing solutions that so often are used as a vehicle for many IV drugs).

120. The answer is c. (*Brunton, pp 344, 353f, 360–361; Craig, p 305; Katzung, pp 402–404.*) Recall that nitrous oxide has an MAC (minimum alveolar concentration) of about 105%. Achieving that concentration in an inspired gas mixture is physically impossible at normal atmospheric pressure. Even if we could safely give pure nitrous oxide (we obviously cannot), and we rounded the MAC to 100%, the drug would (1) cause abolition of a painful response in only 50% of subjects (this is one element of the definition of MAC), and (2) be lethal, since 100% nitrous oxide means no (0%) oxygen at normal atmospheric pressures. This very effective analgesic gas is poorly soluble in the blood, so equilibration between alveolar and blood concentration and the onset of its central effects are quite rapid.

Even at the usual concentrations (typically 80% of the inspired), and whether used only with air (as in dental practice) or with other inhaled anesthetics (common in surgery), nitrous oxide causes little or no bronchospasm nor significant cardiac depression.

121. The answer is b. (*Brunton, pp 464, 474–479, 535; Craig, p 402; Katzung, p 474.*) The question describes common and necessary interventions for managing neuroleptic malignant syndrome, which is characteristically associated with older antipsychotics—chlorpromazine and other "low potency" antipsychotics to a degree, but occurs more so with haloperidol (butyrophenone). Signs and symptoms include muscle tetany/rigidity ("lead pipe rigidity"), profound fever, rapid swings of heart rate, rhythm, blood pressure (autonomic instability), electrolyte abnormalities and dehydration. None of the other agents are associated with this syndrome, whether acutely or with long-term therapy or at therapeutic or toxic serum levels, nor would the interventions described be indicated.

122. The answer is c. (*Brunton, pp 535–536; Craig, p 369; Katzung, pp 452–453, 459.*) This is a question about a drug you may not have learned about explicitly, but given the description of its mechanism, which should be quite familiar to you, you should have no problem arriving at the right answer. Ropinirole (a related drug is pramipexole) directly activates striatal dopamine receptors. It is one of several "dopaminergic" drugs that can be used to initiate therapy of early Parkinson's disease. Dyskinesias and hypotension are relatively common side effects, as also applies to alternatives such as levodopa and bromocriptine (or pergolide). Ropinirole also causes drowsiness or sleepiness; either would render the drug unsuitable for managing daytime anxiety (a), but that is not an indication for the drug, nor is management of hypersomnia (b). The dopaminergic action of ropinirole may exacerbate signs and symptoms of schizophrenia (d); like many other antiparkinson drugs it may lower the seizure threshold in patients with epilepsy, and so would be irrational for managing status epilepticus (e). It has no clinically useful analgesic activity (f).

123. The answer is e. (*Brunton, pp 436t, 447–451; Craig, pp 356–357t; Katzung, pp 272, 360.*) Buspirone is an attractive drug for managing mild short-term anxiety. Among the reasons (and especially when compared with more traditional anxiolytics, such as benzodiazepines) are a lack of sedation (buspirone is not a CNS depressant); very little or no potentiation of the effects of other CNS depressants, including alcohol; no known abuse potential (it is not regulated by the Controlled Substances Act); or tendency for development of tolerance; and no major withdrawal syndrome. One major drawback is a slow onset of symptom relief (a week or two), and typically it takes about a month from the onset of therapy for antianxiety effects to stabilize. (Knowing this slow onset, one should resist the temptation to titrate the dosage upwards, to hasten or increase the drug's effects, prematurely.)

You should recall that long-term benzodiazepine administration is associated with withdrawal phenomena (and, depending on the use, dose, exact drug, and other patient-related factors, the syndrome can be severe). Thus, one can envisage a switch from a benzodiazepine to buspirone. Because buspirone lacks CNS depressant effects and its effects take some time to develop, one should start the buspirone several weeks before stopping the benzodiazepine and then taper the benzodiazepine dose once it's time to stop the drug.

124. The answer is b. (*Brunton, pp 403t, 504, 523; Craig, p 383; Katzung, pp 394–395, 397–398.*) Intravenously administered lorazepam is generally regarded as the drug of choice for initial treatment of status epilepticus. (It has surpassed diazepam because of a faster onset of action and less venous irritation, among other things.) Lorazepam, like the benzodiazepines in general, increases the apparent affinity of the inhibitory neurotransmitter GABA for binding sites on brain cell membranes. The anticonvulsant effects of lorazepam are relatively short-lasting. Therefore, immediately after giving the lorazepam either phenytoin or fosphenytoin should be given to provide longer seizure suppression and "coverage" because the effects of lorazepam wear off in a short time. None of the other drugs listed in the question are appropriate for initial therapy of status epilepticus, despite their widespread use for oral therapy of seizure disorders long-term. Phenobarbital might be used for seizures refractory to any of the preferred initial drugs, however.

125. The answer is e. (*Brunton, pp 369–371f, 376; Craig, pp 330–334; Katzung, pp 426–427.*) This may seem like a trick question, or perhaps a picky one if you've been taught the main properties of only one or two prototypic local anesthetics—for example, lidocaine as the prototype amide and prototype local anesthetic overall; and perhaps procaine as the prototype of the ester class. Nonetheless, there are a couple of important points here, and they revolve around a fundamental difference between amides and esters, and so knowing the class to which a particular local anesthetic belongs: (1) allergic reactions of various severities are more common with esters than with amides; (2) there is class-based cross-reactivity, meaning that if a patient has had a true immunologic reaction to any ester, he or she is at risk for a similar reaction from subsequent exposure to any ester; and (3) there is no cross-reactivity between esters and amides, such that use of an amide in an "ester-sensitive" patient is not likely to pose problems of allergenicity.

Now, the learning "trick," if you haven't learned it before: how to tell whether a local anesthetic (one you've learned about, or not) is an ester or amide. Look at the drug's *generic* name; if there are two occurrences of the letter "i" in it, it's an amide; if not, it's an ester. Thus, we have such esters as cocaine, chlor(o)procaine, procaine itself, and tetracaine, which is the correct answer for this question. The others we listed are amides.

126. The answer is c. (*Brunton, pp 188, 201, 204, 211–214, 538–540; Craig, p 371; Katzung, pp 1010–1011.*) Initial recommended therapy includes use of acetylcholinesterase inhibitors such as tacrine, donepezil, galantamine (which are reversible cholinesterase inhibitors), or rivastigmine (irreversible). These drugs are not cures, but they appear to slow symptoms of brain pathology in some patients. None appears to be invariably superior to any other. Their actions almost certainly involve activation of central muscarinic receptors (indirectly, by inhibiting metabolism of ACh released from viable nerves, of course) because drugs with central antimuscarinic actions reduce their efficacy. Selegiline (MAO-B inhibitor) and high doses of vitamin E (antioxidant) apparently slow neurodegenerative processes, but so far there are no convincing data that they slow cognitive decline, and they are not first-line therapies.

127. The answer is b. (*Brunton, pp 533t, 537; Craig, pp 369–370; Katzung, pp 454–455.*) Trihexyphenidyl (and the related drug benztropine) cause significant antimuscarinic (atropine-like) actions in the CNS—hence, these drugs have been classified as "centrally acting antimuscarinics." These drugs are quire lipophilic and enter the CNS well (this accounts for the drug's marked sedative effects, too) to block muscarinic receptors there. That helps adjust the dopamine-ACh imbalance that appears to be a main biochemical underpinning of parkinsonism. Diphenhydramine can be used instead of trihexyphenidyl or benztropine, but it causes more drowsiness in most patients. Nonetheless, none of these drugs is used to counteract CNS depression caused by other antiparkinson drugs.

Diphenhydramine does help alleviate cutaneous allergy symptoms (e.g., urticaria; d), but those are rare with any of the common antiparkinson drugs (and we did not specify which "other" drug was given). None of these drugs affect manic/hypomanic episodes that might occur with, say, high doses of levodopa. They do not reverse antipsychotic-induced tardive dyskinesias (e); no drug does that effectively.

128. The answer is d. (*Brunton, pp 173, 239, 240t, 449, 537; Craig, pp 391–393; Katzung, pp 493, 1120–1121.*) Many drugs (but not amphetamines, a; barbiturates, b; benzodiazepines, c; or morphine or related opioid analgesics, e) participate in significant interactions with certain foods or beverages. However, when you read phrases along the lines of those noted in the question—"severe and sometimes fatal hypertension from consuming such foods as cheeses and processed meats"—you should automatically be thinking of the older, nonselective (MAO-A/B) monoamine oxidase inhibitors. These drugs have been used for severe hypertension or depression, but due to the potentially lethal interactions with tyramine-containing foods or beverages, their use has dwindled because the risks are too great. (Nonetheless, you need to know your pharmacology for such drugs as pargyline, phenelzine, and tranylcypromine.) Recall that tyramine is a catecholamine-releasing drug with sympathomimetic actions in its own right. When we consume tyramine-rich foods or beverages much of that sympathomimetic is metabolized by hepatic MAO before it reaches the systemic circulation (first-pass metabolism), and so its effects are slight. In the presence of a nonselective MAO inhibitor, however, the metabolic inactivation does not occur and significant amounts of the drug reach the circulation to cause more intense and potentially very intense effects that involve adrenergic receptor activation. In addition, catecholaminergic (e.g., adrenergic) nerves in the MAO-treated patient can be considered "loaded" with an abundance of the neurotransmitter due to inhibited intraneuronal metabolism of the neurotransmitter. Although the neurotransmitter may not be released physiologically, in response to an action potential (at least in the peripheral sympathetic nervous system), it can be released by such drugs as tyramine or by such drugs as pseudoephedrine and ephedrine (mixed-acting sympathomimetics) or amphetamines (indirect-acting sympathomimetics), which can then trigger possibly fatal hypertensive crisis, profound cardiac stimulation, and the consequences thereof. These problems led to the development of MAO inhibitors (e.g., selegiline) that have preferential effects on MAO in the brain (MAO-B) and far less an effect on MAO forms in the liver and peripheral nervous system (MAO-A). Nonetheless, as stated in the question, there is a new nonselective MAO inhibitor that has just been approved for use, for depression, in the form of a transdermal delivery system (skin patch).

129. The answer is d. (*Brunton, pp 578–579, Craig, p 327, Katzung, pp 512, 1070t.*) Dextromethorphan is, indeed, chemically related to codeine, but it lacks many effects you probably associate with codeine or other opioids, except one: it has excellent antitussive activity. This cough-suppressant effect presumably occurs via some ill-defined central mechanism, but does not involve agonist actions on opioid receptors. Dextromethorphan does not have analgesic effects (a); alter gut motility (b); or have effects on the bladder musculature that might relieve nocturia. Very high doses of dextromethorphan can cause CNS depression, but regardless of the dose it is not used as a sedative or other agent for controlling symptoms of ADD/ADHD. Finally, unlike codeine and most other opioids, dextromethorphan lacks addictive properties or potential.

130. The answer is e. (*Brunton, pp 347–349, 416t; Craig, pp 294–295; Katzung, pp 353–359.*) Thiopental can be considered the prototype of the thiobarbiturates (in contrast with such oxybarbiturates as phenobarbital). It is often used as a preanesthetic induction adjunct because of its ability to cause unconsciousness in a matter of seconds. This occurs because the drug is very lipophilic, quickly concentrating in the brain and spinal cord. However, the drug also has a very short duration of action, with patients awaking within minutes unless repeated doses or other CNS depressants are administered afterwards. This is because thiobarbiturates rapidly distribute out of the CNS to other tissues following their rapid CNS uptake. The brief duration is not due to prompt hepatic metabolism (c); in reality, the plasma half-life of thiopental is on the order of 10 to 12 h—a value that not only reflects further redistribution from tissues, but rather slow metabolism. None of the barbiturates cause clinically useful analgesia (a) at dosages that could be considered safe. Thiopental and other barbiturates (at sufficiently high CNS levels) routinely decrease, not increase (b), cerebral metabolic rates. This effect is often beneficial. Seizures are rare with any of the barbiturates; indeed phenobarbital (and some related drugs as metharbital and mephobarbital) are used long-term as anticonvulsants; and induction of a "barbiturate coma" with thiopental or other barbiturates might be used to manage seizures refractory to more first-line anticonvulsants.

131. The answer is a. Whether you have learned or read about this specifically in a pharmacology class or text, for medicolegal and societal (and board-related?) reasons you should be aware of the growing problem of illicit "meth labs" that use pseudoephedrine ("pseudo") as the starting point for a rather easy chemical synthesis of this highly addictive and dangerous CNS stimulant. None of the other drugs listed can be synthesized using this common indirect-acting sympathomimetic as a starting point.

132. The answer is c. (*Brunton, pp 220–222; Craig, pp 342–345; Katzung, pp 105, 430–433, 435.*) Pancuronium is a curare-like nondepolarizing neuromuscular blocker that is commonly used to induce or maintain skeletal muscle paralysis for surgery. It has no effects on brain functions such as levels of consciousness or sensations such as of pain. The drug prevents depolarization of nicotinic receptors on skeletal muscle (it is a competitive antagonist), thereby preventing normal skeletal muscle activation and causing flaccid paralysis. The onset and duration of this effect depends on the actual drug being administered.

Clonidine (a), hopefully familiar to you as a centrally acting oral antihypertensive drug (α agonist in the CNS) can be used parenterally, preoperatively, to cause sedation and an anxiolytic effect. It also has some intrinsic analgesic effects (via α-adrenergic receptors in spinal cord nociceptive pathways), and seems to reduce the need for otherwise high doses of typical analgesics. A clonidine formulation with a trade name different from the formulation used for hypertension is marketed for pain relief. It is usually infused via an intrathecal catheter with an opioid, and can be used not only preoperatively but also to manage severe, intractable pain (as in patients with terminal cancer).

Droperidol (b) is a haloperidol-like neuroleptic drug. It causes drowsiness and sedation in its own right. In some instances it is administered with fentanyl to cause neurolept analgesia (a calming effect, indifference to pain and surroundings); or with fentanyl and nitrous oxide for greater pain control (neurolept anesthesia). The main limitation to using droperidol is its tendency to prolong ventricular repolarization, which renders patients with "long QT syndrome" at risk of serious arrhythmias.

Propofol (d) is an intravenous drug that causes prompt sedation or loss of consciousness (dose-dependent) and can be used for such purposes as induction of anesthesia or sedation for a variety of purposes (patients on ventilators, those undergoing endoscopy, or other noninvasive procedures). Propofol's duration of action is short, and the drug lacks analgesic effects. As such, it is much like thiopental (e), but it is not, chemically, a barbiturate. The main risks with either propofol or thiopental are hypotension and/or ventilatory depression. These usually arise from administering too high a dose, or injecting the drug too quickly.

133. The answer is a. (*Brunton, pp 432t–436t, 438–440; Craig, pp 389–391; Katzung pp 484, 488–490.*) The mention of menstrual irregularities, galactorrhea, and what appears to be extrapyramidal side effects, should be a tip-off that we are dealing with a drug that interacts with dopamine receptors—specifically, by blocking them. Amoxapine, the correct answer, is a tricyclic antidepressant (secondary amine). It is rather unique among all the tricyclics (other secondary amines, and tertiary amines such as the more familiar amitriptyline and imipramine) in several respects. For one thing it inhibits neuronal dopamine and norepinephrine reuptake (the others affect mainly norepinephrine and serotonin). That, however, does not readily explain the amenorrhea-galactorrhea, and extrapyramidal side effects. What provides the explanation or mechanism relates to another rather unique property of amoxapine: one of its metabolites is a strong dopamine receptor antagonist, an action not shared by any of the other tricyclics; the SSRIs (e.g., citalopram, fluoxetine, sertraline; answers b, c, and d); and the monoamine oxidase inhibitors (e.g., tranylcypromine, e; or phenelzine).

You should recall that such antipsychotic drugs as the phenothiazines and haloperidol may also cause amenorrhea-galactorrhea, and extrapyramidal side effects, by the same dopaminergic receptor-blocking mechanism. Conversely, drugs that activate dopamine receptors in one way or another (e.g., bromocriptine) can be used to manage these endocrine dysfunction. Amoxapine's dopamine receptor blockade also seems to account for why the drug exerts some antipsychotic properties, theoretically making it useful for patients with both psychosis and depression.

134. The answer is c. (*Brunton, pp 450, 570; Craig, pp 322–323, 392–393; Katzung, pp 499t, 511, 1120t–1121t.*) Meperidine appears to be rather unusual among the common opioid analgesics in terms of its ability to inhibit neuronal reuptake of serotonin. The MAO inhibitor has increased synaptic levels of serotonin (and other endogenous monoamines) in the central synapses, and so the presence of the opioid has enabled massive overstimulation of serotonin receptors. We have caused the "serotonin syndrome." None of the other drugs listed participate in such an interaction. However, other important drugs not listed in the question certainly do. They include, especially, both tricyclic and SSRI–type antidepressants; and the serotonin agonists commonly referred to as "triptans" (e.g., sumitriptan.)

135. The answer is b. (*Brunton, pp 403–412, 424, 516; Craig, pp 296, 357t; Katzung, pp 357, 359–360, 364.*) The generic name for rohypnol is fluni-trazepam, a very lipophilic and potent benzodiazepine that manifests a typ-ical but unusually strong benzodiazepine-ethanol interaction. Given the unfortunate frequency with which this drug is used illegally (there are some legal uses outside United States), you need to know about it, and we suspect you know that flumazenil is a competitive benzodiazepine receptor antago-nist used to reverse (or diagnose) benzodiazepine overdoses. If you said that flumazenil has no effect on ethanol-induced CNS depression you would be absolutely correct, but our patient has consumed little alcohol; her prob-lems are due to the excessive benzodiazepine effects and their simultaneous interaction with the alcohol. Diazepam (a) and triazolam (e) being in the same class as the offending drug in this situation, are likely to exacerbate the clinical problems. Ketamine, a dissociative anesthetic (b; see Question 101 for more) would be inappropriate. Naltrexone (d) is an opioid antagonist, much like the prototype naloxone, but is used orally for uses somewhat dif-ferent than those for naloxone. Naloxone's specificity is for opioid receptors, and so it would have no good or bad impact on our patient's symptoms.

136. The answer is c. (*Brunton, pp 450–451, 616, 731; Craig, p 388; Katzung, pp 484i, 487t, 489t, 493t.*) One of the most noteworthy actions of bupropion, compared with tricyclics or other common antidepressants, is arguably the lowest incidence of sexual dysfunction. In males there is no antimuscarinic action (e) that might interfere with erection, and no periph-eral α-adrenergic blockade (d) that might interfere with ejaculation or cause orthostatic hypotension. In fact, the drug seems to enhance sexual drive and performance. This is clinically useful when the drug has been used to counteract the suppressed sexual desire caused by many of the SSRI antidepressants, and most of the tricyclics. Women with depression who report a decreased interest in intercourse also seem to benefit from this drug more than others. Bupropion has structural similarities with amphet-amine and so is largely nonsedating (and so a is incorrect); and tends to suppress, rather than increase, appetite (b). The drug lacks any effects on monoamine oxidase (f). However, bupropion's metabolism is dependent on MAO, and it should not be given within about 2–3 weeks of stopping MAO inhibitor therapy to minimize risks of toxicity—the main and most serious of which is a predisposition to seizures.

You may also remember that bupropion is marketed as a smoking cessation aid, under a different trade name than the one labeled for use for depression. It is in situations such as this, where the same active ingredient is sold under two different trade names for two decidedly different uses, that accidental overdoses can occur if both products are inadvertently prescribed for the same patients.

137. The answer is b. (*Brunton, pp 474–479, 535; Craig, p 402; Katzung, p 474.*) Neuroleptic malignant syndrome is thought to be a severe form of an extrapyramidal syndrome that can occur at any time with any dose of a neuroleptic agent. However, the risk is higher when so-called "high-potency antipsychotics" (see Question 109) are used in high doses, especially if given parenterally. Mortality from NMS is greater than 10%. Allergic reactions (a) to haloperidol are rare. While haloperidol overdoses (c) may trigger NMS, that is not a prerequisite for the development of the syndrome. Haloperidol clearly causes a parkinsonian-like clinical presentation (d) and tardive dyskinesias (e); but the fever, elevations of CK, and diminishing level of consciousness would be inconsistent with such findings.

138. The answer is a. (*Brunton, pp 375–377; Craig, p 335; Katzung, pp 419–422.*) Lidocaine and bupivacaine both exert their main effects by blocking sodium channels, not only on neurons but also in cardiac tissue. With lidocaine, the cardiac sodium channel blockade is relatively short-lived, not cumulative (dependent on infusion duration), and largely present during systole. With bupivacaine the block is more persistent (strong even during diastole) and appears to be cumulative even if absolute blood levels do not rise further as administration continues, and even if we attempt to keep the cumulative dose low. The outcome can be serious ventricular arrhythmias, often accompanied by a fall of cardiac output due to a negative inotropic effect; the incidence and severity are much higher than with equianalgesic doses of lidocaine (or most other parenteral local anesthetics for that matter; and successful treatment is difficult.

Answer b is incorrect; bupivacaine's efficacy for causing sensory block is greater than its effects on somatic nerves. Bupivacaine, lidocaine, and the rest, depress contractile activity of all smooth muscles, airway smooth muscle included, and so bronchoconstriction or spasm (c) is not at all likely.

Relaxation of vascular smooth muscle, even in the absence of any cardiac negative inotropic effects, lowers rather than raises blood pressure (d). Nephrotoxicity (e) due to a direct effect of either local anesthetic is quite unlikely, if not frankly rare.

139. The answer is d. (*Brunton, p 534; Craig, pp 367–367; Katzung, pp 448–450.*) Carbidopa is used as an adjunct to levodopa. It works by inhibiting dopamine decarboxylation, and subsequent metabolism of levodopa to dopamine, in the gut. This is important because the majority of an orally administered dose of levodopa is metabolized to dopamine in the gut, and dopamine in the systemic circulation does not cross the blood-brain barrier (and so never reaches the striatum to cause desired antiparkinson effects). Amantadine (a) works in the CNS to promote dopamine release from functional dopaminergic nerves. Benztropine (b) works centrally to block muscarinic receptors, thereby helping to "normalize a dopamine-ACh imbalance" that seems to be important in parkinsonism. Bromocriptine (c) works centrally as a direct dopamine receptor agonist. Selegiline (e) is a centrally acting MAO-B inhibitor that works by reducing metabolic inactivation of dopamine.

140. The answer is e. (*Brunton, pp 574–575; Craig, pp 325–326; Katzung, pp 505–507, 509.*) Adding pentazocine to an analgesic regimen involving morphine or another "pure" opioid agonist will counteract key effects of morphine. In this case, the patient's pain will grow worse, not become less; and such other effects as ventilatory depression will be counteracted also. Under the circumstances described in the question, the worsening of pain is far more likely to occur than seizures, which have been reported "occasionally."

To answer this question you need to remember that pentazocine is classified as a partial μ agonist (or mixed agonist-antagonist); and that morphine causes the following effects by acting as a "pure" agonist on μ receptors: analgesia, respiratory depression, euphoria, sedation, physical dependence, and decreased gut motility. Pentazocine, given alone, causes analgesia, sedation, and decreased gut motility by acting as an agonist on κ receptors. However, it is a weak agonist. But it antagonizes the actions of morphine on μ receptors in a concentration-dependent fashion, and so pain returns in this patient.

141. The answer is b. (*Brunton, pp 174, 299, 443, 529, 533–537; Craig, p 369; Katzung, pp 453.*) Selegiline inhibits MAO-B, thus inhibiting the metabolic breakdown of dopamine and making more neuronally released dopamine available for its postsynaptic receptor activation. It increases the effectiveness of both endogenous and pharmacologically administered L-dopa. Benztropine (a) and trihexyphenidyl (c) are cholinergic muscarinic antagonists that mainly act in the CNS. They have no effect on dopamine metabolism, release, or direct receptor-mediated agonist actions. Bromocriptine (d) is a dopamine receptor agonist. Chlorpromazine (e) is an antipsychotic drug with antiadrenergic properties, and it also competitively blocks dopamine receptors in both the CNS and in the periphery.

142. The answer is c. (*Brunton, pp 474, 641, 1004; Craig, pp 400–401; Katzung, p 469.*) Chlorpromazine, the prototype phenothiazine antipsychotic drug, is also indicated for managing nausea and vomiting, in both adults and children, from a number of causes. The drug can be administered orally, rectally, or intramuscularly for this very purpose. (Some phenothiazines with better antiemetic activity, such as prochlorperazine or promethazine, are usually used instead.) Regardless, the antiemetic mechanism appears to involve blockade of dopaminergic receptors in the chemoreceptor trigger zone of the brain's medulla.

Chlorpromazine (and most other antipsychotics) can lower the brain's seizure threshold, thereby potentially increasing the risk of seizures (a) in susceptible patients. It tends to lower blood pressure (b; by blocking α-adrenergic receptors in the vasculature) and so probably would aggravate preexisting hypotension. Most of the phenothiazines also cause significant antimuscarinic effects, which would aggravate bladder hypomotility (d) and xerostomia (e; and other conditions involving reduced exocrine gland secretions). The antimuscarinic effects would inhibit activation of the bladder's detrusor muscle and inhibit relaxation of the sphincter, thereby aggravating problems with micturition in such patients as the elderly man with an enlarged prostate.

Note: In general, phenothiazines are not used often for managing emesis or nausea. That is, in part, because of the risk of excessive sedation, extrapyramidal reactions, orthostatic hypotension, and occasional cholestatic jaundice (hepatitis) or blood dyscrasias. Nowadays we tend to turn to other dopamine antagonists (e.g., metoclopramide), a cannabinoid (dronabinol), or a serotonin receptor blocker (ondansetron; a 5-HT$_3$—selective blocker).

143. The answer is b. (*Brunton, pp 66, 161, 239, 377, 620–621; Craig, pp 407–410; Katzung, pp 78, 137, 425, 521–523.*) Cocaine, an ester of benzoic acid, has local anesthetic properties; it can block the initiation or conduction of a nerve impulse. It is metabolized by plasma esterases to inactive products. Most important, cocaine (and tricyclic antidepressants) blocks the neuronal reuptake of norepinephrine and other monoamines (e.g., dopamine). This action produces CNS stimulant effects including euphoria, excitement, and restlessness. Peripherally, the blocked norepinephrine reuptake cause sympathomimetic effects including tachycardia and vasoconstriction. Death from acute overdose can be from cardiac failure, stroke (hypertensive crisis), seizures, or apnea during the seizures. Cocaine does not directly activate adrenergic (a) or cholinergic receptors; it has no effect on catecholamine metabolism (c); tachycardia and vasoconstriction, not the opposite (d) are expected responses; and cocaine has local anesthetic activity and so actually suppresses the conduction of a variety of neuron types.

144. The answer is a. (*Brunton, pp 479, 535, 1500; Craig, p 369; Katzung, pp 451–453.*) Central dopamine receptor classifications include D_1 and D_2 receptors. Bromocriptine, a selective D_2 agonist, is useful in the treatment of parkinsonism and hyperprolactinemia. It produces fewer adverse reactions than do less selective dopamine receptor agonists. The antipsychotic activity of such drugs as chlorpromazine (b), fluphenazine (c), haloperidol (d), and promethazine (e), are better correlated with blockade of D_2 receptors.

145. The answer is a. (*Brunton, pp 472t, 474, 477; Craig, pp 399–403; Katzung, pp 466–468.*) Of all the antipsychotics the incidence and severity of these adverse responses are highest with the phenothiazines, of which chlorpromazine can be considered the prototype. Clozapine (b) blocks α–adrenergic, histamine (H_1), ACh (muscarinic) receptors, but the affinity for those receptors is very low in comparison with dopamine and serotonin receptor blockade. Haloperidol has considerable dopamine receptor-blocking activity, and little effect on muscarinic receptors that might account for the side effects described here. (See Question 109 for more on fundamental differences between "high potency" and "low potency" antipsychotics, especially as they predict the relative incidence of peripheral autonomic and central (extrapyramidal) side effects.) Olanzapine (d) is pharmacologically most similar to clozapine, except for the fact that the risk of agranulocytosis is quite low. Sertraline (e) is an SSRI, and you should recall that SSRIs (e.g., the prototype, fluoxetine) lack clinically significant antimuscarinic effects.

146. The answer is b. (*Brunton, pp 552t, 566, 572–573, 1848t; Craig, pp 323–324, 409–412; Katzung, pp 510, 519–520.*) Methadone is a slow, long-acting opioid receptor (μ and κ) agonist. It is used as an analgesic (for long-term pain control when an opioid is indicated) and for maintenance therapy of individuals dependent on opioids. It has greater oral bioavailability than morphine, especially when oral therapy is started. (Recall that morphine is subject to extensive first-pass hepatic metabolism, and only with repeated oral administration can we saturate its drug-metabolizing enzymes such that bioavailability is improved enough to get good analgesia. That's why if our analgesic of choice is morphine, we start treatment with parenteral administration.) Methadone's long biologic half-life accounts for the milder but more protracted abstinence syndrome when the drug is stopped. Methadone does not possess opioid antagonist properties (whether μ or k) and, thus, would not precipitate withdrawal symptoms in a heroin addict, as would naloxone or naltrexone, so long as we administer sufficient doses of the methadone, and that is precisely what we do with methadone maintenance therapy or when we switch a patient to it from another opioid. Excessive doses of methadone can cause typical opioid-related ventilatory depression.

147. The answer is c. (*Brunton, pp 506, 513–514, 523; Craig, pp 292, 295–296, 357; Katzung, pp 390–391, 396–397.*) The symptoms describe absence seizures, for which ethosuximide is very effective (and, according to many, the drug of choice). Phenytoin may aggravate absence seizures. None of the other drugs are effective or indicated for long-term therapy of epilepsy.

148. The answer is b. (*Brunton, pp 308–311, Katzung, pp 276–277.*) Ergotamine has for years been considered a mainstay of aborting migraine headaches. Its likely mechanism involves antagonizing cerebral vasodilation. It activates $5\text{-}HT_3$ receptors, which in turn causes cerebral vasoconstriction. This ergot alkaloid also can cause significant and long-lasting systemic vasoconstriction *via* α–adrenergic receptor activation. While normal coronary vessels aren't uniquely sensitive to this effect, those of patients who are prone to developing coronary vasospasm (Prinzmetal's or variant angina) are at greater risk, and that is likely what this patient had.

(Perhaps you've heard of "St. Anthony's Fire"—what we now call ergotism—that occurred in the Middle Ages. It was characterized by gangrene and "bloodless" loss of the fingers and toes [among other problems], and was due to intense vasoconstriction caused by eating spoiled grains laden with a fungus that produced large amounts of ergot alkaloids.)

Bromocriptine (a), another ergot alkaloid, has little effect on 5-HT or adrenergic receptors. However, it is an efficacious dopamine D_2 agonist and that provides the basis for its use for parkinsonism, hyperprolactinemia, and treatment of some prolactin-secreting pituitary tumors. Morphine (c) is not likely to cause hypertension, and would produce myocardial ischemia (of a global nature) only when such high doses are given that hypotension (and ventilatory depression) ensues.

Phenoxybenzamine (d) blocks 5-HT receptors (and ACh and histamine receptors too), which explains its rather infrequent use for carcinoid syndrome—a tumor that secretes large amounts of serotonin and peptides that stimulate smooth muscles (primarily in the airways and GI tract). However, its main pharmacologic effect is long-lasting and noncompetitive blockade of α-adrenergic receptors, and the related use is adjunctive management of catecholamine-secreting tumors (i.e., pheochromocytoma). Thus, it lowers blood pressure and also would block coronary vasoconstriction or spasm mediated by α–adrenergic activation. Dosages needed to block 5-HT receptors are much higher than those needed to block serotonin receptors.

Phenytoin (e), an important anticonvulsant, has no ability to cause hypertension (nor any other significant increase of blood pressure), nor to cause or exacerbate coronary vasospasm.

149. The answer is a. (*Brunton, pp 506, 513–514; Craig, pp 381–382; Katzung, pp 390–391.*) Ethosuximide is especially useful in the treatment of absence seizures. Although it may act at several sites, the principal mechanism of action at relevant concentrations is on T-type Ca currents in thalamic neurons. This blocks the pacemaker current that affects the generation of rhythmic cortical discharge associated with an absence attack.

150. The answer is e. (*Brunton, p 462, Craig, pp 399–403, 454; Katzung, pp 467–468, 472–473, 1052.*) Promethazine, like most other phenothiazines, tends to cause dose-dependent CNS depression. Of the answers given here, the most likely outcome of that effect is ventilatory depression and apnea, and that is precisely the reason why the FDA bolstered the warnings for children. Like most other phenothiazines, promethazine has significant antimuscarinic activity, and that would not cause heart block (a) or diarrhea (d). It has α-adrenergic blocking activity, which would lower, rather than raise, blood pressure (b). Promethazine may, indeed, cause parkinsonian-like side effects (c), but they are not likely to be a cause of death unless the patient develops neuroleptic malignant syndrome that goes undiagnosed and improperly treated until it is too late.

151. The answer is c. (*Brunton, pp 373–374; Craig, p 331; Katzung, pp 422–423.*) For the key to the simple answer, consider the British term for local anesthetics: regional analgesics. Pain is typically the first sensation to go, the last to return. For a more detailed explanation: The primary effect of local anesthetics is intraneuronal blockade of voltage channel-gated Na channels. Progressively increasing concentrations of local anesthetics result in an increased threshold of excitation, a slowing of impulse conduction, a decline in the rate of rise of the action potential, a decrease in the height of the action potential, and eventual obliteration of the action potential. Local anesthetics first block small unmyelinated or lightly myelinated fibers (pain), followed by heavily myelinated but small-diameter fibers, and then larger-diameter fibers (proprioception, pressure, motor). At high serum concentrations autonomic nerve function can be affected. At toxic concentrations other excitable tissues (cardiac, smooth, skeletal muscle) can be affected.

152. The answer is b. (*Brunton, pp 227–228, 356; Craig, pp 342, 344; Katzung, pp 410–411.*) Although a rare occurrence, halothane and other inhaled volatile liquid anesthetics may cause malignant hyperthermia, the signs and symptoms of which we have described in the question. Apparently, this occurs mainly in genetically susceptible individuals (whether a personal or familial history, as the predisposition seems to be heritable). The prevalence of the reaction is increased by concomitant use of succinylcholine. Indeed, the halothane-succinylcholine interaction is most commonly cited as the main cause of malignant hyperthermia.

153. The answer is c. (*Brunton, pp 503–506, 523; Craig, p 381; Katzung, p 387.*) Vigabatrin (γ-vinyl GABA) is useful in partial seizures. It is an irreversible inhibitor of GABA aminotransferase, an enzyme responsible for the termination of GABA action. This results in accumulation of GABA at synaptic sites, thereby enhancing its effect.

154. The answer is e. (*Brunton, p 481; Katzung, p 387.*) Vigabatrin can induce psychosis. It is recommended that it not be used in patients with preexisting depression and psychosis. None of the other drugs listed are associated with this phenomenon.

155. The answer is d. (*Brunton, pp 509–510; Craig, pp 382–383; Katzung, p 398.*) Folic acid supplementation is generally thought to be important for all pregnant women, but it is particularly important during therapy with such anticonvulsants as phenytoin. The purpose is to reduce the risk of spina bifida and other neural tube defects (and some other teratogenic consequences). The scenario describes no reason to add valproic acid (or add or switch to any other anticonvulsant, including phenobarbital) if the mother is kept seizure-free during pregnancy. Valproic acid is in pregnancy class D; most others are C, and so it appears to carry the highest risk of teratogenic effects of all the common anticonvulsants. Discontinuing all anticonvulsants during pregnancy is inappropriate in this and most circumstances, as it carries the risk of seizure recurrence than can be more dangerous to the mother and the fetus than continuing effective therapy and providing good prenatal care.

156. The answer is b. (*Brunton, pp 463t, 474; Craig, pp 400–402; Katzung, pp 466t, 468, 473.*) Chlorpromazine, of all the drugs listed, has strong α–adrenergic receptor-blocking activity. This accounts for a relatively high incidence of orthostatic hypotension, and explains why measuring the patient's blood pressure in both the supine and standing positions is important. At clinically relevant dosages, buspirone (a) has no significant autonomic or cardiovascular effects. Diphenhydramine strongly blocks both muscarinic and H_1 histamine receptors, and neither action would likely cause hypotension. Haloperidol (d), a butyrophenone antipsychotic, causes few peripheral autonomic side effects, including those noted in the question. Zolpidem (e) is a benzodiazepine-like hypnotic that lacks appreciable peripheral autonomic side effects.

157. The answer is a. (*Brunton, pp 360–361, 403–411; Craig, pp 357–360; Katzung, pp 356–359.*) Midazolam, a benzodiazepine, lacks analgesic effects (b). Fentanyl tends to cause bradycardia and hypotension, not tachycardia or hypertension, and midazolam has no direct effects on these cardiovascular responses. Both midazolam and fentanyl, given individually, can cause ventilatory depression if dosages are sufficiently high, and this is the major concern with coadministration of these drugs. In short, the purpose of using midazolam in part due to its generalized CNS-depressant and anxiety-relieving effects, but more so due to its ability to cause antegrade amnesia such that the patient has little recall of the disturbing procedure.

158. The answer is a. (*Brunton, pp 194, 313, 462–466; Craig, pp 399–402; Katzung p 470.*) Clozapine causes agranulocytosis in 1–2% of treated patients—perhaps a small number in an absolute sense, but far more common and potentially serious with other drugs that might be used in lieu of this unusual antipsychotic. It is generally reversible on discontinuation of the drug but this, of course, depends on frequent blood tests to detect the problem early on. Monitoring for this adverse response is so critical that the initial prescription for the drug, and refills for continued therapy, cannot be filled without proof of blood counts that are within "acceptable" levels. Other concerns with clozapine, for which monitoring is important, include the development of seizures; weight gain (it is common and the patient may put on an extra 10 or 20 pounds); rises of blood glucose levels (perhaps with the development of new-onset diabetes, and so answer c is incorrect); and myocarditis. Extrapyramidal side effects (b) are rare, in contrast with typical antipsychotics, because of clozapine's low affinity for dopamine D_2 receptors. Hypotension (d) and ventilatory depression (e) are not at all common with this drug.

159. The answer is e. (*Brunton, pp 510, 523–524; Craig, pp 377–378; Katzung, pp 381–383.*) Phenytoin, given throughout pregnancy, can inhibit hepatic synthesis (activation) of vitamin K-dependent clotting factors *in utero.* (Phenobarbital and several other anticonvulsants can do the same, and so vitamin K prophylaxis applies to their use as well.) None of the other drugs listed is associated with such an effect. Note, finally, that naloxone (d) is a parenteral opioid antagonist, and it is beyond the realm of possibility that it would be administered "throughout pregnancy."

160. The answer is b. (*Brunton, pp 484–485; Craig, pp 399–400; Katzung, pp 447, 458, 469.*) We are describing some of the symptoms and signs of Gilles de la Tourette's syndrome. Of the drugs listed, haloperidol probably would be tried first. (If patients do not respond well or do not tolerate haloperidol, they might be switched to pimozide, not listed as a potential answer.) Clozapine (a) is not likely to be efficacious for Tourette's, and it carries great risk of causing agranulocytosis and seizures. Levodopa (c) is likely to exacerbate the described signs and symptoms, as may methylphenidate (d), an amphetamine-like drug that is contraindicated in Tourette's. Phenobarbital (e) can be used long-term as an anticonvulsant (mainly as an alternative to phenytoin), but would not be appropriate or effective for this patient.

161. The answer is b. (*Brunton, pp 174, 536–537; Craig, p 370; Katzung, p 454.*) Entacapone is a COMT inhibitor. COMT normally is a minor player in the metabolism of levodopa, but when the major pathway for levodopa metabolism to dopamine (via dopa decarboxylase) is inhibited, as it is with administration of carbidopa, COMT plays a more important role. It helps form 3-O-methyldopa, which competes with levodopa for uptake into the brain. So, when we have poor responses to levodopa (alone or in combination with carbidopa), or when levodopa therapy has been ongoing for so long that the patient develops acute or chronic refractoriness to its effects (e.g., the "on-off" or the "wearing off" phenomena), adding entacapone (or a similar drug, tolcapone) might be reasonable. Donepezil (a) and tacrine (d) are centrally acting cholinesterase inhibitors with no effect on dopamine metabolism. Selegiline (c) is a selective inhibitor of dopamine metabolism by MAO in the brain (MAO-B). Trihexyphenidyl (e) is a centrally acting muscarinic receptor blocking drug. Related drugs are benztropine and diphenhydramine.

162. The answer is c. (*Brunton, pp 593, 602–603, 613; Craig, pp 412–415; Katzung, pp 375, 1119t.*) This is a classic description of an alcohol-disulfiram interaction. Disulfiram is sometimes used in controlling alcohol abuse. It acts by inhibition of aldehyde dehydrogenase, resulting in the accumulation of acetaldehyde. This "acetaldehyde syndrome" is characterized by the signs and symptoms described in the question. The onset of symptoms is almost immediately following ingestion of alcohol and may last for several hours in some patients. None of the other drugs listed in the answers can cause these outcomes. Naltrexone (a), an opioid antagonist, would have no effect on the responses to ethanol. Diazepam (b) and phenobarbital (d), both CNS depressants that clearly have their depressant effects potentiated by alcohol, would not lead to the described effects. Tranylcypromine (e) is an older nonselective MAO inhibitor. MAO plays no role in the metabolism or responses to alcohol.

163. The answer is c. (*Brunton, pp 447–448, 450–451, 616, 731; Craig, pp 386–388; Katzung, pp 483–484, 486, 490.*) Fluoxetine (and related SSRI antidepressants such as sertraline, fluvoxamine, citalopram, and escitalopram) selectively inhibits neuronal serotonin uptake, with minimal effects on other monoamines. The tricyclics (imipramine) and venlafaxine inhibit serotonin and norepinephrine reuptake (and, apparently to a small degree, dopamine). Bupropion affects reuptake of both norepinephrine and dopamine.

164. The answer is d. (*Brunton, pp 410t–411t, 601; Craig, pp 359–408, 411–412; Katzung, pp 520–521.*) Benzodiazepines (particularly those with prompt and significant sedating activity) are considered good choices for alleviating barbiturate withdrawal symptoms. The anxiolytic effects of buspirone (a) take several days to develop, rendering it unsuitable for acute, severe withdrawal signs and symptoms. In addition, it causes little or no CNS depression in most patients. Chloral hydrate (b) and ethanol interact by inhibiting the metabolism of each other, with the main result being profound CNS depression. We would not want to give chloral hydrate to any patient who still may have alcohol in the circulation. Chlorpromazine (c) is used mainly for psychosis, and is not likely to beneficially affect the signs and symptoms that our patient has. Trazodone (e) is an atypical antidepressant; it weakly inhibits neuronal serotonin reuptake and seems to increase serotonin release from serotoninergic nerves. It would not be suitable for the immediate management of this patient.

165. The answer is b. (*Brunton, pp 593, 600; Craig, pp 64, 66t; Katzung, pp 375–377, 989, 993.*) Methanol is metabolized by the same enzymes that metabolize ethanol, but the products are different: formaldehyde and formic acid in the case of methanol. Headache, vertigo, vomiting, abdominal pain, dyspnea, and blurred vision can occur from accumulation of these metabolic intermediates. However, the most dangerous (or at least permanently disabling) consequence in severe cases is hyperemia of the optic disc, which can lead to blindness. The rationale for administering ethanol to treat methanol poisoning is fairly simple. Ethanol has a high affinity for alcohol and aldehyde dehydrogenases and competes with methanol as a substrate for those enzymes, reducing metabolism of methanol to its more toxic products. Important adjunctive treatments include hemodialysis to enhance removal of methanol and its products; and administration of systemic alkalinizing salts (e.g., sodium bicarbonate) to counteract metabolic acidosis. None of the other drugs listed would be appropriate. They may alleviate some of the signs and symptoms resulting from methanol poisoning, but they would have no beneficial effects on the crux of the problem—the metabolism of the methanol.

166. The answer is c. (*Brunton, pp 560, 571–574, 577–578; Craig, pp 317, 323, 326–327; Katzung, pp 498i, 512–513, 984.*) Naloxone is given parenterally. It specifically blocks opioid receptors that are activated by such agonists as morphine, heroin, and fentanyl (among many others). Diazepam (a) and other benzodiazepines (e.g., lorazepam) have no effects on opioid receptors. Flumazenil (b) is a specific benzodiazepine antagonist. It may be life-saving in cases of benzodiazepine overdoses, but has no effects on the responses to opioids. Naltrexone (d) is an opioid receptor antagonist (as is naloxone), but it is given orally, has a slow onset of action, and so will be of little benefit in this acute, life-threatening situation. Fentanyl is unlikely to cause seizures. Phenytoin (e) is an anticonvulsant; it would be inappropriate to administer, and if the administered doses were sufficiently high it might contribute to the CNS and ventilatory depression caused by the fentanyl.

167. The answer is b. (*Brunton, pp 432t, 446–447, 450–451; Craig, pp 389–391; Katzung, pp 486–489t, 493t.*) Imipramine, a tricyclic antidepressants, causes strong peripheral antimuscarinic effects. In the context of our patient, recall that muscarinic receptor activation contracts the detrusor muscle of the bladder, and relaxes the bladder sphincter. Imipramine blocks those effects, and that seems to explain its effects in managing nocturnal enuresis—especially in children. The drug, and other members of its class, does relieve depression signs and symptoms. However, they are due to inhibition, not increase of (a) monoamine neurotransmitter reuptake. Imipramine and its group members tend to cause sedation (c), but that is not likely to reduce the frequency of enuresis. These drugs also have α–adrenergic blocking activity, and one consequence of that would most likely be an increase, not a decrease, of renal blood flow and GFR. Tricyclic antidepressants, nor other major classes of antidepressants, have any important effects on the release of antidiuretic hormone or the responses of the renal tubules to ADH.

168. The answer is a. (*Brunton, pp 436t, 447–448, 453, 616, 731; Craig, p 388; Katzung, pp 484i, 487t, 489t, 493t.*) Bupropion is marketed, under different trade names, for two main purposes: anxiety relief, and suppression of the cravings for nicotine. Since too many physicians prescribe by brand-name products, and ignore the active generic drug, such problems as the one we described in our scenario, due to accidental duplication and overdoses of a drug, are more common than you'd like to believe. One of the main consequences of bupropion overdose is seizures. Chlordiazepoxide (b) is a benzodiazepine that is not indicated for depression or as a stop-smoking aid. If anything, the drug will suppress, rather than cause, seizures. Fluoxetine (c) and imipramine (d) are antidepressants, but they are not normally prescribed as smoking-cessation aids, nor are they marketed in products approved for that use. Lithium (e) is a mood-stabilizing drug used in bipolar illness. It is not at all likely to have been approved for managing depression or for smoking cessation.

169. The answer is c. (*Brunton, pp 537–538, Craig, pp 366–367, Katzung, pp 447–448, 454–456.*) At first blush it would seem that choosing any "antiparkinson" drug would be appropriate for this man. However, if you think about the etiology of schizophrenia and of parkinsonism (especially drug-induced), and the mechanisms of action of the drugs listed, you should select benztropine (or a related drug, trihexyphenidyl, or diphenhydramine, neither of which was listed) as the best choice.

Phenothiazines (chlorpromazine), and especially butyrophenones (haloperidol, e), relieve schizophrenia signs and symptoms largely by blockade of central dopamine D_2 receptors, particularly in the mesolimbic-mesocortical system. Simultaneously, D_2 blockade in the nigrostriatum, and concomitant unmasking of opposing muscarinic-cholinergic effects, seems to account for the extrapyramidal/parkinsonian side effects that have surfaced in patients like the one we describe. Recall that despite the imprecision of the terminology, "high potency" antipsychotics such as haloperidol are associated with a much higher incidence of extrapyramidal side effects than are the "low potency" antipsychotics (i.e., the phenothiazines), due to their stronger central D_2 blockade, and so switching from chlorpromazine to haloperidol would not at all alleviate this patient's parkinsonian side effects: It would likely worsen them.

In idiopathic Parkinson's disease there is deterioration of dopaminergic neurons and, inferentially, a decrease of central dopamine content or release. That pathophysiology provides a rationale for pharmacologically boosting dopaminergic influences: increasing central dopamine synthesis (levodopa, alone or with carbidopa; d); inhibiting dopamine's metabolic inactivation with either a COMT inhibitor (tolcapone, a; or entacapone) or an MAO inhibitor (e.g., selegiline, not listed); or using such other strategies as dopamine-releasing or -mimetic agents (amantadine, bromocriptine).

In this situation of drug-induced parkinsonism, however, dopamine receptors are blocked by the antipsychotic. While we could try to overcome that blockade (since it is surmountable and competitive antagonism we are dealing with), that approach is not likely to be effective nor tolerable to the patient, since we would have to try very large doses of a dopaminergic drug—doses sufficient to cause, in all likelihood, significant side effects.

So what we do, therefore, is attack the dopamine-ACh imbalance from the "other side"—administer a centrally-acting antimuscarinic drug. Note that since we are dealing with symptoms arising from a relative excess of cholinergic influences, a centrally acting cholinesterase inhibitor (donepezil or tacrine, b) would worsen the problems by making even more ACh available at central muscarinic synapses.

170. The answer is b. (*Brunton, pp 354–358; Craig, pp 303–304; Katzung, pp 410–411.*) One of the main reasons why halothane is used infrequently in adult anesthesias is because of the risk of renal and hepatic toxicity. Such halothane-related problems are uncommon in children, and rare in either children or adults anesthetized with the more commonly used drug, isoflurane. Neither halothane nor isoflurane tend to raise blood pressure (a). Isoflurane seems to lower blood pressure mainly as a result of vasodilation; with halothane, both cardiac depression and vasodilation seem to cause hypotension. Another limitation to the use of halothane is its arrhythmogenic effects, which occur by two main mechanisms: (1) it sensitizes the myocardium to catecholamines; and (2) prolongs ventricular repolarization by prolonging the Q-T interval, thus predisposing susceptible patients to ventricular tachycardia, Torsades de Points, or other potentially lethal ventricular arrhythmias. The risks are far lower with isoflurane. Finally, while both halothane and isoflurane are potent anesthetics (they have MACs < 2%), these drugs both lack sufficient analgesic and skeletal muscle-relaxing effects to be used routinely without other appropriate adjuncts (e.g., nitrous oxide, neuromuscular blocking drugs).

171. The answer is d. (*Brunton, pp 479, 535, 1500; Craig, p 369; Katzung, p 452.*) Bromocriptine mimics the action of dopamine in the brain but is not as readily metabolized and inactivated as the endogenous neurotransmitter. It is especially useful in parkinsonism that is unresponsive to L-dopa. Apomorphine (b) is also a dopamine receptor agonist, but its side effects (mainly emesis) preclude its use for parkinsonism. Selegiline (e) is an MAO-B inhibitor. Belladonna preparations (c) are atropine and atropine-like antimuscarincs. Centrally-acting antimuscarinics such as benztropine and trihexyphenidyl are important drugs for managing some patients with parkinsonism, but they work not by enhancing the effects of dopamine but rather by blocking the central effects of ACh. Amantadine (a) is an antiviral agent that also is useful in some cases of parkinsonism. It either (or both) enhances the synthesis or inhibits neuronal reuptake of dopamine. It is not a dopamine receptor agonist.

172. The answer is d. (*Brunton, p 479; Craig, pp 401–402; Katzung, pp 451–452.*) Bromocriptine, an ergot derivative, is a direct-acting dopamine receptor agonist. Its main uses are for adjunctive management of Parkinson's disease, and for management of amenorrhea and infertility (and, if present, galactorrhea) due to hyperprolactinemia. It is also used, long-term, for management of some pituitary adenomas. However, it has gained acceptance as an important adjunct (usually along with dantrolene, as noted in the question) for management of neuroleptic malignant syndrome (NMS). Recall that NMS is a rare but potentially fatal response to traditional neuroleptic/antipsychotic drugs (phenothiazines such as chlorpromazine, and butyrophenones such as haloperidol). The newer, atypical antipsychotics (clozapine, olanzapine, and risperidone) may also cause NMS, but the clinical presentation seems not to include muscle rigidity that is usually an accompaniment of NMS caused by phenothiazines or butyrophenones.

The Cardiovascular System

Agents for heart failure
Antianemics
Atianginals
Antiarrhythmics
Anticoagulants

Antihyperlipidemics
Antihypertensives
Antiplatelet agents
Thrombolytics/Fibrinolytics

Questions

DIRECTIONS: Each item contains a question or incomplete statement that is followed by several responses. Select the **one best** response to each question.

173. The figure below shows typical cardiovascular responses to the intravenous injection of four adrenergic drugs into a normal, resting subject. Assume the doses of each are sufficient to cause expected effects, but not so high that toxic effects occur. No other drugs are present, and sufficient time has been allowed to enable complete dissipation of the effects of any prior drugs, and a return to normal resting hemodynamic status. The dashed line between the systolic and diastolic pressure traces represents mean arterial pressure.

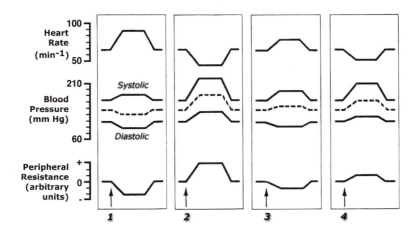

Abbreviations used, and potential answer choices, are

- EPI, epinephrine
- ISO, isoproterenol
- NE, norepinephrine
- PHE, phenylephrine
- PHN, phentolamine
- PRO, propranolol

Which of the following letter answers indicates the drugs that are ordered in the sequence shown (1, 2, 3, 4)?

a. EPI, NE, PHE, ISO
b. ISO, EPI, NE, PHE
c. ISO, PHE, EPI, NE
d. NE, ISO, PHE, EPI
e. PHE, EPI, NE, PRO
f. PHE, ISO, NE, EPI
g. PRO, PHN, PHE, ISO

174. A 65-year-old man with severe congestive heart failure (CHF) is unable to climb a flight of stairs without experiencing shortness of breath. After several years of therapy with first-line drugs for heart failure, we empirically try digoxin to improve cardiac muscle contractility. Within 4 weeks, he has a marked improvement in his symptoms. Which of the following best describes the main cellular action of digoxin that accounts for its ability to improve his overall wellness and his cardiovascular function in particular?

a. Activates β_1-adrenergic receptors
b. Facilitates GTP binding to specific G proteins
c. Increases mitochondrial calcium (Ca^{2+}) release
d. Inhibits sarcolemmal Na^+-K^+-ATPase
e. Stimulates cyclic adenosine 5'-monophosphate (cAMP) synthesis

175. A patient has periodic episodes of paroxysmal supraventricular tachycardia (PSVT). Which of the following drugs would be most suitable for *outpatient prophylaxis* of these worrisome electrophysiologic events?

a. Adenosine
b. Lidocaine
c. Nifedipine
d. Nitroglycerin
e. Verapamil

176. We prescribe a β-adrenergic blocker for a patient with chronic-stable ("effort-induced") angina, and the incidence and severity of anginal attacks are reduced. Which of the following best explains the pharmacologic action by which the β blocker does this?

a. Decreases myocardial oxygen demand
b. Dilates the coronary vasculature
c. Exerts antiplatelet/antithrombotic effects
d. Reduces total peripheral resistance
e. Slows AV nodal conduction velocity

177. Your patient is a 50-year-old man with well-controlled Type 2 diabetes and normal renal function (and no microalbuminuria). Which of the following drugs would be the most rational first choice for starting his antihypertensive therapy?

a. Angiotensin-converting enzyme (ACE) inhibitor or angiotensin receptor blocker
b. β-adrenergic blocker
c. Nifedipine
d. Thiazide diuretic
e. Verapamil or diltiazem

178. We have a 50-year-old man with asymptomatic hyperuricemia, and we are about to start therapy for newly diagnosed essential hypertension (BP 136/90 mm Hg, based on repeated measurements with the patient supine and at rest). Which of the following antihypertensive drugs is most likely to increase his serum uric acid levels further, and possibly precipitate a gout attack?

a. Captopril
b. Hydrochlorothiazide
c. Labetalol
d. Losartan
e. Verapamil

179. We've just diagnosed essential hypertension in a 58-year-old female patient. She tends to be tachycardic. Notes written by her ophthalmologist indicate that she has chronic open-angle glaucoma. Which of the following drugs would be the most rational choice for this woman, given only the information presented in this question?

a. Captopril
b. Diltiazem
c. Hydrochlorothiazide
d. Timolol
e. Verapamil

180. Our newly diagnosed hypertensive patient has a history of vasospastic angina. Which of the following drugs or drug classes would be the most rational for starting antihypertensive therapy because it exerts antihypertensive effects, directly lowers myocardial oxygen demand and consumption, and also tends to inhibit cellular processes that otherwise favor coronary vasospasm?

a. Angiotensin-converting enzyme (ACE) inhibitor or angiotensin receptor blocker
b. β-Adrenergic blocker
c. Nifedipine
d. Thiazide diuretic
e. Verapamil (or diltiazem)

181. We have a patient with newly diagnosed essential hypertension, and start them on a commonly used antihypertensive drug at a dose that is considered to be therapeutic for the vast majority of patients. Soon after starting therapy the patient experiences crushing chest discomfort. EKG changes show myocardial ischemia. Studies in the cardiac cath lab show episodes of coronary vasospasm, and it is likely the antihypertensive drug provoked the vasoconstriction. Which of the following antihypertensive drugs or drug class most likely caused the ischemia and the angina?

a. Atenolol
b. Diltiazem
c. Hydrochlorothiazide
d. Losartan
e. Metolazone

182. A 28-year-old woman is receiving drug therapy for essential hypertension. She subsequently becomes pregnant. We realize that the drug she's been taking for her high blood pressure can have serious, if not fatal, effects on the fetus (it is in pregnancy category X). As a result, we stop the drug and substitute another that is deemed to be equally efficacious in terms of her blood pressure, and safer for the fetus. Which of the following drugs was she most likely taking before she became pregnant?

a. α-Methyldopa
b. Captopril
c. Furosemide
d. Labetalol
e. Verapamil

183. We have just diagnosed Stage 1 essential hypertension in a 30-year-old man who has a history of asthma. He regularly uses an inhaled corticosteroid, which seems to work well, but does need to use an albuterol inhaler about once every 3 weeks for suppression of asthma attacks. Which antihypertensive drug or drug class poses the greatest risk of exacerbating the patient's asthma and counteracting the desired pulmonary effects of the albuterol, even though it might control his blood pressure well?

a. Diltiazem
b. Hydrochlorothiazide
c. Labetalol
d. Ramipril
e. Verapamil

184. We treat a patient with a drug that affects the clotting-thrombolytic systems for a time sufficient to let the drug's effects and blood levels stabilize at a therapeutic level. We then isolate platelets from a blood sample and test their *in vitro* aggregatory responses to ADP, collagen, PAF, and thromboxane A_2. Aggregatory responses to ADP are inhibited; responses to the other platelet proaggregatory agonists are unaffected. Which drug did we most likely administer to this patient?

a. Aspirin
b. Bivalirudin
c. Clopidogrel
d. Heparin
e. Warfarin

185. A healthy adult subject is given an intravenous injection of a test drug. Both blood pressure and total peripheral resistance rise promptly. This is followed immediately by a reduction of heart rate. In repeated experiments we find that the vasopressor response is not affected by pretreatment with prazosin. However, pretreatment with atropine prevents the cardiac chronotropic response. The test drug was most likely which of the following?

a. Angiotensin II
b. Dobutamine
c. Isoproterenol
d. Norepinephrine
e. Phenylephrine

186. You are reviewing the medication history of a 59-year-old man. He has been taking ramipril, pravastatin, and metformin for the last 5 years; and escitalopram for the last 12 months to help manage his depression. At his last clinic visit, a year ago, he was told to continue his current medications but also started on slow-release niacin because diet, exercise, and other lifestyle modifications, and his current medications, were not adequate. What was the most likely reason for adding the niacin?

a. Counteract deficiencies of B-vitamin absorption caused by the antidepressant
b. Counteract polyphagia, and overeating, caused by the metformin
c. Lower triglyceride levels that did not respond adequately to the statin
d. Prevent statin-induced neuropathy
e. Slow the progression of diabetic nephropathy caused by the ACE inhibitor

187. Quinidine is ordered for a patient with recurrent atrial fibrillation and who refuses any interventions other than drugs in an attempt to terminate and control the arrhythmia. Which of the following is the most likely effect of quinidine?

a. Is likely to increase blood pressure *via* a direct vasoconstrictor effect
b. Is contraindicated if the patient also requires anticoagulant therapy
c. Slows spontaneous SA nodal depolarization as its predominant effect
d. Tends to slow electrical impulse conduction velocity through the AV node
e. Will increase cardiac contractility (positive inotropic effect) independent of its antiarrhythmic effects

188. A patient who has been taking an oral antihypertensive drug for about a year develops a positive Coombs' test. Which of the following drugs is the most likely cause?

a. Captopril
b. Clonidine
c. Labetalol
d. Methyldopa
e. Prazosin

189. A patient presents with severe hypertension and tachycardia. Blood chemistry results, MRI findings, and the overall clinical presentation point to pheochromocytoma. The tumor appears operable, but the patient will have to wait a couple of months for the surgery. We prescribe phenoxybenzamine in the interim, with the goal of suppressing some of the major signs and symptoms caused by the tumor. Which of the following best summarizes what phenoxybenzamine does, or how it acts?

a. Controls blood pressure by blocking α-adrenergic receptors in the peripheral vasculature
b. Controls heart rate by selectively blocking β_1-adrenergic receptors
c. Inhibits catecholamine synthesis in the adrenal (suprarenal) medulla
d. Lowers blood pressure by inhibiting angiotensin converting enzyme and bradykininase
e. Stimulates catechol-O-methyltransferase, thereby facilitating epinephrine's metabolic inactivation

190. We want to compare and contrast the cardiac and hemodynamic profiles of immediate-acting dihydropyridine-type calcium channel blockers (CCBs) and the nondihydropyridines, verapamil, and diltiazem (benzothiazepines). Which of the following best summarizes how verapamil or diltiazem differs from nifedipine?

a. Are suitable for use in conjunction with a β blocker or digoxin
b. Cause a much higher incidence of reflex tachycardia
c. Cause significant dose-dependent slowing of AV nodal conduction velocity
d. Cause significant venodilation, leading to profound orthostatic hypotension
e. Have significant positive inotropic effects

191. Digoxin affects a host of cardiac electrophysiologic properties. Some of its effects are caused directly by the drug. Others are indirect: they may involve increasing "vagal tone" to the heart or other compensations that arise when cardiac output is improved in a patient with heart failure. For some parameters the direct and indirect effects may be qualitatively (but not quantitatively) opposing, but one will predominate over the other. Which of the following is an expected and predominant effect of the drug?

a. Increased rate of SA nodal depolarization
b. Reduced atrial automaticity
c. Reduced ventricular automaticity
d. Slowed AV nodal conduction velocity
e. Slowed conduction velocity through the atrial myocardium and His-Purkinje system

192. A patient has Stage III essential hypertension. After evaluating the responses to several other antihypertensive drugs, alone and in combination, the physician places the patient on oral hydralazine. Which of the following adjunct(s) is/are likely to be needed to manage the expected and unwanted cardiovascular side effects of the hydralazine?

a. Captopril plus nifedipine
b. Digoxin plus spironolactone
c. Digoxin plus vitamin K
d. Hydrochlorothiazide and a β blocker
e. Nitroglycerin
f. Triamterene plus amiloride

193. We administer a drug with the intent of lowering a patient's elevated LDL and total cholesterol levels, and raising HDL levels. The drug we choose inhibits cholesterol synthesis by inhibiting 3-hydroxy-3-methylglutaryl-coenzyme A (better known as [HMG CoA] reductase). Which of the following drugs best fits this description and works by the stated mechanism of action?

a. Clofibrate
b. Gemfibrozil
c. Lovastatin
d. Nicotinic acid (niacin)
e. Probucol

194. We have a patient who is taking a tricyclic antidepressant (e.g., imipramine), which blocks neuronal catecholamine reuptake. We now have to start him on antihypertensive drug therapy. If we continue the tricyclic, which of the following drugs will most likely have its antihypertensive effects inhibited?

a. Diazoxide
b. Guanadrel
c. Hydralazine
d. Prazosin
e. Propranolol

195. We are administering nitroprusside intravenously for control of severe hypertension during surgery. The dose has gotten too high, and the drug has been administered too long. Refractoriness to the antihypertensive effects has occurred. Blood pressure is rising, and other signs and symptoms of potentially severe toxicity develop. What is the main nitroprusside metabolite that accounts for these problems?

a. A highly efficacious α-adrenergic agonist
b. An extraordinarily potent and irreversible Na-K-ATPase inhibitor
c. An irreversible agonist for angiotensin II receptors
d. Cyanide
e. Nitric oxide

196. A 64-year-old man with coronary atherosclerosis and "mild" heart failure has been treated with digoxin and several other drugs. He complains of nausea, vomiting, and diarrhea. His EKG reveals a bigeminal rhythm and second-degree heart block. A drug-drug interaction is suspected. Which of the following coadministered drugs most likely provoked the problem?

a. Captopril
b. Cholestyramine
c. Furosemide
d. Lovastatin
e. Nitroglycerin

197. At high (but not necessarily toxic) blood levels, a cardiovascular drug with which you should be familiar causes many signs and symptoms that resemble what you see with "low-grade" aspirin toxicity (salicylism): lightheadedness, tinnitus, and visual disturbances such as diplopia.

What is the most likely drug that caused these responses?

a. Atropine
b. Captopril
c. Dobutamine
d. Propranolol
e. Quinidine

198. We have a patient who is diagnosed with variant (vasospastic) angina. Which of the following drugs would be most appropriate, and generally regarded as most effective, for long-term therapy aimed at reducing the incidence or severity of the coronary vasospasm?

a. Aspirin
b. Atorvastatin
c. Diltiazem
d. Nitroglycerin
e. Propranolol

199. It is generally acceptable and common to administer unfractionated heparin along with other classes of drugs that affect some aspect of the coagulation or thrombolytic processes. The proviso, of course, is to monitor closely all drug dosages, the appropriate blood tests, and the patient's responses overall, since the main risk is uncontrolled or excessive bleeding, if not frank hemorrhage.

There is one main exception. With which one of the following drugs is concomitant administration of heparin contraindicated because of an extremely high risk of excessive bleeding or frank hemorrhage?

a. Alteplase (t-PA)
b. Aspirin
c. Clopidogrel
d. Streptokinase
e. Warfarin

200. A 56-year-old man has heart failure. His family doctor, who has been caring for him since he was a young lad, has been treating him with digoxin, furosemide, and triamterene for several years. The patient now develops atrial fibrillation, and so his doctor starts quinidine and warfarin. Which of the following is the most likely outcome of adding the quinidine?

a. Development of signs and symptoms of quinidine toxicity (cinchonism)
b. Hyponatremia due to quinidine's ability to enhance diuretic-induced sodium loss
c. Onset of signs and symptoms of digoxin toxicity
d. Precipitous development of hypokalemia
e. Prompt suppression of cardiac contractility, onset of acute heart failure

201. You pass a room where a cardiologist is talking about various antiarrhythmic drugs. You stop and listen just as he comments on antiarrhythmics in Vaughan-Williams Class I-c. Which of the following is the most likely correct and clinically relevant "take home" message about antiarrhythmics in this class?

a. Are only given for arrhythmias during acute myocardial infarction
b. Are particularly suited for patients with low ejection fractions
c. Are preferred drugs (drugs of choice) for relatively innocuous ventricular arrhythmias
d. Cause pulmonary fibrosis and a hypothyroid-like syndrome when given long term
e. Have a significant pro-arrhythmic effect (induction of lethal arrhythmias)

202. A 44-year-old obese man has extremely high plasma triglyceride levels, but cholesterol levels are within normal limits. Following treatment with a drug specifically indicated for hypertriglyceridemia, triglyceride levels decrease to almost normal. Which of the following agents is most likely to have caused this desired change?

a. Atorvastatin
b. Cholestyramine
c. Colestipol
d. Ezitemibe
e. Gemfibrozil

203. A patient has received excessive doses of nitroprusside, and toxic manifestations are developing. Which of the following drugs should we administer to help nitroprusside's metabolism proceed to the formation of a less toxic metabolite?

a. Epinephrine
b. Sodium thiosulfate
c. Thrombin
d. Vitamin C
e. Vitamin E
f. Vitamin K

204. Nicotinic acid (niacin), in large doses that are used to treat hyper triglyceridemia, causes an often-disturbing cutaneous flush. Which one of the following mechanisms most likely contributes to the vasodilatory response and the flushing?

a. Activation of α-adrenergic receptors
b. Calcium channel activation in vascular smooth muscle
c. Production of local prostaglandins
d. Release of angiotensin II
e. Release of histamine

205. A patient with Stage 2 essential hypertension is treated with usually effective doses of an ACE inhibitor. After a suitable period of time blood pressure has not been lowered satisfactorily. The patient has been compliant with drug therapy and other recommendations (e.g., weight reduction, exercise). A thiazide is added to the ACE inhibitor regimen. Which of the following is the most likely and earliest untoward outcome of this drug add-on, for which you should monitor closely?

a. Fall of blood pressure sufficient to cause syncope
b. Hypokalemia due to synergistic effects of the ACE inhibitor and the thiazide on renal potassium excretion
c. Onset of acute heart failure from depression of ventricular contractility
d. Paradoxical hypertensive crisis
e. Sudden prolongation of the P-R interval and increasing degrees of heart block

206. A 52-year-old woman with essential hypertension, hypercholesterolemia, and chronic-stable angina develops severe constipation. It is attributed to one of her medications. Which was the most likely cause?

a. Atorvastatin
b. Captopril
c. Labetalol
d. Nitroglycerin
e. Verapamil

207. Angiotensin-converting enzyme (ACE) inhibitors are among the first-line drugs for managing essential hypertension (prehypertension or Stage 1 hypertension). However, in contrast with the main alternatives (thiazide or thiazide-like diuretics, β blockers, or calcium channel blockers), the ACE inhibitors are associated with a comparatively high incidence of a rather unusual adverse reaction. Which of the following is that?

a. Bradycardia, often involving AV block
b. Hepatitis
c. Hirsutism
d. Hypokalemia
e. Proteinuria, renal insufficiency

208. A 45-year-old man postmyocardial infarction (MI) is being treated with several drugs, including intravenous unfractionated heparin. Stool guaiac on admission was negative, but is now four, and he has had an episode of hematemesis. Which of the following would be the best drug to administer to counteract the effects of excessive heparin remaining in the circulation?

a. Aminocaproic acid
b. Dipyridamole
c. Factor IX
d. Protamine sulfate
e. Vitamin K

209. A patient with multiple cardiovascular disorders present in your clinic. His primary complaints are fever and arthralgia, and other "flu-like symptoms." These findings, plus a facial "rash" and results of blood work, all point to a drug-induced lupus-like syndrome. Heart rate, BP, and all other cardiovascular findings are completely normal. Which of the following drugs is the most likely cause of these findings?

a. Aspirin ("low dose") for its cardioprotective/antiplatelet effects
b. Atorvastatin for primary prevention of CAD
c. Captopril for hypertension and heart failure
d. Carvedilol for hypertension, heart failure, and angina prophylaxis
e. Furosemide as adjunctive management of his heart failure
f. Nitroglycerin, sublingual, for effort-induced angina
g. Procainamide for atrial fibrillation

210. A 45-year-old man asks his physician for a prescription for sildenafil to improve his sexual performance. Because of risks from a serious drug interaction, this drug should not be prescribed, and the patient should be urged not to try to obtain it from other sources, if he is also taking which of the following drugs?

a. An angiotensin-converting enzyme inhibitor
b. A β-adrenergic blocker
c. A nitrovasodilator (e.g., nitroglycerin)
d. A statin-type antihypercholesterolemic drug
e. A thiazide or loop diuretic

211. A physician is preparing to administer a drug for which there is a label warning: "do not administer this drug to patients with second-degree or greater heart block, or give with other drugs that may cause heart block." Which of the following findings would be specifically indicative of heart block and second-degree heart block in particular?

a. Auscultation of the precordium reveals an irregular rhythm
b. Blood pressure is low
c. Heart rate is abnormally low (bradycardia), but there is normal sinus rhythm
d. The EKG reveals ventricular ectopic beats
e. The EKG shows a prolonged PR interval, and some P waves are not followed by a normal QRS complex
f. The EKG shows abnormally widened QRS complexes

212. A 70-year-old woman is treated with sublingual nitroglycerin for occasional bouts of effort-induced angina. Which of the following best describes the mechanism by which nitroglycerin causes its desired antianginal effects, or a mediator involved in it?

a. Blocks α-adrenergic receptors
b. Forms cyanide, much like the metabolism of nitroprusside does
c. Increases local synthesis and release of adenosine
d. Raises intracellular cGMP levels
e. Stimulates phosphodiesterase

213. A 67-year-old patient complains of muscle aches, pain, and tenderness. These affect the legs and trunk. There is no fever, bruising, or any recent history of muscle trauma or strains (as from excessive exercise). There is myoglobinuria, a clinically significant fall of creatinine clearance, and a rise of serum creatine kinase (CK) to levels nearly 10 times the upper limit of normal. Which of the following drugs is the most likely cause of these findings?

a. Aspirin ("low dose") for its cardioprotective/antiplatelet effects
b. Captopril for hypertension and heart failure
c. Carvedilol for hypertension, heart failure, and angina prophylaxis
d. Furosemide as adjunctive management of his heart failure
e. Nitroglycerin, sublingual, for effort-induced angina
f. Pravastatin to control his hypercholesterolemia and the associated risks

214. We use invasive hemodynamic techniques to measure or calculate the effects of various drugs on such parameters as arterial pressure, total peripheral resistance, and central venous (right atrial) pressures. Our goal is to evaluate whether the drug primarily causes arteriolar or venular dilation, or affects both sides of the circulation. Which one of the following drugs exerts vasodilator effects in both the arterial and venous circulations?

a. Diazoxide
b. Hydralazine
c. Minoxidil
d. Nitroprusside
e. Nifedipine

215. A 20-year-old varsity hockey player is referred to you by his coach. The young athlete has excessive bruising after a very physical match 2 days before. His knee had been bothering him, so he took two 325-mg aspirin tablets several hours before the contest. He got checked hard into the boards 10 times during the game, but denies any excessive or unusual trauma. As you ponder the etiology you order several blood tests. Which test or finding do you most likely expect to be abnormal as a result of the prior aspirin use?

a. Activated partial thromboplastin time (APTT)
b. Bleeding time
c. INR (International Normalized Ratio)
d. Platelet count
e. Prothrombin time

216. A patient in the coronary care unit develops episodes of paroxysmal AV nodal reentrant tachycardia (PSVT). Which of the following would generally be considered a first-line drug for promptly stopping the arrhythmia?

a. Adenosine
b. Digoxin
c. Edrophonium
d. Phenylephrine
e. Propranolol

217. A 60-year-old man, hospitalized for an acute myocardial infarction, is treated with warfarin (among other drugs). What is the main mechanism by which warfarin is causing the effects for which it is given?

a. Increase in the plasma level of Factor IX
b. Inhibition of thrombin and early coagulation steps
c. Inhibition of synthesis of prothrombin and coagulation Factors VII, IX, and X
d. Inhibition of platelet aggregation in vitro
e. Activation of plasminogen
f. Binding of Ca^{2+} ion cofactor in some coagulation steps

218. An 83-year-old man has been effectively treated with hydrochlorothiazide to control his elevated blood pressure. He has had a recent onset of weakness. Blood chemistry analysis reveals hypokalemia. Another drug is added, and 1 month later his serum K⁺ is normal. Which of the following drugs most likely helped normalize his serum potassium levels?

a. Acetazolamide
b. Amiloride
c. Furosemide
d. Metolazone
e. Mannitol

219. A 66-year-old woman with heart failure and mild hearing loss is given a diuretic as part of a regimen that includes a β blocker and an ACE inhibitor. In the course of treatment she develops an AV conduction defect and is found to be hypocalcemic and hypomagnesemic. She also reports what she describes as some worsening of her hearing, characterized mainly by an inability to distinguish between similarly sounding words. Audiometry confirms the hearing loss. The signs and symptoms noted here abate when the drug is stopped. Which of the following drugs most likely contributed to these findings?

a. Acetazolamide
b. Amiloride
c. Furosemide
d. Hydrochlorothiazide
e. Mannitol

220. A 30-year-old pregnant woman requires heparin for prophylaxis of thromboembolism. Which of the following best summarizes heparin's main mechanism of action?

a. Activates plasminogen
b. Increases the plasma level of Factor IX
c. Inhibits platelet aggregation in vitro
d. Inhibits synthesis of prothrombin and coagulation Factors VII, IX, and X
e. Inhibits thrombin and early coagulation steps
f. Lyses platelets

221. A 42-year-old man with an acute MI is treated with alteplase. Which of the following most accurately describes how this drug exerts its intended effect?

a. Blocks platelet ADP receptors
b. Inhibits platelet thromboxane production
c. Inhibits synthesis of vitamin K–dependent coagulation factors
d. Prevents aggregation of adjacent platelets by blocking Glycoprotein IIb/IIIa receptors
e. Promotes conversion of plasminogen to plasmin

222. A patient with atrial fibrillation is placed on long-term arrhythmia control with amiodarone. In addition to "standard" monitoring, periodic assessments of which of the following should be made in order to detect adverse effects that are unique to this drug?

a. Blood glucose, triglyceride, cholesterol, and sodium concentrations
b. Hearing thresholds (audiometry) and serum albumin concentration
c. Prothrombin time and antinuclear antibody (ANA) titers
d. Pulmonary function and thyroid hormone status
e. White cell counts and serum urate concentration

223. A 64-year-old woman has had several episodes of transient ischemic attacks (TIAs). Aspirin would be a preferred treatment, but she has a history of severe "aspirin sensitivity" manifest as intense bronchoconstriction and urticaria. Which of the following would you consider to be the best alternative to the aspirin?

a. Acetaminophen
b. Aminocaproic acid
c. Clopidogrel
d. Dipyridamole
e. Streptokinase

224. A patient, who has excessively slow AV nodal conduction rates that unfortunately haven't been recognized, is started on a drug. As soon as blood levels climb towards the usual therapeutic range the patient goes into complete heart block. Which of the following drugs most likely provoked this further prolongation of the P-R interval, ultimately leading to the complete heart block?

a. Captopril
b. Losartan
c. Nifedipine
d. Nitroglycerin
e. Prazosin
f. Verapamil

225. A patient with heart failure, Stage 2 essential hypertension, and hyperlipidemia (elevated LDL cholesterol and abnormally low HDL-C) is taking furosemide, captopril, atenolol, and simvastatin (an HMG CoA reductase inhibitor).

During a scheduled physical exam, about a month after starting all the above drugs, the patient reports a severe, hacking, and relentless cough. Other vital signs, and the overall physical assessment, are consistent with good control of both the heart failure and blood pressure and indicate no other underlying disease or abnormalities. Results of blood tests are not yet available.

Which of the following is the most likely cause of the cough?

a. An expected side effect of the captopril
b. An allergic reaction to the statin
c. Dyspnea due to captopril's known and powerful bronchoconstrictor action
d. Excessive doses of the bumetanide, which led to hypovolemia
e. Hyperkalemia caused by an interaction between bumetanide and captopril
f. Pulmonary edema from the bumetanide

226. A 60-year-old woman with deep-vein thrombosis (DVT) is given a bolus of heparin, and a heparin drip is also started. Thirty minutes later she is bleeding profusely from the intravenous site. The heparin is stopped, but the excessive bleeding continues. You decide to give protamine sulfate to reverse the adverse effect of heparin. Which statement best describes the mechanism of action of this antidote?

a. Activates the coagulation cascade, overriding the action of heparin
b. Causes hydrolytic inactivation of heparin
c. Causes platelet aggregation, thereby providing a natural hemostatic effect
d. Changes the conformation of antithrombin III to prevent binding to heparin
e. Combines with heparin as an ion pair, thus neutralizing it

227. A patient with a history of hypertension, heart failure, and peripheral vascular disease has been on oral therapy with drugs suitable for each for about 3 months. He runs out of the medication and plans to have the prescriptions refilled in a week or so.

Within a day or two after stopping his medications he experiences an episode of severe tachycardia accompanied by tachyarrhythmias, and an abrupt rise of blood pressure to 240/140 mm Hg—well above pretreatment levels. He complains of chest pain, anxiety, and a pounding headache. Soon thereafter he suffers a hemorrhagic stroke.

Which of the following drugs or drug groups, the man suddenly stops taking, most likely causes these responses?

a. ACE inhibitors
b. Clonidine
c. Digoxin
d. Furosemide
e. Nifedipine (a long-acting formulation)
f. Warfarin

228. A patient has been receiving otherwise "proper" doses of a drug for 5 days straight. Dosing was done correctly, starting with usual maintenance doses; no loading dose strategy was used. Then, and rather precipitously, they develop signs and symptoms of widespread thrombotic events; platelet counts decline significantly concomitant with the thrombosis. The patient dies within 24 h of the onset of signs and symptoms. Which is the most likely cause?

a. Abciximab
b. Clopidogrel
c. Heparin (unfractionated)
d. Nifedipine
e. Warfarin

229. Your patient has bipolar illness, hypercholesterolemia, chronic-stable angina, and Stage I essential hypertension. He has been taking lithium and an SSRI for the bipolar illness. Cardiovascular drugs include atorvastatin, diltiazem, sublingual nitroglycerin, captopril, and hydrochlorothiazide. Which of the following outcomes, due to interactions involving these drugs, would you most likely expect?

a. Development of acute psychosis from an ACE inhibitor-antipsychotic interaction
b. Development of a hypomanic state from antagonism of lithium's action by the nitroglycerin
c. Lithium toxicity because of hyponatremia caused by the hydrochlorothiazide
d. Loss of cholesterol control from antagonism of the HMG CoA reductase inhibitor by the antipsychotic
e. Worsening of angina because the antipsychotic counteracts the effects of the calcium channel blocker
f. Worsening of angina because the lithium antagonizes the effects of the nitroglycerin

230. A patient is hospitalized and waiting for coronary angiography. His history includes angina pectoris that is brought on by "modest" exercise, and is accompanied by transient electrocardiographic changes consistent with myocardial ischemia. There is no evidence of coronary vasospasm. In the hospital he is receiving nitroglycerin and morphine (slow intravenous infusions), plus oxygen via nasal cannula.

He suddenly develops episodes of chest discomfort. Heart rate during these episodes rises to 170–190 beats/min; blood pressure reaches 180–200/110–120 mm Hg, and prominent findings on the EKG are runs of ventricular ectopic beats that terminate spontaneously, plus ST-segment elevation.

Although there are several things that need to be done for immediate care, administration of which one of the following is most likely to remedy (at least temporarily) the majority of these signs and symptoms and pose the lowest risk of doing further harm?

a. Aspirin
b. Captopril
c. Furosemide
d. Labetalol
e. Lidocaine
f. Nitroglycerin (increased dose as a bolus)
g. Prazosin

231. A first-year house officer notices that a patient is experiencing significant and rapidly rising blood pressure (currently 180/120 mm Hg). One of the medications the patient had been taking is immediate-acting nifedipine oral capsules. There is a dose of this nifedipine formulation at the bedside, so the MD pricks the capsule open and squirts the contents into the patient's mouth. This technique avoids "first-pass" metabolism of the drug and causes rapid absorption and all the effects associated with this calcium channel blocker. Which of the following is the most likely outcome, given the scenario?

a. AV nodal block
b. Further rise of heart rate, worsening of the ventricular arrhythmia
c. Hypotension and bradycardia
d. Normalization of blood pressure and heart rate
e. Return of blood pressure toward normal, no significant effect on heart rate or the EKG

232. A patient with multiple cardiovascular diseases is being treated with digoxin, furosemide, triamterene, atorvastatin, and nitroglycerin—all prescribed by the family physician he's had for decades. The patient now experiences nausea, vomiting, and anorexia, and describes a "yellowish-greenish tint" to white objects and bright lights. These signs and symptoms are most characteristic of toxicity due to which one of the following drugs?

a. Atorvastatin
b. Digoxin
c. Furosemide
d. Nitroglycerin
e. Triamterene
f. The triamterene-furosemide combination (drug interaction)

233. Your patient has severe (Stage 4) hypertension that is being controlled with a combination of hydralazine, furosemide, and carvedilol. He also has had bouts of atrial fibrillation that are being managed long term with quinidine and warfarin for prophylaxis of thromboembolism. He presents with fever, chills, arthralgia, and a purplish discoloration on the face. The diagnosis is a drug-induced lupus-like syndrome. Which drug in the regimen noted above is most likely to have accounted for this finding?

a. Carvedilol
b. Furosemide
c. Hydralazine
d. Quinidine
e. Warfarin

234. We have a 28-year-old female patient with Stage II essential hypertension, tachycardia, and occasional palpitations (ventricular ectopic beats). Normally we might consider prescribing a β blocker to control the blood pressure and cardiac responses, but our patient also has asthma, and she is trying to get pregnant. Which of the following drugs would be the best alternative to the β blocker in terms of likely efficacy on pressure and heart rate, and in terms of relative safety?

a. Diltiazem
b. Enalapril
c. Furosemide
d. Phentolamine
e. Prazosin

235. A patient presents with what was initially thought to be Stage 2 hypertension. The actual underlying cause—a pheochromocytoma—is not looked for nor detected in the initial work-up. An oral antihypertensive drug is prescribed. We soon find that the patient's blood pressure has risen to levels above pretreatment levels—so much so that we are worried about imminently dangerous effects from the drug-induced worsening of hypertension. Concomitant with the drug-induced rise of blood pressure the patient develops signs and symptoms of heart failure. Which of the following drugs was most likely administered?

a. Captopril
b. Hydrochlorothiazide
c. Labetalol
d. Losartan
e. Propranolol
f. Verapamil

236. A patient on long-term warfarin therapy arrives at the clinic for her weekly prothrombin time measurement. Her INR is dangerously prolonged, and the physical exam reveals petechial hemorrhages. She's had episodes of epistaxis over the last 2 days. We are going to stop the warfarin until the INR becomes acceptable (and perhaps admit the patient for follow-up). However, we are concerned with her ongoing bleeding. Which of the following drugs would you most likely administer to counteract the warfarin's excessive effects?

a. Aminocaproic acid
b. Epoetin alfa
c. Ferrous sulfate
d. Phytonadione (vitamin K)
e. Protamine sulfate

237. A patient with hypertension and heart failure has been treated for 2 years with carvedilol and lisinopril. He has just had hip replacement surgery, and because he is not ambulating, he is started on unfractionated heparin, postoperatively, for prophylaxis of deep venous thrombosis. Oral antacids and ranitidine (H_2 antagonist) have been added for prophylaxis of acute stress ulcers. Five days postop he experiences sudden onset dyspnea and electrocardiographic and other indications of an acute MI. The patient's platelet counts are dangerously low. Which of the following is the most likely underlying problem?

a. Accidental substitution of low-molecular-weight heparins (LMWH) for unfractionated heparin
b. Accidental/inadvertent aspirin administration
c. Hemolytic anemia from a carvedilol-ACE inhibitor interaction
d. Heparin-induced thrombocytopenia
e. Reduced heparin effects by increased metabolic clearance (caused by ranitidine)

238. For many hypertensive patients we can prescribe either lisinopril (or an alternative in the same class) or losartan. Which one of the following statements correctly summarizes how losartan differs from lisinopril or its related drugs?

a. Lisinopril competitively blocks catecholamine-mediated vasoconstriction, losartan does not
b. Lisinopril effectively inhibits synthesis of Angiotensin II, losartan does not
c. Losartan causes a higher incidence of bronchospasm and hyperuricemia
d. Losartan is preferred for managing hypertension during pregnancy, whereas captopril is contraindicated
e. Losartan is suitable for administration to patients with heart failure, whereas captopril and related drugs should be avoided

239. A 46-year-old man has Stage II essential hypertension, primary hyper-cholesterolemia, and modestly elevated fasting glucose levels (130 mg/dL) measured on several occasions. His cholesterol levels (total, HDL, LDL) have not been acceptably modified by dietary changes and daily use of a "statin." The physician adds ezetimibe to the regimen. Which of the following statements is correct about ezetimibe's actions, or what might be expected in response to its use?

a. Exerts profound cardiac negative inotropic effects that pose a risk of heart block
b. Frequently causes orthostatic hypotension that in turn triggers reflex cardiac stimulation
c. More likely than other drugs to increase the risk of severe statin-induced myopathy
d. Reduces intestinal cholesterol uptake, has no direct hepatic effect to inhibit cholesterol synthesis
e. Significantly increases risk of atherosclerotic plaque rupture

240. A 58-year-old man presents with a myocardial infarction—his first episode of ACS. Angioplasty and stenting are not possible because the cardiac cath lab is busy with other high-priority patients, so administration of a thrombolytic drug is the only option. Which one of the following is the most important determinant, overall, of the success of thrombolytic therapy in terms of salvaging viable cardiac muscle?

a. Choosing a "human" (cloned) plasminogen activator (e.g., t-PA), rather than one that is bacterial-derived
b. Infarct location (i.e., anterior wall of left ventricular vs. another site/wall)
c. Presence of collateral blood vessels to the infarct-related coronary artery
d. Systolic blood pressure at the time the MI is diagnosed
e. Time from onset of infarction to administration of the thrombolytic agent

241. A patient with coronary artery disease takes excessive doses of sublingual nitroglycerin in an attempt to abort chest discomfort from an ischemic episode. By the time help arrives he is dead from an overdose of the very drug he took to seek relief. Which of the following best describes the most likely mechanism by which this antianginal/anti-ischemic drug led to the patient's death?

a. Caused fatal bronchospasm
b. Caused generalized convulsive seizures, with death arising from apnea
c. Caused hemorrhagic stroke from hypertension
d. Provoked coronary vasospasm
e. Worsened myocardial ischemia

242. A patient presents in the emergency department with acute hypotension that requires treatment. Hypovolemia is ruled out as a cause or contributor, and information gathered from the patient and family indicates the cause is overdose of an antihypertensive drug.

One approach to treatment is to administer a pharmacologic (ordinarily effective) dose of phenylephrine, an α-adrenergic agonist. You do just that, and blood pressure fails to rise at all—and a second dose doesn't work either. On which antihypertensive drug did the patient most likely overdose?

a. Captopril or another ACE inhibitor
b. Hydralazine
c. Prazosin
d. Thiazide diuretic (e.g., hydrochlorothiazide)
e. Verapamil

243. An elderly male patient who has just been referred to your practice has been taking a drug for symptomatic relief of benign prostatic hypertrophy. In addition to its effects on smooth muscles of the prostate and urethra, this drug can lower blood pressure in such a way that it reflexly triggers tachycardia, positive inotropy, and increased AV nodal conduction. The drug neither dilates nor constricts the bronchi. It causes the pupils of the eyes to constrict and interferes with mydriasis in dim light. Initial oral dosages of this drug have been associated with a high incidence of syncope. Which prototype is most similar to this unnamed drug in terms of the pharmacologic profile?

a. Captopril
b. Hydrochlorothiazide (prototype thiazide diuretic)
c. Labetalol
d. Nifedipine
e. Prazosin
f. Propranolol
g. Verapamil

244. You are contemplating starting ACE inhibitor therapy for a patient with essential hypertension. Which of the following patient-related condition(s) contraindicates use of an ACE inhibitor and so should be ruled out before you prescribe this drug?

a. Asthma
b. Heart failure
c. Hyperlipidemia, coronary artery disease
d. Hypokalemia
e. Is a woman who is pregnant or may become pregnant

245. A patient develops sinus bradycardia. Heart rate is dangerously low, and an effective and safe drug needs to be given right away. Which of the following would be the best choice?

a. Atropine
b. Amiodarone
c. Edrophonium
d. Lidocaine
e. Phentolamine

246. A patient is started on therapy with abciximab. Which one of the following best describes how this drug causes its desired effects?

a. Blocks thrombin receptors selectively
b. Blocks ADP receptors
c. Blocks glycoprotein IIb/IIIa receptor
d. Inhibits cyclooxygenase
e. Inhibits prostacyclin production

247. We administer reserpine on a daily basis, at usual effective doses, for a time sufficient for the drug to exert its maximal and expected effects. Which of the following effects would most likely occur?

a. Accumulation of NE in synapses, leading to vasoconstriction and tachycardia
b. Depletion of intraneuronal NE stores leading to reduced blood pressure, heart rate, and contractility
c. Dry mouth, blurred vision, constipation, and urinary retention
d. Further metabolism of NE to epinephrine, development of a pheochromocytoma-like tumor
e. Subsensitivity of pre- and post-synaptic α-adrenergic receptors

248. A patient with angina is started on a nitroglycerin transdermal delivery system ("skin patch") for prophylaxis of his angina. He wears the patch 24 h a day, 7 days a week, except for the few minutes when he showers each day. Which of the following is the main concern with "around-the-clock" administration of this or other long-acting formulations of nitrovasodilators?

a. Cyanide poisoning
b. Development of tolerance to their vasodilator actions
c. Gradual development of reflex bradycardia in response to successive doses
d. Onset of delayed, characteristic adverse responses including thrombosis and thrombocytopenia
e. Paradoxical vasoconstriction leading to hypertension

249. A patient presents in the emergency department (ED) with severe angina pectoris, and acute myocardial ischemia is confirmed by electrocardiographic and other clinical indicators. Unknown to the ED team is the fact that the ischemia is due to coronary vasospasm, not to coronary occlusion with thrombi. Given this etiology, which one of the following drugs, administered in usually effective doses, may actually make the vasospasm, and the resulting ischemia, worse?

a. Alteplase (t-PA)
b. Aspirin
c. Captopril
d. Nitroglycerin
e. Propranolol
f. Verapamil

250. Many clinical studies have been conducted to investigate the benefits of daily aspirin use in the primary prevention of coronary heart disease and sudden death in adults. The results have been somewhat inconsistent, in part because different dosages were studied, and there were important differences in the populations that were studied. Nonetheless, many (if not most) of the studies have revealed that for some at-risk patients, aspirin increased the incidence of a particularly unwanted adverse response, even when dosages were kept within the range of dosages typically recommended for cardioprotection (81 mg/day). Which of the following is the most likely adverse response associated with the drug?

a. Centrolobular hepatic necrosis
b. Hemorrhagic stroke
c. Nephropathy
d. Tachycardia and hypotension leading to acute myocardial ischemia
e. Vasospastic angina

251. A patient with essential hypertension has been treated with a fixed-dose combination product that contains hydrochlorothiazide and triamterene. Blood pressure and serum electrolyte profiles have been kept within acceptable limits for the last 18 months. Now, however, blood pressure has risen to the point where the physician wants to add a third antihypertensive drug. The drug is started; after several weeks blood pressure falls into an acceptable range, but the patient has become hyperkalemic. Which one of the following drugs was added and was most likely responsible for the desired blood pressure fall and the unwanted rise of serum potassium levels.

a. Diltiazem
b. Prazosin
c. Propranolol
d. Ramipril
e. Verapamil

252. A patient has supraventricular tachycardia. We inject a drug and heart rate falls to a normal or at least more acceptable level. Although this drug caused the desired response, it did so without any direct effect in or on the heart. Which of the following drugs was most likely used?

a. Edrophonium
b. Esmolol
c. Phenylephrine
d. Propranolol
e. Verapamil

253. A 69-year-old man presents with NYHA Stage II ("mild") heart failure. He is placed on usual therapeutic doses of digoxin and furosemide. At a follow-up exam 3 months later we find good symptomatic relief of the heart failure. Serum electrolytes and all other lab tests are within normal limits. At this time, which electrocardiographic change would you expect to see in response to the digoxin's expected effects, compared with a baseline (pretreatment) EKG?

a. P waves widened, amplitude increased
b. P-R intervals prolonged
c. QRS complexes widened
d. R-R intervals shortened
e. S-T segments elevated

254. A 23-year-old nonpregnant woman has been using a preparation of oral ergotamine to manage her frequent migraine headaches. She consumes an excessive dose of the drug while trying to abort a particularly severe and refractory attack. Which of the following adverse cardiac or cardiovascular consequences are most likely to occur as a result of the ergot overdose?

a.   Myocardial and peripheral (e.g., limb) ischemia due to intense vasoconstriction
b.   Renal failure secondary to rhabdomyolysis
c.   Spontaneous bleeding due to direct inhibition of platelet activation/aggregation
d.   Syncope secondary to acute hypotension
e.   Tachycardia, tachyarrhythmias from β_1 adrenergic receptor activation

255. A patient presents with severe hypertension (BP is 220/120) and tachycardia (96 beats per minute) despite usually effective antihypertensive drug therapy. Further work-up indicates the patient has a rare cause of these and other signs and symptoms: pheochromocytoma. You realize that β-adrenergic blockers are useful as antihypertensive drugs, and for helping to normalize heart rate in patients with sinus tachycardia. As a result of the diagnosis, and your knowledge, you administer a usually effective dose of a nonselective (β_1/β_2) β blocker. Which of the following is the most likely outcome of doing this?

a.   Blood pressure falls promptly, followed by reflex tachycardia
b.   Epinephrine release from the tumor is suppressed, hemodynamics normalize
c.   Heart rate and cardiac function rise quickly because the β blocker has triggered additional epinephrine release from the tumor
d.   Left ventricular afterload is decreased; cardiac output rises via increases of both left ventricular stroke volume and heart rate
e.   Total peripheral resistance rises, cardiac output falls, the patient goes into heart failure

256. A 59-year-old man presents in the emergency department with crushing chest discomfort. An EKG indicates a transmural infarction, and prompt cardiac catheterization and assessment of prior lab results indicate significant hypercholesterolemia. The patient is given all the drugs listed, for both immediate management of the ischemia and its symptoms and for long-term prevention of a subsequent, and potentially fatal, MI. Which one of the following drugs provides immediate relief of the consequences of myocardial ischemia but has no long-term effects to reduce the risk of sudden death or ventricular dysfunction from another MI?

a. Aspirin
b. Atorvastatin
c. Captopril
d. Nitroglycerin
e. Propranolol

257. A 65-year-old normotensive woman is transferred to the thoracic surgery ICU after cardiac surgery. She has diffuse rales bilaterally, a pulse of 110/min, an elevated venous pressure, and a blood pressure of 160/98 mm Hg. The surgery resident wants to inject an otherwise correct dose of an IV drug to control heart rate and blood pressure, but grabs a syringe that contains the wrong drug. The patient's heart rate increases to 150/min and her blood pressure rises to 180/106 mm Hg.

Which one of the following drugs was most likely given?

a. Dobutamine
b. Esmolol
c. Neostigmine
d. Propranolol
e. Verapamil

258. A 50-year-old man is well aware of the benefits of aspirin in terms of reducing the risk of death from an acute myocardial infarction, mainly because he has seen and carefully studied many of the ads and internet posts about this. He notices that the usual recommended dose of aspirin for cardioprotection is 81 mg/day, but reasons that the bigger the dose, the bigger the protective effect. He has taken "at least" 1000 mg of aspirin twice a day for the last 6 months. While he is fortunate in terms of having no apparent gastrointestinal adverse effects, he suffers an MI. Autopsy results show considerable platelet occlusion of several coronary vessels. Which of the following most likely explains the mechanism by which aspirin triggered these events?

a. Acetylated platelet glycoprotein IIb/IIIa receptors, triggering aggregation
b. Favored adhesion of platelets to the vascular (coronary) endothelium
c. Ruptured atherosclerotic plaque in the coronaries, exposing platelets to collagen
d. Suppressed hepatic synthesis of vitamin K–dependent clotting factors
e. Triggered excessive activation of platelets by ADP

259. You are in a debate with a colleague over which α blocker to use, adjunctively, to control blood pressure in a pheochromocytoma patient. Your colleague correctly states that phenoxybenzamine is the "preferred" drug. You state that prazosin would be a better choice. Which of the following statements about prazosin is correct in comparison with phenoxybenzamine, and might actually support your proposal that it would be the better choice?

a. Causes not only peripheral α-blockade but also suppresses adrenal epinephrine release
b. Has a longer duration of action, which enables less frequent dosing
c. Has good intrinsic β-blocking activity, phenoxybenzamine does not
d. Overdoses, and the hypotension it may cause, are easier to manage pharmacologically
e. Will not cause orthostatic hypotension, which is a common consequence of phenoxybenzamine

260. A man has an aneurysm in the aortic root, a consequence of Marfan's syndrome. He experiences a hypertensive crisis that requires prompt blood pressure control. Nitroprusside will be infused for its immediate antihypertensive effects. Which of the following drugs must we administer along with the nitroprusside to minimize the risk of aneurysm rupture as blood pressure falls?

a. Atropine
b. Diazoxide
c. Furosemide
d. Phentolamine
e. Propranolol

The Cardiovascular System

Answers

173. The answer is c. (*Brunton, pp 243–244; Craig, pp 97–98, 100–102; Katzung, pp 129–132.*) ISO, PHE, EPI, NE. Yes, responses to some of these drugs are variable, largely depending on the dose and the speed of administration. Nonetheless, the responses shown are typical.

ISO, a β_1/ β_2 agonist, lowers peripheral resistance (and diastolic blood pressure) via β_2-mediated peripheral vasodilator actions. That fall of diastolic pressure is greater than the rise of systolic pressure (which occurs because of a direct cardiac positive inotropic/β_1-activating effect), so mean pressure falls a bit. The combined reflex response to a fall of mean pressure (albeit slight), plus the drug's direct positive chronotropic effect, leads to significant tachycardia.

PHE, which activates only (and all) α-adrenergic receptors, causes only a vasopressor response that accounts for the changes of pressures and peripheral resistance. These changes activate the baroreceptor reflex, leading to reflex bradycardia. The drug has no β agonist activity.

EPI, injected in (reasonably) low doses in normal humans, can cause the effects shown here (and certainly no other drug listed as a possible answer could do the same). The fall of peripheral resistance and diastolic pressure reflects predominant β_2-mediated vasodilation; the rise of systolic pressure is a melding of both peripheral vasoconstriction (α) and direct cardiac stimulation (β_1). Heart rate also reflects direct changes (β_1), as there is no appreciable baroreceptor influence because there is no sudden or significant blood pressure change. Responses to epinephrine are arguably more variable than those of any other drugs listed. Clearly, when large doses are given to a hypotensive patient (e.g., in anaphylaxis), the predominant and wanted vascular effect is a pressor response, much greater than what we see here.

NE, lacking any β_2 activity but being quite effective as an α and β_1 agonist, causes typical responses like those shown here. Peripherally, there is no vasodilation; just constriction. Diastolic, mean, and systolic pressures rise. The rise is sufficient to reflexly slow heart rate; that is, it is sufficient to overcome NE's direct positive chronotropic effects.

174. The answer is d. (*Brunton, pp 886–887; Craig, p 154; Katzung, pp 205–207.*) Digoxin inhibits the sarcolemmal Na^+, K^+-ATPase ("sodium pump"). This reduces the active (ATP–dependent) extrusion of intracellular Na^+. The relative excess of intracellular Na^+ competes with intracellular Ca^{2+} for sites on a sarcolemmal 2Na–Ca exchange diffusion carrier, such that less Ca^{2+} is extruded from the cells. The net result is a rise of free $[Ca^{2+}]_i$ and greater actin-myosin interactions (i.e., a positive inotropic effect that increases cardiac output through an increase of stroke volume).

175. The answer is e. (*Brunton, pp 832–838, 914; Craig, pp 171t, 183t, 192–193; Katzung, pp 227–228, 235–236.*) Verapamil, a nondihydropyridine calcium channel blocker (CCB), depresses both the SA node and the AV node and would be effective for prophylaxis of paroxysmal atrial or supraventricular tachycardia. Nifedipine (c), the prototypic dihydropyridine CCB, has little effect on SVT because it and the other dihydropyridines lack cardiac depressant effects. Moreover, if we chose a fast-/immediate-acting dosage form of nifedipine, we would probably trigger substantial reflex cardiac stimulation. The increased sympathetic tone to the heart could worsen the PSVT. Nitroglycerin (d) is mainly a venodilator, but it can cause falls of arterial blood pressure sufficient to trigger reflex cardiac activation that would exacerbate the tachydardia. Adenosine (a) may be useful in diagnosing whether ventricular tachycardia is of supraventricular or ventricular origin, because it effectively slows AV nodal conduction. It is also used as acute therapy for PSVT. However, it is a fast-and-short-acting parenteral drug, which renders it unsuitable for the condition we stated: outpatient prophylaxis. Lidocaine (b) is mainly used for ventricular tachyarrhythmias, not those of supraventricular origin. Both adenosine and lidocaine are parenteral drugs with short half-lives; neither property makes them suitable for outpatient prophylactic use.

176. The answer is a. (*Brunton, pp 271–276, 838; Craig, pp 200–203; Katzung, pp 151–157, 197–199.*) β-Adrenergic receptor blockers slow resting heart rate and reduce contractility, both of which reduce myocardial oxygen demand. They also blunt cardiac stimulatory effects, such as those triggered by exercise and that increase oxygen demand, whenever the sympathetic nervous system is activated (e.g., in response to exercise or drugs that tend to cause reflex sympathetic activation). Recall, too, that coronary blood flow occurs during diastole. By slowing heart rate they prolong diastole, thereby indirectly allowing more time for the myocardium to be perfused.

These drugs have no antiplatelet/antithrombotic effects; they do not cause coronary vasodilation (and may favor constriction, which can become clinically significant in patients with variant angina; see Question 198); and they may increase total peripheral resistance by blocking dilation in some vascular beds (the effect is usually slight and insignificant). The β blockers do slow AV nodal conduction velocity, but that effect per se contributes little to the reduced oxygen demand that is mainly derived from the drugs' effects on overall rate and contractility.

177. The answer is a. (*Brunton, pp 858–860; Craig, p 212; Katzung, pp 177–179.*) ACE inhibitors are generally the preferred drugs for hypertensive patients who also have diabetes mellitus—provided their renal function is satisfactory (specifically, no severe bilateral renal arterial stenosis or adequate blood flow to one kidney if the other was removed). These drugs do not cause any problems with glucose regulation or the responses to antidiabetic drugs, and they seem to exert some protective effect that slows or delays diabetes-related nephropathy.

β-Adrenergic blockers would not be a good choice if hypertension is accompanied only by diabetes mellitus. Should the diabetic patient experience an episode of hypoglycemia (more of a concern with Type I diabetes than with Type II), a β blocker may delay recovery of blood glucose levels, mask tachycardia that is one symptom of hypoglycemia development, and interact with some antidiabetic drugs (even those used for Type II; excessive blood glucose-lowering). (If the diabetes is well controlled, and if the patient has other disorders for which benefits of β blockade may outweigh potential problems, such as mild-moderate heart failure or recent myocardial infarction, then a β blocker may be considered.)

Thiazides can elevate blood glucose levels, or at least antagonize the desired effects of antidiabetic drugs (probably by reducing parenchymal cell responsiveness to insulin). Nonetheless, they usually would not be a first-choice in the setting of diabetes.

Verapamil, diltiazem, and nifedipine seem not to complicate blood glucose regulation or interact with antidiabetic drug therapy. Nonetheless, they lack other benefits offered by ACE inhibitors (especially the renal-protective effects) in the setting of diabetes and so would not be a first choice or of special value.

178. The answer is b. *(Brunton, pp 753–757, 847–850; Craig, pp 246, 441–442; Katzung, pp 178–180, 249–251.)* Thiazide diuretics tend to raise serum uric acid levels. This may be of little concern for patients with no history of hyperuricemia or gout, but for those with such a history it can be a problem that is not associated with any of the other answer choices given. Thiazides can be administered to hyperuricemic/gouty patients, but that usually requires another drug (allopurinol; xanthine oxidase inhibitor) to counteract diuretic-induced rises of urate levels. If we can avoid the problems by avoiding the thiazide, and the possible need for adding a second drug to counteract the hyperuricemia, why not do just that?

None of the other answer choices have any appreciable desired or untoward effects on serum urate levels, renal handling of urate, or the incidence or severity of gout.

179. The answer is d. *(Brunton, pp 290, 1721t–1723; Craig, pp 114–116, 232–233; Katzung, pp 151–153, 161–162, 170–172.)* Timolol is a nonselective β-adrenergic blocker. Oral dosage forms are approved for managing essential hypertension (and angina). A topical ophthalmic dosage form is indicated for managing some cases of chronic open-angle glaucoma. β Blockers are not only likely to control blood pressure, and help lower intraocular pressure, but also to reduce catecholamine-induced cardiac stimulation (the tachycardia).

Verapamil or diltiazem (b, e), both calcium channel blockers (CCBs) of the nondihydropyridine class, will not only lower blood pressure but also tend to modulate the tachycardia (through direct but β-receptor-independent processes). However, they don't lower intraocular pressure. All other things being equal, then, the β blocker would still be a better choice for the hypertensive, tachycardiac, glaucomatous patient. Thus, we get three potential benefits from β blockade and only two with verapamil or diltiazem.

ACE inhibitors such as captopril (a) and thiazide diuretics (c), have no actions that would make them particularly suitable for hypertensive patients who are tachycardic, have glaucoma, or both.

180. The answer is e. *(Craig, pp 201–202, 220–221; Brunton, pp 837–840; Katzung, pp 176, 192–196.)* The vascular calcium channel–blocking actions of verapamil or diltiazem (nondihydropyridine class) will not only lower systemic blood pressure, but also tend to counter coronary arterial calcium influx that favors vasospasm. Thus, in this setting we can expect both antihypertensive and antianginal effects from one drug.

One might argue that nifedipine (answer c) would be a reasonable alternative. However, recall that the dihydropyridines (which is the class to which nifedipine belongs) lack cardiac depressant actions. Rapidly acting formulations of a dihydropyridine, even if given orally, are likely to lower blood pressure (the desired antihypertensive effect), but lacking cardiac-depressant actions are liable to trigger reflex (sympathetic/baroreceptor) cardiac stimulation. The resulting increases of either or both cardiac rate and contractility (mediated, reflexly, by sympathetic activation) necessarily may raise myocardial oxygen demand sufficient to cause myocardial ischemia, and/or may trigger coronary vasospasm. (The degree to which a dihydropyridine will cause unwanted reflex cardiac stimulation depends on the drug, the dose, and even the dosage form [e.g., immediate-acting vs. extended-acting].) Nonetheless, a nondihydropyridine would have a much better overall profile of cardiac/vascular actions.

ACE inhibitors or an ARB (a), or a thiazide (d), might cause no particular problems for a patient with vasospastic angina, but they also have no actions that would help that comorbidity. Why select one of them when a nondihydropyridine calcium channel blocker might be beneficial for both problems.

β Blockers (b) would be a poor choice. Recall that the coronary vasculature constricts in response to α-adrenergic influences, while β-receptor activation tends to cause coronary vasodilation. Patients with vasospastic angina depend on β-mediated vasodilatory influences, and are at greater risk of ischemic events if the β receptors are blocked.

181. The answer is a. (*Brunton, pp 143t, 272–275, 824–826, 837–840; Craig, pp 114–116, 202–203; Katzung, pp 197–199.*) β blockers (represented in this question by atenolol) should not be administered (especially by a systemic route) to patients with vasospastic angina unless for a medical emergency that requires β blockade as a life-saving measure. Recall the dual roles of adrenergic receptors in the coronary vasculature. Activation of β_2-adrenergic receptors causes vasodilation. Activation of α-adrenergic receptors in the coronary (and other) vasculature favors vasoconstriction or—in the setting of variant angina—vasospasm. Normally these receptors are bathed with circulating epinephrine, which causes the opposing vasodilator (β_2) and vasoconstrictor (α) effects. Norepinephrine is also activating α-adrenergic receptors. Block only the β (vasodilator) effects in the coronaries and the constrictor (and spasm-favoring) effects of the α receptors are left unopposed.

Diltiazem (b), a nondihydropyridine calcium channel blocker, would not only lower blood pressure but also suppress the tendency for coronary vasoconstriction by blocking vascular smooth muscle calcium influx. Hydrochlorothiazide (c) is a thiazide diuretic, and metolazone (e) is thiazide-like in terms of its pharmacologic profiles. Neither is likely to cause or favor vasoconstriction in the coronary vessels or elsewhere. Losartan (d) is an angiotensin receptor blocker. It not only has good antihypertensive activity, but also is apt to suppress any coronary vasoconstrictor influences of circulating angiotensin.

182. The answer is b. (*Brunton, p 809; Craig, pp 212–213; Katzung, p 178.*) ACE inhibitors (and angiotensin receptor blockers, ARBs, e.g., losartan) are contraindicated in pregnancy (category X), and should not be administered to "women of childbearing potential"—not just women who are pregnant—in the first place. Normal *in utero* development of the kidneys and other urogenital structures seems to be angiotensin-dependent. ACE inhibitors, or ARBs, given during the second or third trimesters (not the first) have been associated with severe and sometimes fatal developmental anomalies of these structures. Cranial hypoplasia, and neonatal hyperkalemia and hypotension, have also been reported.

α-Methyldopa (a) is considered one of the preferred antihypertensive drugs for pregnant women. It not only controls maternal blood pressure well, but also is remarkably free of adverse effects on the fetus. (Indeed, it is the most likely drug that we would prescribe for this hypertensive and now pregnant woman.)

β Blockers such as labetalol (d) are sometimes used during pregnancy, posing no specific or significant risks to the mother or the fetus provided adequate perinatal care is given and blood pressure doesn't fall excessively. None of the calcium channel blockers (including verapamil, e) seems to have any significant benefits or risks during pregnancy, compared with other drugs. (Verapamil, for example, is in pregnancy category c.) One theoretical concern with verapamil and diltiazem is a prolongation of labor as parturition draws near, due to suppression of uterine contractility.

There are concerns with using diuretics during pregnancy. Furosemide (c) or other loop diuretics pose significant fetal risks. However, that is related to potential maternal hypovolemia and hypotension, which may lead to placental underperfusion. There is no teratogenic or embryopathic risk on par with that associated with the angiotensin modifiers. Moreover, when the goal is treating essential hypertension in the absence of hypervolemia, edema, ascites, and so on, loop diuretics seldom are used. Instead, thiazide or thiazide-like diuretics are the ones usually chosen. Nevertheless, the thiazides also pose a risk of placental underperfusion, and so they are not preferred or ideal antihypertensives for the pregnant woman.

183. The answer is c. (*Brunton, pp 287–288; Craig, pp 115–116; Katzung, pp 151, 157.*) No β blocker ordinarily should be administered to patients with asthma, because of a great risk of severe and potentially fatal bronchoconstriction or bronchospasm (unless the β blocker is being given for a medical emergency that requires β blockade). This applies to all classes of β blockers: nonselective, like propranolol; $β_1$ "selective," that is, atenolol or metoprolol; those with intrinsic sympathomimetic/partial agonist activity, such as pindolol; and those that also have α-blocking activity, that is, labetalol and carvedilol. The contraindication applies to all administration routes, including topical (ophthalmic); there are clinical reports of fatal bronchospasm induced by topical ophthalmic administration of "just one drop" of β blockers.

The reason? Airways of persons with asthma are exquisitely sensitive to a host of bronchoconstrictor stimuli and exquisitely dependent on the bronchodilator effects of circulating epinephrine ($β_2$ receptors). Block those β receptors, and that sets the stage for bronchoconstriction or bronchospasm. Another important factor is that this patient needs albuterol for occasional relief of bronchospasm. The drug works, of course, by activating $β_2$-adrenergic receptors in the airways. Any or all of the available β blockers will antagonize albuterol's desired effects.

Diltiazem (a) and verapamil (e), both nondihydropyridine calcium channel blockers, might be a good choice for this patient. They not only lower blood pressure by blocking calcium influx into vascular smooth muscle, but also (theoretically, at least) do the same in airway smooth muscle, thereby preventing bronchoconstriction. Hydrochlorothiazide possibly could exacerbate the problems by causing excessive fluid loss (which could favor bronchoconstriction), but the chances of this problem are low. (Loop diuretics such as furosemide would be of more concern, owing to their greater efficacy in terms of causing loss of circulating fluid volume.) There are no specific concerns with using ramipril, an angiotensin converting enzyme inhibitor. (Remember: drugs with generic names ending in "-pril" are ACE inhibitors, so even if you learned about only captopril as an ACE inhibitor, you should have realized that ramipril is in the same class.)

184. The answer is c. *(Brunton, pp 1468f, 1482f–1483; Craig, pp 262–263; Katzung, p 554.)* Clopidogrel (and the lesser-used drug ticlopidine), is a noncompetitive antagonist of ADP. This prodrug (it must be metabolically activated) causes largely irreversible (i.e., for the lifetime of the platelet) inhibition of platelet aggregation by blocking ADP binding to the G_i-coupled P2Y(AC) receptor. It has no effect on platelet activation and amplification caused by such other proaggregatory agonists as collagen, thromboxane A2, thrombin, PAF, serotonin, or epinephrine.

Aspirin (a) inhibits platelet aggregation caused by thromboxane A2 (TXA2) only, and does so only by inhibiting TXA2 synthesis via cyclooxygenase, not by blocking TXA2 receptors.

Bivalirudin (b) is a synthetic hirudin derivative (you may recall that hirudin is produced by the medicinal leach, *Hirudo medicinalis*). It is classified as an anticoagulant, not as an antiplatelet drug. It is a direct-acting inhibitor of free and clot-bound thrombin, which leads to two main effects: (1) decreased conversion of fibrinogen to fibrin and (2) reduced activation of Factor XIIIa, which in turn decreases conversion of soluble fibrin monomers to insoluble (polymerized) fibrin.

Bivalirudin is given IV as an alternative to heparin (both drugs bind to free thrombin, but bivalirudin also interacts with clot-bound thrombin), mainly along with aspirin for patients with unstable angina who are undergoing angioplasty. It is also used to help treat heparin-induced thrombocytopenia and seems to be more effective than heparin when given post-myocardial infarction A–related drug is argatroban.

Heparin and warfarin (d, e) are anticoagulants, and have no direct effects on platelets. (You should also recall that since warfarin's site of action is the liver, it has no anticoagulant effects when tested *in vitro*.)

185. The answer is a. *(Brunton, pp 795–800; Craig, pp 208–211; Katzung, pp 283–284.)* The bradycardia caused by the unknown drug is reflex, mediated by baroreceptor activation in response to the rise of blood pressure. Angiotensin II, by activating vascular A-II receptors, raises blood pressure and peripheral resistance, and that response would not be inhibited by pretreatment with prazosin (selective α_1 adrenergic antagonist), nor any other adrenergic blocker (antagonist) for that matter.

The bradycardia, of course, involves reflex parasympathetic activation (and relative and simultaneous withdrawal of sympathetic tone to the heart), release of ACh from the vagus and activation of muscarinic receptors on the

SA node. Atropine pretreatment indeed prevents that response, as described in the question—regardless of whether the original pressor response was caused by A-II or any other vasopressor drug for that matter.

Dobutamine (b) doesn't fit the bill; it is largely a selective β_1 agonist. For all practical purposes it causes no vasoconstriction (an α_1 response if we limit things to adrenergic drugs), and via the β_1 activation will directly increase heart rate, contractility, automaticity, and electrical impulse conduction (e.g., through the AV node). No α activation occurs (rises of blood pressure, if they occur in response to dobutamine, are due to the positive inotropic effect), and so prazosin would have no direct effect on responses to dobutamine. Isoproterenol (c) can be ruled out for largely similar reasons; it activates both β_1 and β_2 receptors; and lacks vasoconstrictor activity, whether due to activation of α-adrenergic receptors or by other mechanisms.

Could norepinephrine (d) be a reasonable answer? It certainly causes a vasopressor response and reflex bradycardia (at usual doses). However, the question stated that the unknown drug's pressor response is *not* inhibited by α-blockade. Since a major element of NE's pressor effect depends on α activation, it's not a reasonable choice. The same applies to phenylephrine (e): this nonselective α-agonist also causes a pressor response that *would be* reduced or blocked altogether by prazosin pretreatment.

186. The answer is c. (*Brunton, pp 955–956; Craig, pp 272–273; Katzung, pp 570–571.*) Answering this question correctly indeed depends on your knowledge of several drugs, and their prototype or representative agents, that goes beyond "cardiovascular." If you correctly assumed the answer was in the cardiovascular area (because the question is in this cardiovascular chapter), you may have been at some earned advantage.

Nonetheless, niacin (nicotinic acid; vitamin B_3) is used—in dosages higher than those used for vitamin supplementation—mainly to lower serum triglyceride levels. Pravastatin and other statins (HMG CoA reductase inhibitors), while mainly used for hypercholesterolema, often concomitantly lower serum triglyceride levels adequately. When they don't, and when lifestyle modifications fail to control triglyceride levels adequately, adding niacin may be considered. Two related things to remember, although not pertinent to answering this question correctly, are: (1) Immediate-acting niacin preparations, used at dosages typically used for hypertriglyceridemia, tend to facial flushing, headache, and related consequences of vasodilation. (The incidence and severity of these problems can be reduced by prescribing slow-release niacin formulations, or by having the patient take an aspirin tablet before the niacin. This suggests that the vasomotor responses are somehow prostaglandin-mediated, since aspirin inhibits prostaglandin synthesis.) (2) Niacin is one of the lipid-lowering drugs that can increase the risk of statin-induced hepatic or skeletal muscle damage.

Citalopram (a), escitalopram, and other SSRI–antidepressants, have no known effects on altered vitamin absorption or on the cardiovascular system. Metformin (b), the prototype biguanide often used for managing Type II diabetes mellitus, typically suppresses (not increases) appetite. Statins do not cause peripheral neuropathy (d); and ACE inhibitors (ramipril and others; e) do not cause diabetic nephropathy, although they are clearly contraindicated for patients with severe bilateral renal arterial stenosis, such as that associated with severe and poorly controlled diabetes mellitus.

187. The answer is c. (*Brunton, pp 928–929; Craig, pp 170–173; Katzung, pp 226–228.*) Quinidine's main beneficial effect in supraventricular arrhythmias is a suppression of spontaneous depolarization of the SA node.

Concomitantly, the predominant effect on the AV node is an increase of nodal electrical impulse conduction velocity (not a slowing, as noted in d). This is the main reason why, when quinidine therapy is to be started and atrial rates are still high, we pretreat the patient with a dose of a drug that "blocks down" the AV node: often digoxin, sometimes verapamil or diltiazem, and occasionally a β blocker. The main reason why ventricular rates aren't identical (or close to) atrial rates during atrial fibrillation is because the AV node cannot transmit impulses at such high rates. This protective effect depends on AV nodal refractoriness and a relative inability to transmit too many impulses per time. If we did not suppress the AV node before giving quinidine, the AV nodal effects of the quinidine might increase AV nodal transmission; ventricular rates might rise to dangerous levels as atrial rate slows in response to the quinidine.

Quinidine is not likely to increase blood pressure, or worsen pre-existing hypertension. Quite the contrary: the predominant vascular effect of the drug is dilation, probably due to some α-adrenergic blocking activity. Likewise, quinidine exerts a negative inotropic effect—not a positive one—on ventricular myocardial tissue.

For long-term management of a patient with atrial fibrillation, anticoagulants are important for prophylaxis of thrombosis. The use of quinidine does not preclude or complicate proper oral anticoagulant therapy.

Note: We acknowledge that the use of quinidine, and many other antiarrhythmic drugs, is dwindling as the use of internal defibrillators and pacemakers, and ablative therapies, rises. Nonetheless, don't be surprised if you are asked questions about such classic antiarrhythmics as quinidine on tests.

188. The answer is d. (*Brunton, pp 852–854; Craig, pp 235–236; Katzung, p 166.*) Among all the common oral antihypertensives, a Coombs-positive test is associated with methyldopa. It occurs in up to about 20% of patients taking this drug long term. Although rare, it may progress to hemolytic anemia. The cause is formation of a hapten on erythrocyte membranes, which induces an immune reaction (IgG antibodies) directed against and potentially lysing the red cell membrane. Other drugs with the potential to cause an immunohemolytic anemia are penicillins, quinidine, procainamide, and sulfonamides.

189. The answer is a. (*Brunton, pp 267–268; Craig, p 112; Katzung, pp 144–147.*) Phenoxybenzamine is a long-acting and noncompetitive α-adrenergic blocker. It works by alkylating the α-adrenergic receptors, thereby rendering them incapable of interacting with α-adrenergic agonists such as epinephrine (which is being released in abundance by the pheochromocytoma). The drug has no ability to block β-adrenergic receptors (b), inhibit catecholamine synthesis (c), inhibit angiotensin converting enzyme or bradykininase (d), or affect any of the major enzymes involved in catecholamine degradation (COMT, answer e; or MAO).

190. The answer is c. (*Brunton, pp 832–836; Craig, pp 219–220, 220t; Katzung, pp 192–196.*) In a nutshell, this question summarizes some of the main and important differences between the dihydropyridine CCBs (e.g., nifedipine, and especially in immediate-release formulations, plus many others) and the nondihydropyridines (diltiazem and verapamil). The dihydropyridines are relatively "selective" for their vascular effects. They cause significant arteriolar dilation, which usually activates the baroreceptor reflex that increases sympathetic influences on the heart: positive inotropy, positive chronotropy (reflex tachycardia can be severe), and increased automaticity and conduction velocity (dromotropic effects).

In contrast, diltiazem and verapamil cause not only arteriolar dilation (via calcium channel blockade there), but also direct cardiac depressant effects (due to calcium channel blockade in cardiac tissues). These cardiac effects oppose, or blunt, reflex sympathetic cardiac activation: such problems as reflex tachycardia and positive inotropy are much less—often nonexistent—with the nondihydropyridines. In fact, when reflex cardiac stimulation caused by other drugs (e.g., nitroglycerin) is problematic and must be controlled, either verapamil or diltiazem may be a reasonable alternative to the traditional agents for blocking the unwanted cardiac responses: the β-adrenergic blockers. Moreover, a nondihydropyridine CCB is usually the drug of choice for controlling cardiac stimulatory responses when a β blocker is contraindicated (e.g., in asthma). Note that combined use of diltiazem or verapamil with a β blocker is risky due to possibility of additive inhibitory effects on cardiac rate, contractility, and perhaps especially AV nodal function.

191. The answer is d. *(Brunton, pp 886–889, 921–923; Craig, p 192; Katzung, pp 206–208.)* Of the effects listed here, you would expect to find slowed AV nodal conduction velocity. This is a common and, in many situations useful, effect. For example, when we give the drug as part of the pharmacologic management of atrial fibrillation or flutter, the main desired response is not suppression of the arrhythmia per se, but rather to "block down" the AV node so that as atrial rates fall (but are still high), the AV node will be unable to transmit the same frequency of impulses to the ventricles. That is, we "protect" the ventricles from excessive acceleration by inducing a degree of AV block. In terms of more specific effects on the AV node, digoxin slows conduction velocity and increases AV nodal refractory periods.

Other "predominant" effects on the heart—all concentration-dependent—include increases of both atrial and ventricular automaticity and of conduction velocity through those structures and the His-Purkinje system.

192. The answer is d. *(Brunton, pp 860–862; Craig, pp 155, 228–229; Katzung, pp 172–174.)* Hydralazine predominately dilates arterioles, with negligible effects on venous capacitance. It typically lowers blood pressure "so well" that it can trigger the following two unwanted cardiovascular responses that need to be dealt with:

1. Reflex cardiac stimulation (involving the baroreceptor reflex) is common, and it is typically managed with a β-adrenergic blocker (unless it is contraindicated). An alternative approach would be to use either verapamil or diltiazem (but not a dihydropyridine-type calcium channel blocker such

as nifedipine, which would not suppress—and, in fact might aggravate—the reflex cardiac stimulation).

2. The renin-angiotensin-aldosterone system is activated. One consequence of this unwanted compensatory response would be increased renal sodium retention that would expand circulating fluid volume and counteract hydralazine's blood pressure–lowering effects. This is typically managed with a diuretic. A thiazide often is sufficient to combat the renal sodium retention, but a more efficacious diuretic (loop diuretic) may be necessary.

Captopril (or another ACE inhibitor, or an angiotensin receptor blocker such as losartan) might be a suitable add-on (it would cause synergistic antihypertensive effects and prevent aldosterone-mediated renal effects). However, combining it with nifedipine (dihydropyridine) is irrational. As noted above, given the "pure" vasodilator actions of nifedipine and no cardiac-depressing activity whatsoever (as we get with verapamil or diltiazem), the net effect on heart rate would be either no suppression of the tachycardia or a worsening of it.

Digoxin, alone or with virtually any other drug, is not rational. There is no indication that there is need for inotropic support in this patient.

Spironolactone, alone or with digoxin, would be of little benefit. One could argue that by virtue of the spironolactone's ability to induce diuresis by blocking aldosterone's renal tubular effects, it would counteract hydralazine's ability to lead to renal sodium retention. That may be true, but spironolactone (with or without digoxin) will do nothing desirable to the unwanted tachycardia.

Nitroglycerin would add to hydralazine's antihypertensive effects, but it would probably aggravate the reflex cardiac stimulation and also increase the unwanted renal response (via a hemodynamic mechanism).

Both triamterene and amiloride are potassium-sparing diuretics. The combination of two diuretics in this class is generally irrational (it can lead to hyperkalemia). Either might beneficially combat a propensity for renal sodium retention in response to hydralazine. But, as with any diuretic alone, either or both would do little if anything to control the cardiac response.

Vitamin K was included as a foil. If you are associating hydralazine with some vitamin-related problem, you should be thinking of vitamin B_6 (pyridoxine): hydralazine can interfere with B_6 metabolism, causing such symptoms as peripheral neuritis, and so prophylactic B_6 supplementation is often used along with long-term hydralazine therapy.

193. The answer is c. *(Brunton, pp 948–953; Craig, pp 269–271; Katzung, pp 568–570.)* Simvastatin (and atorvastatin and all the other "statins") decreases cholesterol synthesis in the liver by inhibiting HMG CoA reductase, the rate-limiting enzyme in the synthetic pathway. This results in an increase in LDL receptors in the liver, thus reducing blood levels for cholesterol. These drugs, like other lipid-lowering agents, are best used as adjuncts to exercise and proper diet. They are considered essential components in the primary prevention of coronary heart disease. Some have been shown to lower mortality from cardiovascular causes (MI, stroke, etc.).

194. The answer is b. *(Brunton, pp 171–173; Craig, pp 233–234; Katzung, pp 168–169.)* Guanethidine is occasionally used for severe or refractory hypertension. It must be taken up by adrenergic nerve endings in order for it to exert its effects. This requires intraneuronal transport by the same mechanism by which released norepinephrine reenters the neuron (the so-called amine pump), and that process is blocked by tricyclic antidepressants (e.g., amitriptyline, imipramine) and by cocaine. Once it is in the adrenergic nerve terminal it gradually displaces and then replaces norepinephrine. It is then released into the synaptic cleft by usual processes (e.g., an action potential). However, unlike the native neurotransmitter guanadrel lacks efficacy to activate any adrenergic receptors. This "sympatholytic" effect accounts for reduced vasoconstriction, reduced blood pressure, reduced cardiac rate and contractility and a host of other side effects.

Amine pump blockers such as the tricyclic antidepressants have no pharmacodynamic effects on the other drugs listed, as they do not require neuronal uptake to work. Diazoxide (a) and hydralazine (c) act directly on blood vessels (or their endothelia); prazosin (d) and propranolol (e) exert postsynaptic blocking effects on α- and β-adrenergic receptors, respectively.

195. The answer is d. *(Brunton, pp 863–865; Craig, pp 230–231; Katzung, p 175.)* Cyanide is the ultimate toxic metabolite of nitroprusside sodium. The drug is initially metabolically reduced to nitric oxide, which is responsible for the arteriolar and venular dilation. However, it is another metabolite, CN^- (and to a lesser extent the next metabolite, thiocyanate) that is the main cause of or contributor to toxicity.

When CN^- accumulates to sufficiently high levels (as from excessive or excessively prolonged administration of the drug), the vasculature develops what amounts to a tolerance to the drug's vasodilator effects, and so blood pressure usually starts to rise despite the presence of high drug levels. Toxic cyanide accumulation can also lead to severe lactic acidosis: the CN^- reacts with Fe^{3+} in mitochondrial cytochrome oxidase, inhibiting oxidative phosphorylation. Other characteristic signs and symptoms of the toxic syndrome include a cherry red skin (because mitochondrial oxygen consumption is blocked, venous blood remains oxygenated and as "bright red" as normal arterial blood), hypoxia, and, ultimately, hypoxic seizures and ventilatory arrest.

196. The answer is c. (*Brunton, pp 886–889, 921–923; Craig, pp 154, 246; Katzung, pp 208, 212, 254.*) Hypokalemia due to the effects of potassium-wasting diuretics such as furosemide increase susceptibility to digoxin toxicity, and they are probably the most common cause of it. Captopril (a) has no effects on digoxin's actions. (We might add that an ACE inhibitor such as captopril, along with a β blocker and a diuretic, now is considered the preferred therapy for most patients with heart failure—not digoxin.) Cholestyramine (b), a cholesterol-binding resin, interacts with concomitantly administered (oral) digoxin to reduce digoxin absorption. It would not increase the risk of digoxin toxicity; quite the opposite, it would reduce digoxin's therapeutic effectiveness. Lovastatin (d; an HMG CoA reductase inhibitor/"statin") and nitroglycerin (e) are not likely to cause the observed toxicity either.

197. The answer is e. (*Brunton, pp 690, 928; Craig, pp 172, 429; Katzung, pp 227, 581–582.*) Many of the signs and symptoms of salicylism are similar to those caused by high blood levels of quinidine (antiarrhythmic) or quinine (mainly used as an antimalarial). Quinidine, quinine, and related drugs are called cinchona alkaloids, and the low grade toxicity syndrome caused by these drugs is called cinchonism. (These drugs were originally obtained from a plant known, generically, as *Cinchona*.) Aspirin and the cinchona alkaloids are chemically similar in some important chemical and pharmacologic ways. The common signs and symptoms include light-headedness, tinnitus, and visual disturbances such as diplopia.

198. The answer is c. (*Brunton, p 837; Craig, pp 202–203, 221; Katzung, pp 196–197.*) The etiology involves coronary vasospasm, and that can be blocked well with a calcium channel blocker (CCB): diltiazem, verapamil, or dihydropyridines (e.g., nifedipine, for which slow-/extended-acting oral formulations are used). The CCBs block coronary vascular smooth muscle influx of calcium, which is a critical process in triggering vasospasm.

Nitroglycerin seems to be marginally effective in terms of long-term symptom relief, although it may be the only rapidly acting drug that will be efficacious for acute angina and self-medication.

Aspirin, through its antiplatelet aggregatory effects, would be beneficial, prophylactically, if coronary thrombosis were part of the etiology of variant angina, but thrombosis isn't the main problem with coronary vasospasm.

Atorvastatin (or other statins) are useful for primary prevention of coronary heart disease, but coronaries that undergo spasm may be remarkably free of atherosclerotic plaque, and the statins have no antispasmodic effects per se.

The β blockers, which are important drugs for many patients with ischemic heart disease, can do more harm than good in vasospastic angina. In essence, β-receptor activation in the coronaries tends to cause vasodilation, an effect that to a degree counteracts simultaneous α-mediated constriction. Block only the β receptors and the α-mediated constrictor effects—vasospasm-favoring effects—are left unopposed. Variant angina, then, is likely to be made worse, not better, with β blockers. (You might ask whether a combined α/β blocker like labetalol or carvedilol might be better than a nonselective or cardioselective β blocker. Perhaps in theory, but not in practice. Remember that the α-blocking effects of these drugs are comparatively weak; their β-blocking, spasm-favoring effects may predominate.)

199. The answer is d. *(Brunton, pp 1472, 1480–1481; Craig, pp 259–260, 264–265; Katzung, pp 552–553.)* Streptokinase (SK) has been aptly described as "non-clot-specific" in terms of its sites of action. It forms an SK–plasminogen complex that converts plasminogen into plasmin, which degrades the fibrin network that holds clots intact. That is the basis of its thrombolytic effects. However, the site of action of this prototype thrombolytic drug is not "confined" to clots, as is the case with such drugs as alteplase (a) or tenecteplase (and several others synthesized using recombinant DNA techniques). The systemic formation of plasmin caused by SK leads to degradation or otherwise decreased levels of fibrinogen and other essential clotting factors throughout the circulatory system. This leads to a markedly increased risk of hemorrhage. There is an increased risk of bleeding when heparin is used with any thrombolytic, but proper dosing and monitoring can reduce the risks dramatically. The risks are too great, however, to use heparin concomitant with SK.

It should be obvious that aspirin (b), clopidogrel (c), and warfarin (e) exert anticoagulant effects, and concomitant use of aspirin may increase the bleeding risk. However, with proper (and necessary) monitoring of coagulation parameters, and proper adjustments of doses, these drugs can be safely used with aspirin, as they often are.

200. The answer is c. (*Brunton, pp 921–923, 929; Craig, pp 172–173, 816–818, 870–871; Katzung, pp 205, 1119.*) Digoxin toxicity is likely to occur within 24 to 48 h unless the digoxin dose is adjusted down. The reason is that quinidine will reduce the renal excretion of digoxin (digoxin's main elimination route). This is probably due to some mechanism by which quinidine inhibits P-glycoprotein transport of digoxin in the kidneys.

There is no "reverse interaction"—that is, an ability of digoxin to cause signs and symptoms of quinidine toxicity (a). Quinidine has no significant impact on the renal actions of any diuretics, whether these actions are expressed in terms of urine output (volume or concentration) or renal handling of sodium or potassium or other electrolytes or solutes (b, d).

Quinidine-induced digoxin toxicity may suppress cardiac contractility, but that would not be a direct effect of an interaction on the inotropic state of the myocardium. Rather, it would be secondary to potential digoxin-induced arrhythmias, and it would not occur "promptly."

Quinidine does cause some drug-drug interactions by pharmacokinetic mechanisms. It is a potent inhibitor of CYP2D6, and can, for example, inhibit the analgesic effects of codeine by inhibiting its metabolism to morphine. However, this mechanism does not apply to the quinidine-digoxin interaction; digoxin is eliminated completely by the kidneys, with no prior metabolism.

201. The answer is e. (*Brunton, pp 911–915; Craig, pp 169, 180–181; Katzung, pp 231–232.*) Flecainide, propafenone, and to a degree moricizine, the class I-C antiarrhythmics, are associated with a higher incidence of severe proarrhythmic events than virtually any other antiarrhythmics in other classes. This risk partially explains why, when these drugs were first approved, they were indicated only for life-threatening ventricular arrhythmias that failed to respond to all other reasonable (and safer) alternatives. (This risk also contributed to why another I-C agent, encainide, was withdrawn from the market.)

Nowadays, these I-C agents are still used for serious (life-threatening) and refractory ventricular arrhythmias, their efficacy arising from significant sodium channel blockade. However, they also block some potassium channels, which accounts for modestly growing interest in and use of these drugs for some atrial arrhythmias. Regardless of whether the use is for an atrial or ventricular arrhythmia, the proarrhythmic effects should be of concern.

You may have learned that when these drugs (and others) were evaluated in the Cardiac Arrhythmia Suppression Trial (the CAST study) many years ago, the risks of proarrhythmic effects and sudden death from I-C drugs were quite prominent in patients with previous myocardial infarction and ventricular ectopic activity. Indeed, patients receiving some of the I-C drug had a higher rate of sudden cardiac death than placebo-treated patients. These drugs are not indicated for arrhythmias during an acute MI. They are poor choices for any patient with low ejection fractions or cardiac output, mainly because they can suppress cardiac contractility further.

Pulmonary fibrosis and alterations of thyroid hormone status (typically, a hypothyroid-like state) are uniquely associated with amiodarone (among all the antiarrhythmics), and amiodarone was not one of the answer choices.

Finally, it is probably worth opining that memorizing which antiarrhythmic agents are in which Vaughn-Williams class may not be profitable (except for answering nitpicky and clinically irrelevant exam questions). Among the reasons why: (1) this classification is based largely on electrophysiologic effects of the drugs in largely normal, isolated cardiac cells, not in diseased intact human hearts; (2) some antiarrhythmic drugs have electrophysiologic/ionic mechanisms of action that would reasonably place them in more than one Vaughn-Williams class; (3) belonging to a particular Vaughn-Williams class does not necessarily predict clinical use of the antiarrhythmic; and (4) side effects profiles and toxicities of drugs in the same class—both cardiac and extracardiac—can differ substantially.

202. The answer is e. (*Brunton, p 957; Craig, pp 273–275; Katzung, pp 571–573.*) Gemfibrozil mainly lowers triglycerides and is used specifically for that purpose. This fibric acid derivative is sometimes classified as a peroxisomal proliferator-receptor activator (PPAR). It stimulates lipoprotein lipase synthesis and hydrolysis of triglycerides in chylomicrons and VLDL. The net effect is increased clearance of triglycerides. Clofibrate is a related (but lesser used) fibrate. As you should recall, atorvastatin (a; and other statins) inhibits cholesterol synthesis by inhibiting HMG CoA reductase, and depending on a host of factors they may or may not lower triglycerides; cholestyramine (b) and colestipol (c) are bile acid sequestrants; ezetimibe (d), a relatively new drug, inhibits uptake of dietary cholesterol from the gut. Those other drugs may have beneficial effects on serum triglyceride levels, but they are not first-line drugs for managing hypertriglyceridemia with or without concomitant hypercholesterolemia.

203. The answer is b. (*Brunton, pp 864–865; Craig, pp 230–231; Katzung, p 175.*) Cyanide, whether from nitroprusside metabolism or from other sources (see Question 484 in the toxicology chapter), normally reacts with endogeous sulfur-containing compounds, mainly thiosulfate; under the influence of mitochondrial rhodanese (a trans-sulfurase), relatively nontoxic (less toxic than CN) thiocyanate is formed and is readily excreted in the urine. With excessive exposure to nitroprusside (or CN⁻ from other sources), endogenous sulfur-containing substrate stores are depleted. We manage this, then, by IV infusion of an aqueous sodium thiosulfate solution.

Note: To avoid or at least reduce the risks of nitroprusside-induced cyanide toxicity, some agencies add sodium thiosulfate to the nitroprusside before the drug is administered, thereby providing ample exogenous substrate for the detoxification reaction.

204. The answer is c. (*Brunton, p 956; Craig, pp 272–273; Katzung, pp 570–571.*) The cutaneous flushing and the underlying vasodilation caused by niacin almost certainly involves prostaglandins. We reach that conclusion rather empirically, based on the fact that these responses may be prevented by the prior administration of aspirin, which is known to block prostaglandin synthesis. (Using sustained-release niacin preparations reduces the incidence and severity of these problems too.) α-Adrenergic receptor activation (a) would tend to counteract, not cause or contribute to the vasodilation that is involved in the flush; calcium channel blockers have no effect on the phenomenon, so we rule out answer (b). Similarly, drugs that inhibit angiotensin synthesis or its receptor activation (d), or histamine receptor blockers (e: whether H_1 or H_2) have any effect on the phenomenon.

205. The answer is a. (*Brunton, pp 847–849, 858–859; Craig, pp 211, 214, 245–246, 251–252; Katzung, pp 177–178, 179–180.*) Although combined use of an ACE inhibitor (or angiotensin receptor blocker [ARB], e.g., losartan) and a diuretic is quite common, great care must be taken when adding one of the drugs to therapy that has been started with the other. The reason is that some patients develop a sudden fall of blood pressure that may be sufficient to cause syncope or other complications. Volume (and sodium) depletion seem to be among several probable causative factors.

Answer b is incorrect. The effects of ACE inhibitors (or ARBs) and thiazides on renal handling of potassium are the opposite of one another, not synergistic. ACE inhibitors tend to elevate serum potassium levels (in part, by lowering aldosterone levels); the thiazides (and loop diuretics, e.g., furosemide) are potassium-wasting.

There is no evidence that adding one of these drugs to therapy with the other can cause acute (or chronic) heart failure (c); indeed, such a combination is often an essential component in managing chronic heart failure. Blood pressure will fall, not rise, and certainly not cause hypertensive crisis (d); and slowed AV nodal conduction rates (e) due to this drug combination do not occur.

206. The answer is e. *(Brunton, p 836; Craig, pp 191, 222; Katzung, pp 194–197.)* Constipation is a fairly common and sometimes very bothersome response to many calcium channel blockers. If severe and not managed properly, fecal impaction or other significant intestinal problems can occur. The incidence and severity are greatest with the nondihydropyridines, verapamil and diltiazem, than with dihydropyridines (e.g., nifedipine). The best initial approach—if continued use of the offending drug is needed—is to modify the diet by increasing water and dietary fiber intake.

207. The answer is e. *(Brunton, pp 808–809, 858–859, 879; Craig, p 212; Katzung, pp 178–179.)* One of the adverse responses to ACE inhibitors is impairment of renal function, as evidenced by proteinuria. Fortunately, it is not common, but nonetheless requires periodic monitoring. Elevations of blood urea nitrogen (BUN) and creatinine occur frequently, especially when stenosis of the renal artery or severe heart failure exists. Given the fact that these drugs ultimately inhibit aldosterone release, hyperkalemia is much more likely than hypokalemia. These drugs are to be used very cautiously where prior renal failure is present and in the elderly. Other toxicities include persistent dry cough, neutropenia, and angioedema. Hepatic toxicity has not been reported.

208. The answer is d. (*Brunton, p 1474; Craig, pp 66t, 260–261; Katzung, p 548.*) A slow intravenous infusion of protamine sulfate will quickly reverse the bleeding. Protamine binds to heparin, forming a stable complex that abolishes heparin's anticoagulant activity. It may also have its own anticoagulant effect by binding with platelets and fibrinogen. Aminocaproic acid (a) binds avidly to plasmin and plasminogen, and so is an effective inhibitor of fibrinolysis and an antagonist of fibrinolytic/thrombolytic drugs. Dipyridamole weakly blocks platelet ADP receptors, and has a long but uninspiring history as an antiplatelet drug. Factor IX will not reverse the excessive effects of heparin. Vitamin K is used as an antidote for excessive effects of such drugs as warfarin, and does nothing for heparin overdoses.

209. The answer is g. (*Brunton, pp 926–927; Craig, p 173; Katzung, pp 228–229.*) Procainamide is associated with the development of a lupus-like syndrome. The risk is higher in patients who, because of genetically based drug metabolizing capacity, are "slow acetylators"; that is because it appears that the parent drug, not the main metabolite [N-acetylprocainamide (NAPA)], is the culprit. The precise mechanism by which procainamide-associated lupus occurs is not known. Increases of antinuclear antibodies (ANA) are not uncommon in patients taking the drug, nor does the presence of such an increase require that procainamide therapy be stopped. However, be aware that many patients (estimates are as high as 50%) taking this drug long-term will develop symptoms and signs of a lupus-like syndrome that usually appears first as the characteristic rash and arthralgias.

None of the other drugs listed are associated with a lupus-like syndrome, whether administered alone or in combination with one another, or with other drugs not listed here.

Note 1: There is one other drug traditionally discussed in the cardiovascular section of texts and courses that is linked to a lupus-like syndrome: hydralazine. (Such other drugs as quinidine have caused lupus-like responses, but this is quite rare in comparison with the frequency seen with procainamide or hydralazine.)

Note 2: If carvedilol (d) is not familiar to you, learn that it's a β-adrenergic blocker with α-adrenergic blocking activity. In this respect it is similar to labetalol. It is probably the most widely used β-blocker for long-term management (along with an ACE inhibitor and, usually, a loop diuretic) of heart failure in ambulatory patients.

210. The answer is c. *(Brunton, pp 829–830; Craig, pp 197, 739–740; Katzung, pp 186, 189.)* Nitroglycerin causes its vasodilator effects via a nitric oxide (NO)- and cyclic GMP-dependent mechanism. The NO activates guanylyl cyclase which forms cGMP from GMP. The cGMP, in turn, dephosphorylates myosin light chains, leading to reduced acting-myosin interactions and relaxation of the smooth muscle cells. Normally, this vascular effect is modulated by cGMP degradation (to GMP) by cGMP-specific phosphodiesterases (PDEs).

Sildenafil (and the related drugs tadalafil and vardenafil), inhibit the activity of those PDEs, thereby maintaining cGMP levels and potentiating the vasodilator effects. This interaction may lead to severe excessive effects, including life-threatening hypotension and myocardial and cerebral ischemia. Sildenafil and related drugs also increase the risk of symptomatic hypotension if taken by people who are also being treated with α-adrenergic blockers, including those that selectively block α_1 receptors (e.g., prazosin and doxazosin) and are used for managing hypertension.

Note the important mechanistic links between vasodilation/hypotension, sexual intercourse, and potentially fatal cardiac responses. Sexual arousal—and, especially orgasm—causes a massive activation of the sympathetic nervous system. One consequence of that, α-mediated vasoconstriction that tends to keep blood pressure up, may be too feeble to overcome the hypotensive effects of the sildenafil-nitroglycerin combination. Along with a fall of blood pressure is a fall of coronary perfusion pressure (diastolic blood pressure), that is, reduced myocardial blood flow/oxygen supply. Yet the sympathetic activation concomitantly causes significant increases of cardiac rate and contractility, that is, increased myocardial oxygen demand. Oxygen demand rises, supply falls, and the stage is set for acute myocardial ischemia.

A final point to consider: it is reasonable to assume that if the patient is taking *any* or even several of the drugs listed in the question, he has underlying cardiac disease. However, and in contrast with what some students have suggested, underlying cardiac disease per se does not automatically contraindicate or even excessively increase the risks from sexual intercourse and orgasm. (How severe is the patient's cardiovascular disease? Is it well controlled? What *are* the specific diseases and risks he has?) Similarly, none of the drugs listed other than the nitrovasodilators (and some α blockers mentioned in the previous paragraph) contraindicate the use of any of the ED drugs.

211. The answer is e. *(Brunton, pp 902–904; Craig, p 165; Katzung, pp 221–222.)* Although you may not consider this question a pharmacology question, being able to answer it correctly is important to the rational and safe use of many drugs.

In general, heart block refers to excessively slowed AV nodal conduction, which you assess by measuring the PR interval on the EKG. Recall that this interval gives information on how long it takes for electrical impulses that originate with SA nodal depolarization to pass through the AV node, ultimately leading to ventricular activation (manifest as the QRS complex). Impulse conduction through the atria is normally quick; it is the AV node that has the slowest intrinsic impulse conduction rate anywhere in the heart, and it is arguably the structure that is most susceptible to drug- (or disease-) induced changes of supraventricular conduction that lead to the diagnosis of AV block.

In first-degree heart block, the only manifestation is a prolonged PR interval, but each P wave is followed by a normally generated QRS complex. In second-degree heart block, the PR interval is prolonged and some P waves are not conducted through the AV node, and so are not followed by a QRS triggered by the prior atrial activation. In third-degree (complete) heart block, no P waves are conducted normally through the AV node, and ventricular activation is solely dependent on intrinsic automaticity of the ventricles (or conducting tissue therein).

Auscultation of the heart, the presence of blood pressures that are above or below what is generally regarded as normal, or the presence of a slow sinus rhythm, are not reliable indicators of heart block.

212. The answer is d. (*Brunton, pp 824–826; Craig, pp 198–199; Katzung, pp 186–187.*) Nitric oxide is thought to be enzymatically released from nitroglycerin. It then reacts with and activates guanylyl cyclase to increase GMP, which in turn dephosphorylates myosin light chain kinase, causes calcium extrusion, and suppresses smooth muscle tone. Tolerance may develop in part from a decrease in available sulfhydryl groups. Autonomic receptors are not involved in the primary response of nitroglycerin, but compensatory mechanisms may counter the primary actions.

213. The answer is f. (*Brunton, p 951; Craig, p 272; Katzung, pp 569–570.*) The findings are consistent with statin-induced myositis and myopathy, which seems to have progressed to rhabdomyolysis and renal failure—both potentially fatal. This syndrome (and hepatotoxicity) is the most serious adverse response to the statins. It is more prevalent in older patients, those with multiple illnesses, and especially those with renal or liver disease. Coadministration of most other lipid-lowering drugs (none of which are in the list) increases the risk of rhabdomyolysis, hepatotoxicity, or both. As an aside, the risk of rhabdomyolysis (or lesser skeletal muscle changes) is not too much different between the currently available statins. However, it was (allegedly) such a problem with one relatively recent drug, cerivastatin that the drug was pulled from the market.

214. The answer is d. (*Brunton, pp 857–858, 860–862, 864–865; Craig, p 228; Katzung, pp 172–175.*) Nitroprusside relaxes both arterioles and venules to relatively comparable degrees. It tends not to increase cardiac output (and does not do so through any direct cardiac action), and this property contributes to its usefulness in the management of hypertensive crisis associated with MI. Diazoxide (a), hydralazine (b), minoxidil (c; rarely used because of risks of cardiotoxicity and pulmonary fibrosis), and nifedipine (e) relax arteriolar smooth muscle more so than smooth muscle on the venous side, so their effects on venous capacitance are negligible.

215. The answer is b. (*Brunton, pp 688, 1482; Craig, pp 257f, 262–263, Katzung, pp 316, 574.*) Aspirin inhibits cyclooxygenases I and II. In terms of clotting, the main effect will be inhibition of platelet aggregation by reduced formation of thromboxane A_2. Bleeding time will be prolonged and will remain that way until sufficient numbers of new platelets have been synthesized and released into the bloodstream, because aggregation of those platelets already exposed to the drug will be inhibited for their lifetime. The APTT, which should not be affected by aspirin, is used to monitor effects and adjust the dose of unfractionated heparin (such monitoring is not required with low molecular weight heparin, e.g., enoxaparin). The prothrombin time (and its normalized value, the INR) are used with warfarin. Platelet counts, also not affected by aspirin, are used to assess for the development of thrombocytopenic purpura, which may rarely occur during therapy with, for example, the clopidogrel-like drug ticlopidine, or with heparin when thrombocytopenia is anticipated or suspected.

216. The answer is a. (*Brunton, pp 917, 920; Craig, pp 166–169, 192–193; Katzung, pp 227–228, 236.*) Nowadays, IV injection of adenosine is generally regarded as first choice for terminating PSVT in which reentry phenomena play an important pathophysiologic role. Among other reasons, it is preferred over another reasonable alternative, verapamil, because of a faster onset of action. Adenosine is also a primary drug for managing episodes of ventricular tachycardia, provided there are no cardiac structural defects (aneurysms, damage to papillary muscles of the chordae tendinae, etc.)

Digoxin (b), edrophonium (c; rapidly acting ACh esterase inhibitor), phenylephrine (d; nonselective α-adrenergic agonist), and propranolol or other β blockers (e) , are older therapies falling into relative disuse. In one way or another their effects revolve around causing or unmasking increased parasympathetic influences on the SA and/or AV nodes: digoxin *via* its predominant effects to slow AV nodal conduction; phenylephrine by increasing blood pressure, which triggers a baroreceptor reflex that reduces sympathetic drive and essentially increases or unmasks parasympathetic tone; propranolol, by blocking β_1-mediated sympathetic influences; and edrophonium, which quickly but briefly raises parasympathetic influences on nodal tissues.

217. The answer is c. (*Brunton, pp 1746–1747; Craig, p 261; Katzung, pp 549–551.*) Warfarin is a coumarin derivative that is generally used for long-term anticoagulation, and is wholly unsuitable for immediate anticoagulation because it takes at least 5 days of administration for meaningful inhibition of prothrombin time (reported as the International Normalized Ratio [INR]) to develop and stabilize. It antagonizes the γ-carboxylation of several glutamate residues in prothrombin and the coagulation Factors VII, IX, and X. This process is coupled to the oxidative deactivation of vitamin K. The reduced form of vitamin K is essential for sustained carboxylation and synthesis of the coagulation proteins. It appears that warfarin inhibits the action of the reductase(s) that regenerate the reduced form of vitamin K. The prevention of the inactive vitamin K epoxide from being reduced to the active form of vitamin K results in decreased carboxylation of the proteins involved in the coagulation cascade.

218. The answer is b. (*Brunton, pp 757–759, 763f; Craig, pp 248–249; Katzung, p 256.*) Amiloride is a K-sparing diuretic with a mild diuretic and natriuretic effect. The parent compound is active, and the drug is excreted unchanged in the urine. Amiloride has a 24-h duration of action and is usually administered with a thiazide or loop diuretic (e.g., furosemide) to prevent hypokalemia. The site of its diuretic action is the late distal tubule and collecting duct, where it interferes with Na^+ reabsorption and allows for K^+ retention. Acetazolamide (a), furosemide (c), and metolazone (d) are all potassium-wasting. Although it would be irrational adding them to therapy with hydrochlorothiazide, if that were indeed done the patient's serum potassium levels would most likely fall, not rise or normalize. Mannitol (e) is a parenteral osmotic diuretic, and would not be "added" to long-term therapy.

219. The answer is c. *(Brunton, pp 749–753; Craig, p 250; Katzung, pp 247–248.)* Furosemide can cause hypokalemia by blocking Na^+ reabsorption in the loop of Henle, followed by exchange of K^+ for Na^+ in the principal cells in the distal tubules. Hypokalemia is often associated with and a cause of digoxin toxicity. Furosemide and other loop diuretics (torsemide, bumetanide, ethacrynic acid) also cause a net loss of calcium and magnesium *via* urine. They also can cause or exacerbate hearing loss (they are considered to be ototoxic drugs), especially in people with prior hearing loss and/or renal impairment.

220. The answer is e. *(Brunton, pp 1470–1472; Craig, p 259; Katzung, pp 545–547.)* Heparin binds to antithrombin III (a plasma protease inhibitor), thereby enhancing its activation. The heparin-III complex interacts with thrombin. This inactivates thrombin and other coagulation factors such as VIIa, IXa, Xa, and IIa. Heparin accelerates the rate of thrombin-antithrombin binding, resulting in the inhibition of thrombin. The latter effect is not typically seen with low-molecular-weight heparins (e.g., enoxaparin) that are not of sufficient length to catalyze the inhibition of thrombin.

221. The answer is e. *(Brunton, pp 1469f, 1480–1481; Craig, pp 263–264; Katzung, pp 553–554.)* Alteplase, a thrombolytic drug, is an unmodified tissue plasminogen activator (t-PA). It activates plasminogen that is bound to fibrin (i.e., it is "clot-specific," unlike streptokinase, which acts throughout the circulatory system). The plasmin that is formed in response to the drug acts directly on fibrin. This results in dissolving the fibrin into fibrin-split products, followed by lysis of the clot. Clopidogrel is an example of an antiplatelet drug that works by blocking platelet ADP receptors (a); aspirin exerts antiplatelet effects by inhibiting thromboxane production (b) *via* cyclooxygenase; abciximab is an example of an antiplatelet drug that blocks the platelet Gp IIb/IIIa receptors. Warfarin, an anticoagulant (neither a thrombolytic nor an antiplatelet agent) inhibits hepatic synthesis (activation) of vitamin K-dependent clotting factors (c).

222. The answer is d. *(Brunton, pp 920–921, 1526t, 1527, 1532t; Craig, pp 187–188; Katzung, pp 233–234.)* Pulmonary fibrosis has been reported with long-term amiodarone therapy, but not in response to other antiarrhythmics. Pulmonary function tests may remain normal for months and then decline quickly and to significant degrees as irreversible fibrosis develops. Changes of thyroid hormone status—sometimes reflecting hypothyroidism and, for many other patients, hyperthyroidism—are also uniquely associated with amiodarone: this drug is structurally related to the thyroid hormones and is rich in iodine. Changes of thyroid hormone status may be subclinical and detectable only with suitable blood tests or may lead to typical signs and symptoms of hyper- or hypothyroidism.

Keep in mind that some adverse responses that are unique to other antiarrhythmic drugs were listed as possible answers. For example, low-grade quinidine toxicity (cinchonism) often includes tinnitus (but that manifestation of ototoxicity cannot be detected with audiometry), and procainamide commonly causes a lupus-like syndrome, for which monitoring of ANA titers is important.

Of course, it's likely that a patient with atrial fibrillation will be placed on warfarin (at least for a while), and so monitoring the prothrombin time (reported as the INR) would be essential in that case. And, since this patient may have multiple cardiovascular "risk factors," periodic monitoring of lipid profiles would be essential too. Nonetheless, these do not apply specifically or uniquely to amiodarone.

223. The answer is c. *(Brunton, pp 1481–1483; Craig, p 263; Katzung, p 554.)* Clopidogrel (ticlopidine is a related drug) decreases platelet aggregation by blocking a population of platelet ADP receptors (which dipyridamole, d, also seems to do, but very weakly), thereby inhibiting ADP-induced platelet activation. It has no direct platelet effects involving activation by thromboxane A2, collagen, or other mediators, nor does it inhibit platelet aggregation by any actions on the platelet glycoprotein IIb/IIIa receptors. Acetaminophen (a) has no antiplatelet effects. Aminocaproic acid (b) prevents activation of plasminogen and inhibits plasmin directly. It may be used to counteract the effects of thrombolytic drugs given in relative or absolute overdoses. Streptokinase (e) is a bacterial derived, "non-clot-specific" thrombolytic drug.

224. The answer is f. *(Brunton, pp 834–835, 914, 916t; Craig, pp 191–192; Katzung, pp 235–236.)* In essence, we are asking "which drug can suppress

AV nodal conduction velocity?" Verapamil (and the very similar nondihydropyridine calcium channel blocker, diltiazem) do that. Recall the profile of verapamil and diltiazem: a vasodilator effect plus a direct cardiac "depressant" effect that includes slowing of AV conduction (and potential depression of other cardiac contractile and electrophysiologic phenomena).

(Be sure you can contrast this dual vasodilator/cardiac depressant profile for verapamil and diltiazem with that of the dihydropyridines [e.g., nifedipine; answer c]. The dihydropyridines cause vasodilation, but lack any cardiac depressant actions. Indeed, with dihydropyridine dosages sufficient to lower blood pressure enough, and quick enough, there will be reflex (baroreceptor) activation of the sympathetic nervous system. One consequence of increased norepinephrine release at the heart would be increased (faster) AV nodal conduction velocity, which could be construed as an "unblocking" of the AV node—precisely the opposite of what may happen with verapamil or diltiazem.)

Captopril (ACE inhibitor) and losartan (angiotensin receptor blocker) have no significant effects on AV nodal conduction.

Nitroglycerin (nitrovasodilator) and prazosin (a vasodilator that acts by competitive α_1 blockade) also have no direct effect on the AV node, but are likely to lead to an indirect quickening of AV conduction via baroreceptor activation.

On a final and important note, be sure you understand that all β-adrenergic blockers (including those with some α-blocking activity, e.g., labetalol and carvedilol) can slow AV nodal conduction and can cause or worsen heart block.

225. The answer is a. (*Brunton, pp 808–809, 879; Craig, p 212; Katzung, p 178.*) Captopril, and some of the other ACE inhibitors, may cause severe, hacking, and relentless cough in some patients. It is thought to be due to increased levels of bradykinin in smooth muscles in the throat. (Recall that angiotensin-converting enzyme, which forms angiotensin II, is the same enzyme as bradykininase, which metabolically inactivates bradykinin.) Many patients receiving captopril (or other ACE inhibitors) experience no problems of this sort. Still other patients, mainly taking other ACE inhibitors, may develop swelling of the oropharyngeal mucosae, and some may develop life-threatening angioedema.

There are no likely allergic reactions (b) triggered by any of the drugs, statins included.

Captopril is not a bronchoconstrictor (c). Hyperkalemia is not a likely explanation. Note that by indirectly lowering aldosterone levels (angiotensin II is the main stimulus for aldosterone release, and we have inhibited angiotensin II synthesis), the main renal effects would be increased sodium excretion and increased potassium retention. However, we are administering furosemide (a loop diuretic), which causes renal potassium-wasting. Thus, we would not expect hyperkalemia from this combination of drugs (as we would if the diuretic was a potassium-sparing one such as amiloride, triamterene, or sprionolactone).

Cough is not part of the main side effect/toxicity profile of simvastatin or other HMG CoA reductase inhibitors. Recall that their main toxicities include myositis, myopathy, rhabdomyolysis, renal damage (from the rhabdomyolysis), and hepatotoxicity.

226. The answer is e. (*Brunton, p 1474; Craig, p 260; Katzung, p 545.*) Heparin is a mixture of sulfated mucopolysaccharides and is highly acidic and charged. Protamine is a very basic polypeptide that combines with heparin, rendering a complex that has no anticoagulant activity. Excess protamine does have anticoagulant activity, so just enough should be given to counteract the heparin effect. A single dose of protamine sulfate has duration of action of about 2 hours. Protamine causes no "overall activation" of either the intrinsic or extrinsic clotting pathways (a); does not hydrolyze heparin (b); or trigger platelet aggregation (c). Heparin exerts its anticoagulant effect, in part, though an interaction with antithrombin III (AT-III). However, protamine does not interact directly with AT-III, but rather with the heparin, as noted above.

227. The answer is b. (*Brunton, pp 255–256, 854–855; Craig, p 237; Katzung, pp 31–32, 166–167.*) Abrupt discontinuation of clonidine has been associated with a rapidly developing and severe "rebound" phenomenon that includes excessive cardiac stimulation and a spike of blood pressure that may be sufficiently great as to cause stroke or other similar complications. Recall that clonidine is a "centrally acting α_2-adrenergic agonist." Through its central effects it reduces sympathetic nervous system tone. This, in turn, appears to cause supersensitivity of peripheral adrenergic receptors to direct-acting adrenergic agonists, including endogenous norepinephrine and epinephrine. Once, and soon after, the drug is stopped, endogenous catecholamines trigger hyper-responsiveness of all structures under sympathetic control.

When ACE inhibitors (or angiotensin receptor blockers), furosemide, or nifedipine (long-acting or otherwise) are abruptly stopped, blood pressure (and blood volume, depending on the drug) will begin to rise from treatment levels, but there will be no sudden "spike" of pressure nor an "overshoot" of it.

Digoxin discontinuation is not associated with the symptoms noted in the question. Besides, the half-life of digoxin (about 36 to 40 h if renal function is normal) is such that stopping the drug abruptly would not in all likelihood lead to any significant "withdrawal" events occurring within a day or two of discontinuation.

There is no reason to predict that suddenly stopping warfarin would cause tachyarrhythmias, hypertension, or hemorrhagic stroke—and certainly not within 24 to 48 h.

228. The answer is c. *(Brunton, p 1474; Craig, pp 259–260; Katzung, pp 545–548.)* This brief scenario describes heparin-induced thrombocytopenia (HIT). It is an immune-mediated thrombocytopenia that is accompanied by a paradoxical *increase* in thrombotic events (e.g., in limbs, brain, lungs, heart). It affects about 1–3% of patients receiving heparin for more than about 4 days in a row. The cause appears to involve formation of antibodies that develop to heparin-platelet complexes. This leads to substantial increases of platelet activation that, in turn, leads to, thrombosis, vascular damage, and eventually significant declines in the number of functional circulating platelets (since platelets have been consumed in widespread thrombotic events). This phenomenon is not associated with any of the other drugs listed in the question.

229. The answer is c. *(Brunton, pp 487–488, 753; Craig, pp 393–395; Katzung, pp 256, 475–478.)* There is a clinically important relationship between serum sodium concentrations and the concentration-dependent effects of lithium. In essence, Li^+ and Na^+ compete with one another, such that in the presence of hyponatremia the effects of the lithium may be increased to the point of causing toxicity. (Conversely, hypernatremia can counteract lithium's therapeutic effects.) Of the drugs listed, hydrochlorothiazide (and other thiazides and such thiazide-like agents as metolazone) poses the greatest risk of causing hyponatremia. (And you should consider the ultimate renal effects of ACE inhibition to lower serum Na^+ levels further when used with a diuretic. ACE inhibitors used without a diuretic are not at all as likely to cause hyponatremia.)

There are no clinically significant pharmacodynamic or pharmacokinetic interactions between nitroglycerin or HMG CoA reductase inhibitors and the SSRIs (fluoxetine, sertraline, others) or lithium.

230. The answer is d. *(Brunton, pp 838, 850–851, 884, 914–915; Craig, pp 182–184, 232–233; Katzung, pp 154, 171.)* Labetalol is the best choice. Given its combination of both α- and β-adrenergic (β_1 and β_2) blocking effect, it offers the best approach for managing the hypertension, the tachycardia, the resulting oxygen supply-demand imbalance that leads to both chest discomfort and the ischemic ST-changes, and the ventricular ectopy (which is probably a reflection of excessive catecholamine stimulation of β_1 receptors). If the patient is having an acute myocardial infarction, starting β-blocker therapy early is also decidedly beneficial in the short term and for the long run. (Most any other β blocker might be a suitable alternative, but only labetalol has the combined α/β-blocking actions that are likely to be of greatest benefit. Carvedilol has the same profile, but it is given orally and in this setting that would not be ideal because of slow onset of action.)

Aspirin will do no harm in this situation, but it will also do no good acutely unless there is ongoing platelet aggregation and coronary occlusion. Even if there were, the aspirin would do little to control heart rate, blood pressure, or the EKG changes.

Nothing in the scenario suggests this patient is volume-overloaded or suffering acute pulmonary edema. Therefore, administering the furosemide in such a situation is not appropriate. Moreover, giving it is likely to cause prompt reductions of blood volume and, along with it, of blood pressure. The latter effect is likely to lead to further—and unwanted—reflex sympathetic activation that would make matters worse.

Lidocaine might be suitable for the ventricular ectopy. However, we have identified several other important signs and symptoms that would not be relieved by this antiarrhythmic drug. As noted above, the profile of labetalol offers the greatest likelihood of managing multiple problems with one drug.

Increasing the dose of nitroglycerin (and especially giving it as a bolus) is likely to drop blood pressure acutely, triggering reflex (baroreceptor) stimulation of the heart. The usual "anti-ischemic" effects of the drug would be counteracted by such "pro-ischemic" changes as further rises of heart rate and a probable worsening of the premature ventricular beats.

Prazosin would lower blood pressure nicely. However, once again we have to worry about excessive pressure lowering, triggering the baroreceptor reflex, and worsening many of the already worrisome findings (e.g., heart rate, PVCs).

231. The answer is b. (*Brunton, pp 835–838; Craig, p 222; Katzung, pp 176, 192–195.*) A good way to arrive at the answer is to remember the rather narrow cardiovascular profile of nifedipine, the prototype dihydropyridine calcium channel blocker, and perhaps to compare it with the two main nondihydropyridines, diltiazem, and verapamil.

The nondihydropyridines block vascular smooth-muscle calcium channels, and so cause vasodilation. Any of these drugs, therefore, would help lower this patient's blood pressure.

However, nifedipine (and other dihydropyridines) lack any cardiac-depressant effects. The implication is that as the nifedipine drives blood pressure down (and it will, quite promptly and in an uncontrolled fashion with this sometimes-used but wholly inappropriate and unsafe administration method), there will be intense baroreceptor activation and resulting cardiac stimulation. There are no drug-induced negative inotropic, chronotropic, or dromotropic (conduction velocity) effects to counteract the excessive cardiac stimulation as there would be if we had used either diltiazem or verapamil.

So, in the presence of reflex-mediated increases of catecholamines affecting the heart, AV conduction would increase (not be slowed or blocked); there would be further increases of heart rate (at least; certainly, no fall) to accompany lowering of blood pressure (possibly to hypotensive levels); and the current episodes of ventricular ectopy might convert to longer runs, or to ventricular tachycardia or fibrillation.

232. The answer is b. (*Brunton, p 889; Craig, p 184; Katzung, p 212.*) This collection of signs and symptoms is characteristic of digoxin toxicity, regardless of the cause (e.g., frank overdose or the development of hypokalemia, which increases the risk of digoxin toxicity). Although a probable cause of the hypokalemia is the furosemide, it is not correct to say that furosemide per se is the cause, because signs and symptoms of furosemide toxicity are not similar at all to those described here. Note, too, that we have administered triamterene. The expected effect of that potassium-sparing diuretic is to counteract renal potassium loss from the furosemide (potassium-wasting).

Do recall that the digoxin-induced visual changes described in the question are called chromatopsia.

233. The answer is c. (*Brunton, p 861; Craig, p 229; Katzung, pp 172–174.*) Hydralazine is probably one of the two "main" cardiovascular drugs (procainamide is the other) associated with a somewhat common incidence of medication-related lupus-like syndrome. As with procainamide, acetylation is the first step in the drug's metabolism, and individuals who are genetically predisposed to metabolize the drug slowly (so-called "slow acetylators") are more susceptible to the arthralgia, fever, and other characteristics of the syndrome. The frequency rises for any patient when very high doses of the drug are used long term, as may be done for severe hypertension or (to a lesser degree) heart failure.

234. The answer is a. (*Brunton, pp 832–837, 857–858; Craig, pp 220–221; Katzung, pp 172–174, 179–180, 209.*) Our main goals are to safely lower blood pressure and help normalize heart rate. If we cannot use a β blocker for that, a nondihydropyridine calcium channel blocker, either diltiazem or verapamil, would be an excellent choice. In addition to controlling the cardiovascular problems they are unlikely to exacerbate the asthma.

Enalapril (b), one of many ACE inhibitors, might nicely and gradually lower blood pressure, and should have no adverse effects on airway function. Nonetheless it is unlikely that it or any other ACE inhibitor would have much of a beneficial impact on the tachycardia. More important is the fact that ACE inhibitors, and angiotensin receptor blockers such as losartan, should not be administered to women who are pregnant or likely to become pregnant. Furosemide (c) would transiently lower blood pressure, but our patient has essential hypertension: she is not volume-overloaded, and so this diuretic would not be a good choice. Moreover, if circulating fluid volume fell sufficiently, and sufficiently fast, the baroreceptor reflex might be activated, causing even further rises of heart rate.

Phentolamine (d) and prazosin (e) are both α-adrenergic blocker. Phentolamine is rapidly acting, given parenterally, and nonselectively blocks both α_1 and α_2 (presynaptic) receptors. Even with small doses, the blood pressure fall usually is sufficient to reflexly increase heart rate (and contractility) even more. A parenteral drug such as this simply is not appropriate therapy in this situation. Prazosin is given orally, works relatively slowly, and blocks only α_1 receptors. While its effects are more gradual, perhaps slow enough that the baroreceptors are not activated, this drug will do nothing to control the patient's tachycardia.

235. The answer is e. *(Brunton, pp 143t, 164, 256, 1643; Katzung, pp 146–147, 151.)* Pheochromocytomas—rare causes of hypertension—generally involve excessive levels of circulating catecholamines from tumors of the adrenal (suprarenal) medulla. (In adults, only about 10% of all cases of pheochromocytoma are due to catecholamines released from extra-adrenal sites.) Regardless of the site(s) of the tumor(s), the main factor in leading to an increase of blood pressure and heart rate in this condition is α-mediated vasoconstriction arising from excessive levels of epinephrine, norepinephrine, or both. Epinephrine (but not norepinephrine) will cause β_2-mediated dilation of some vascular beds. However, that vasodilator effect, which might be construed as a mechanism to keep blood pressure from rising too much, is extraordinarily slight in comparison with the opposing vasoconstrictor (α-mediated) influences of the catecholamines elsewhere in the peripheral vasculature. Even if you consider the vasodilator influences to be slight, they will be blocked by propranolol or any other β-adrenergic blocker, such that diastolic and mean blood pressures will rise further, at least initially. (The so-called cardioselective/β_1 blockers such as atenolol and metoprolol will block β_2 receptors in the vasculature, and elsewhere, at blood levels that are not too far above the usual "therapeutic" range.) In essence, blockade of β_2 receptors in the vasculature will leave α-mediated constrictor effects unopposed, and blood pressure will rise (concomitant with suppression of cardiac contractility and rate). The problem is not likely to happen with labetalol; it is, indeed, a β blocker, but it also has intrinsic α-blocking activity that should blunt to some useful degree the vasoconstrictor influences of circulating epinephrine and neuronally released norepinephrine. None of the other drug would raise blood pressure further, and while none of them is indicated as primary therapy for pheochromocytomas, ultimately any of them are more likely to lower blood pressure.

236. The answer is d. *(Brunton, pp 1478, 1485; Craig, pp 66t, 261, 781–782; Katzung, pp 552, 556.)* Phytonadione (vitamin K_1) is the antidote. It overcomes (reverses, antagonizes) warfarin's hepatic anticoagulant effects, which involve inhibited synthesis of clotting factors (VII, IX, X, and prothrombin).

Aminocaproic acid is a backup (to whole blood, packed red cells, or fresh-frozen plasma) for managing bleeding in response to excessive effects of thrombolytic drugs (e.g., alteplase [tPA], streptokinase, tenecteplase). It is not indicated for warfarin-related bleeding. Epoetin alfa is a hematopoietic growth factor that stimulates erythrocyte production in peritubular cells in the proximal tubules of the kidney. Its uses include management of anemias associated with chronic renal failure, chemotherapy (of nonmyeloid malignancies), or zidovudine therapy in patients with acquired immunodeficiency syndrome. It is inappropriate for this patient. Ferrous sulfate (or fumarate or gluconate) is indicated for prevention or treatment of iron-deficiency anemias. It will do nothing to lower the patient's INR or alleviate related symptoms. Protamine sulfate is the antidote for heparin overdoses. It acts electrostatically with heparin, in the blood, to form a complex that lacks anticoagulant activity. It does nothing to the hepatic vitamin K–related problems that are at the root of excessive warfarin effects.

237. The answer is d. (*Brunton, p 1474; Craig, p 260; Katzung, p 547.*) This is a fairly typical presentation of heparin-induced thrombocytopenia (HIT) in terms of both physical findings and time-course of onset. If heparin administration lasts for more than about a week, platelet counts should be checked several times a week for the first month or so and then monthly thereafter, because this is a potentially fatal response. It is immune-mediated: antibodies form against a heparin-platelet complex; platelets are activated (thus, the thrombosis and such complications as pulmonary and/or coronary occlusion, as we described); the vascular endothelia are damaged; and ultimately damaged platelets are cleared (hence the thrombocytopenia). The overall incidence is about 10 times higher with unfractionated heparin than with LMW heparins. Should HIT occur, or be suspected, the approach includes stopping the heparin and substituting other anticoagulants. A good choice would be a direct thrombin inhibitor (e.g., bivalirudin).

Aspirin, by virtue of its antiplatelet effects, should not induce thrombosis. ACE inhibitors and β blockers (carvedilol, any others) do not interact to cause hemolytic anemia or other blood dyscrasias. Ranitidine (or famotidine or nizatidine, the other two H_2 blockers) do not alter the metabolism of other drugs; the prototype H_2 blocker, cimetidine, is a strong mixed function oxidase (P450) inhibitor.

238. The answer is b. (*Brunton, pp 800–805, 813–814; Craig, pp 210–213; Katzung, pp 177–179.*) Losartan, an angiotensin receptor blocker (ARB) has no effect on angiotensin II synthesis (as do the ACE inhibitors such as lisinopril, captopril, and others). Its main antihypertensive actions, therefore, include only blockade of angiotensin II–mediated aldosterone release from the adrenal cortex, and of angiotensin II's vasoconstrictor effects.

Lisinopril and the other ACE inhibitors inhibit angiotensin II synthesis, and that effect accounts (indirectly) for reduced aldosterone release and AII-mediated vasoconstriction. They also inhibit metabolic inactivation of bradykinin, an endogenous vasodilator (bradykininase, angiotensin-converting enzyme, and kininase II are synonyms for essentially the same enzyme).

Neither an ACE inhibitor nor an ARB is associated with an increased incidence of bronchospasm (b; although some ACE inhibitors may cause cough, presumably from locally increased bradykinin levels, and angioedema, perhaps by the same mechanism). Neither elevates serum urate levels.

There is some evidence that angiotensin II enhances (not inhibits) sympathetic-mediated vasoconstriction (by increasing neuronal norepinephrine release and/or blocking neuronal norepinephrine reuptake). Either an ACE inhibitor or an ARB should be equivalent in attenuating that blood pressure–elevating effect.

ACE inhibitors are considered to be an "essential" part of therapy (along with β blockers and a diuretic) for most patients with heart failure. Angiotensin receptor blockers such as losartan may prove to be equally effective alternatives.

By the way: didn't learn explicitly about lisinopril and so didn't recognize its classification? Remember: drugs with generic names that end in "-pril" are ACE inhibitors.

239. The answer is d. (*Brunton, pp 959–960; Katzung, pp 572–573.*) Ezetimibe inhibits absorption of dietary cholesterol through the gut. It has no hepatic or other direct effects that contribute to its clinically desired effect. The drug lacks cardiac effects (a) or vascular effects (b). There is no good evidence that ezetimibe increases the risks of plaque rupture, and the subsequent and often devastating consequences of that. Other lipid-lowering drugs, such as niacin, the fibrates, and perhaps some of the cholesterol-binding resins, seem to increase the risks of statin-induced myopathy, rhabdomyolysis, or liver dysfunction. Such increased risks are the major problems to be faced when statins are used in combination of other lipid-lowering agents. However, this seems not to be a problem with ezetimibe. It is a rational drug to combine with a statin, and one proprietary fixed-dose combination that contains ezetimibe and a statin is available and quite widely used.

240. The answer is e. *(Brunton, pp 831–841, 1480–1481; Craig, pp 263–265; Katzung, pp 572–574.)* "Time is muscle," some say. It is true that choosing alteplase (a) or some other t-PA variant may be associated with a lower risk of bleeding, owing to their clot-specific site of action; and that it is *relatively* safer to use them with heparin. In contrast, streptokinase administration once may lead to antibodies that, if the patient is retreated with the same drug (within about 5 days to 2 years), may either or both neutralize the drug (rendering it ineffective) or trigger an allergic reaction. However, we stated this was our patient's first MI. (You could argue that the patient may already have anti-SK antibodies from a prior *strep* infection, but you didn't think of that, did you?)

The key point, then, is starting thrombolysis as quickly as possible, not which drug is chosen. There seems to be maximum benefit (salvaging tissue, reducing ultimate infarct size, maintaining reasonable cardiac function, and reducing mortality) if a thrombolytic—any thrombolytic—is administered within 1 hr of symptom onset. According to many studies, benefits of thrombolysis become comparable to placebo if the drug isn't started until around 6 hours after symptom onset, and in terms of mortality thrombolytics may actually increase the risk of death if not given after about 12 hours or so.

241. The answer is e. *(Brunton, pp 825–827, 829; Craig, pp 197–200; Katzung, pp 184–189.)* In excess, this "anti-ischemic" drug, which may be lifesaving, can cause myocardial ischemia sufficient to hasten (if not directly cause) death. Remember that ischemia (of any organ) is an imbalance between myocardial oxygen supply and demand. The primary "driving force" that provides the "demand side" of the equation is blood pressure, and for the heart that is diastolic blood pressure. Nitroglycerin and other organic nitrovasodilators cause dose-dependent and generalized vasodilation. At therapeutic doses, there is not a sufficient fall of blood pressure to compromise coronary perfusion; simultaneously, reducing arterial pressure just a little lowers the oxygen demand of the heart (less contractile force need be generated to eject blood during systole). As nitroglycerin blood levels go up and up, as we described for our patient, blood pressure (and, so, diastolic perfusion pressure) fall, ultimately to a point where blood can no longer be driven through coronary vessels. And if those vessels are already stenotic, the effects of reduced pressure on perfusion will become dangerous even at blood pressure capable of perfusing patent vessels.

Nitroglycerin does not cause bronchoconstriction (a) or seizures (b). It is not likely to cause stroke from hypertension (c; remember, this drug lowers blood pressure). It does not provoke coronary vasospasm (d).

Note: Some students have stated that seizures are the main cause of death, and specifically say that is due to the accumulation of cyanide arising from nitroglycerin's metabolism. While nitroprusside indeed is metabolized to cyanide (the nitroprusside molecule is bristling with cyanide groups), nitroglycerin and such related drugs as isosorbide mononitrate or dinitrate neither contain nor are metabolized to cyanide.

242. The answer is c. (*Brunton, pp 254, 269–270; Craig, pp 104–105; Katzung, pp 115, 133–134, 142, 145–148, 1070t, 1071.*) Phenylephrine, as noted, causes vasoconstriction through its agonist activity on α-adrenergic receptors. Prazosin competitively blocks those receptors, and since we have a patient who has taken an excessive dose of the antagonist it should be no surprise that usually effective (or even higher) doses of phenylephrine will not be able to overcome that blockade. None of the other drugs listed have any direct effects on an α-adrenergic receptors, nor the ability of phenylephrine to activate them. (Thiazides probably exert their antihypertensive effects by causing some net sodium depletion, which reduces vascular responsiveness to adrenergic agonists, angiotensin II, and any other vasoconstrictors you may conjure. However, it is highly unlikely that a thiazide would completely eliminate any vasopressor effects of a usual dose of phenylephrine—let alone repeated doses.)

243. The answer is e. (*Brunton, pp 269–271; Craig, pp 94, 111–113, 231–232; Katzung, pp 144t, 145, 147–148, 172.*) This is an apt description of an α-adrenergic blocker, and not at all descriptive of the actions or effects of any other drug listed. Prazosin can be considered the prototype of the α-adrenergic blockers, at least those that selectively block α_1 receptors (in comparison with phentolamine and several other drugs, which block both α_1 and α_2 receptors). It's not likely your patient was taking prazosin itself (or a related drug like doxazosin or terazosin). That is because those drugs not only exert significant inhibitory effects on smooth muscle of the prostate capsule and urethra, but also on the peripheral vasculature. They could be (and sometimes are) used for benign prostatic hypertrophy. If the patient is also hypertensive, one drug may help both conditions. If blood pressure is normal, or controlled well with other antihypertensives, then prazosin or doxazosin may lower pressure too much (unless we change dosages or drugs). More likely your patient is taking tamsulosin. It's clearly in the same class as prazosin, but seems to have more selectivity for smooth muscles in the urinary tract, and fewer or milder peripheral vascular actions that would tend to lower blood pressure and trigger the other responses we noted.

244. The answer is e. *(Brunton, p 809; Craig, pp 210–212; Katzung, pp 177–179, 209.)* ACE inhibitors (and angiotensin receptor blockers, ARBs, e.g., losartan) are contraindicated in women who are pregnant or of child-bearing potential. ACE inhibitors and ARBs do not exacerbate asthma (a); they are considered first-line adjunctive drugs for managing most patients with heart failure (b), which may or may not be an accompaniment of hyperlipidemias or coronary artery disease (c). We might want to normalize serum potassium levels if the patient were hypokalemic (d; it depends on what the absolute serum potassium levels are, and whether the hypokalemia is symptomatic), before we gave an ACE inhibitor, but one would want to be very careful in terms of how to go about doing that. ACE inhibitors and ARBs ultimately lower circulating aldosterone levels, which in turn favors more renal potassium retention. One of these drugs, alone, might correct serum potassium levels. Giving an ACE inhibitor or ARB along with a potassium-sparing diuretic may not merely correct the hypokalemia but, eventually and more likely, cause hyperkalemia.

245. The answer is a. *(Brunton, pp 192, 197; Craig, p 136; Katzung, p 151.)* Sinus bradycardia can be conceptually viewed as an imbalance of two opposing factors on the SA node: (a) too great an influence of the parasympathetic nervous, specifically, of ACh acting on muscarinic receptors; or (b) too little activation of β_1 adrenergic receptors. We can take either, or both, approaches pharmacologically. Of the answer choices given, we went with atropine to block excessive parasympathetic influences, and heart rate should go up. Amiodarone (b) is neither effective nor indicated for sinus bradycardia. It is used as a first-line drug for cardiac arrest; is indicated for managing some serious and life-threatening ventricular arrhythmias; and has gotten growing attention for its apparent efficacy to manage atrial fibrillation—a rather unusual use given the seriousness of the other arrhythmias for which the drug is given. Edrophonium (c) would be among the worse drugs you could give to this bradycardic patient. This rapidly acting ACh esterase inhibitor will cause accumulation of even more ACh at the SA node and elsewhere in the autonomic nervous system where ACh is the neurotransmitter activating smooth muscles and various exocrine glands. If the patient's heart doesn't stop in response to edrophonium, assuming we give a usual dose, it is mere luck. Lidocaine (d) is effective for a host of ventricular arrhythmias, including those associated with an MI. It will do nothing good for the bradycardia. You might argue that phentolamine (e), the prototype α-adrenergic blocker, would work. It might, but probably at great cost to this patient's hemodynamic status. When we inject "usual" doses of phentolamine heart rate indeed goes up. That is mediated by the baroreceptor reflex: we have given enough drug to rapidly and markedly drop blood pressure *via* the drug's vasodilator actions. That, in turn, "withdraws" central parasympathetic tone and causes a relative increase in sympathetic outflow. Both effects would increase heart rate. Unfortunately, our bradycardic patient probably already has a blood pressure and cardiac output that are on the low side of conducive to a long and happy life. Even if he didn't, causing blood pressure to promptly and markedly fall often doesn't lead to a favorable outcome.

246. The answer is c. (*Brunton, pp 1468f, 1483; Craig, p 263; Katzung, p 555.*) Abciximab, and such related drugs as tirofiban and eptifibatide, block the glycoprotein IIb/IIIa receptor on platelets. Abciximab is an antibody raised against the IIb/IIIa receptor. It binds to the receptor, and in doing so blocks the formation of fibrinogen bridges between the IIb/IIIa receptors on adjacent platelets. That is, otherwise, the final critical step in causing platelets to aggregate with their neighbors.

It is also noteworthy that platelet activation can be triggered by thromboxane A_2, thrombin, collagen, ADP, and platelet-activating factor (PAF) (among other agonists). Block the activating effects of just one of those factors (e.g., those of ADP with clopidogrel), and the proaggregatory effects of the other activators are left unchecked. Platelet activation ensues; some platelet-derived activators are released, thereby recruiting the activation of more platelets—the amplification process.

Abciximab, in contrast, blocks the "final step" in aggregation, regardless of the presence or absence of influences from "upstream" activators.

247. The answer is b. *(Brunton, pp 161–162, 173–174, 474, 856–857; Craig, pp 89–92, 94; Katzung, pp 81–90.)* Reserpine blocks NE entry into the intraneuronal storage vesicles, rendering the neurotransmitter vulnerable to inactivation by MAO. Ultimately, neuronal NE stores are depleted. Physiologic activation of postsynaptic structures by adrenergic nerves depends on NE release, and in reserpine-treated individuals the amount of NE available for release is diminished. It appears, then, as if the overall activity of the sympathetic nervous system has been "ratcheted down"—and normally opposing parasympathetic influences become unmasked and predominate, causing such responses as excessive salivation, lacrimation (and secretions from other exocrine glands), constipation, and urinary frequency or incontinence: precisely the opposite of what is described in answer c.

Catecholamine (i.e., NE) depletion in adrenergic nerves, as caused by reserpine, does not drive the metabolism of the neurotransmitter on to form EPI, the primary catecholamine hormone in the adrenal/suprarenal medulla.

We should note that concomitant with NE depletion and reduced physiologic stimulation of adrenergic receptors (due to diminished NE release, for example; or due to long-lasting adrenergic receptor blockade), the postsynaptic adrenergic receptors become supersensitive (not subsensitive; e). Those receptors will have heightened responses (in terms of intensity) to a given dose of an exogenous α or β agonist.

248. The answer is b. *(Brunton, pp 828–829; Craig, pp 197–200; Katzung, pp 190–191.)* Using long-acting nitrovasodilators "24-7" is not at all a good idea, because it ultimately leads to tolerance to the desired vasodilator effects. This is of concern in part because, by definition, when a system or function develops tolerance to a drug, we must increase the dose in order to achieve effects of the same intensity as occurred before. With nitroglycerin patches, or other long-acting nitrovasodilators, increasing the dose to restore the response ultimately accelerates or otherwise intensifies the tolerance, such that further dosage increases seem warranted. More importantly, with the development of tolerance, the vasodilator/antianginal efficacy of sublingual (or transmucosal) nitrate is diminished too. So, should the patient develop angina, usual dosages of immediate-acting drugs may not provide relief of either the symptoms or the underlying myocardial ischemia.

If you thought cyanide poisoning (a) you were probably thinking of nitroprusside toxicity. Cyanide is not a metabolite of nitroglycerin or other drugs traditionally used for angina. Doses of nitrates that are too high, or that otherwise lower peripheral resistance too quickly, may trigger reflex tachycardia. This is, for some patients, a problem early on in therapy with rapidly acting nitrates. It usually becomes less problematic as therapy continues, of if the dosage is titrated down a bit. It is rarely a problem with long-acting nitrates. We do not see bradycardia (c), reflex or otherwise, in response to these drugs. Nitrovasodilators, short- or long-acting, and regardless of the administration route, do not cause thrombosis or affect any other aspects of the coagulation-thrombolysis processes (d). Paradoxical vasoconstriction leading to hypertension (e) does not occur.

249. The answer is e. *(Brunton, pp 143t, 272–275, 824–826, 837–840; Craig, pp 200–203; Katzung, pp 148–151, 197–198.)* In terms of autonomic control of coronary vascular tone, envisage a "balance" between the vasoconstrictor influences of α-adrenergic activation and the opposing vasodilator influences of β-receptor activation. Spasm-prone coronaries appear to be very dependent on the β-mediated vasodilator influences to reduce the incidence and severity of spasm. Any β blocker will remove those favorable influences, and tend to provoke (or intensify or prolong) spasm and the resulting ischemia in distal tissues. This vascular effect is likely to overshadow any beneficial effects attributed to reductions of myocardial oxygen demand via suppression of heart rate and contractility.

You could correctly argue that in the absence of demonstrated coronary occlusion the administration of t-PA (a) would be inappropriate. However, that drug is not likely to make matters worse. Captopril (c), the prototype ACE inhibitor, should have no negative or positive effects on vasospasm. Nitroglycerin (d) might reduce the incidence or severity of spasm through nitric-oxide-mediated vasodilation. Verapamil (f) would probably be one of the most rational drugs to give, since its vascular calcium channel blocking activity would help suppress spasm; its negative inotropic and chronotropic effects would, additionally, reduce myocardial oxygen demand and be beneficial.

250. The answer is b. *(Brunton, pp 688, 1482; Craig, pp 262–263, 428–429; Katzung, pp 298–305, 553–555, 578–582.)* That aspirin might increase the risk of stroke should not be surprising. The same mechanism, by which the drug exerts protective effects against MI, by inhibiting platelet aggregation, explains why some patients who otherwise might develop a cerebral bleed are at increased risk of doing so. There is no good evidence that aspirin ingestion causes hepatotoxicity of any sort (a); tachycardia and/or hypotension (d; other than via blood loss and hypovolemia due to excessive bleeding); nor causes or provokes coronary vasospasm (e). Long-term use of many nonsteroidal anti-inflammatory drugs may cause nephropathy, but that is typically associated with high-dose use, and rarely with aspirin itself.

251. The answer is d. (*Brunton, pp 797–798, 809; Craig, pp 210–212, 214, 246–248; Katzung, pp 209, 246–252, 281–294.*) The patient has been taking two diuretics, one potassium-wasting (the thiazide), the other potassium-sparing. Ramipril is an ACE inhibitor (recall: drugs with generic names ending in "-pril" are members of that class) that ultimately will lower serum aldosterone levels. This will, in essence, counteract the sodium-retaining effects of aldosterone, and also its potassium-wasting effects. So by adding the ACE inhibitor to the regimen we will now be treating the patient with two drugs that tend to elevate serum potassium levels to a degree that cannot be compensated for by the thiazide.

Adding an ACE inhibitor to our patient's regimen would be a good idea (provided there are no contraindications to doing so) in terms of getting additional blood pressure control, but it would probably require eliminating the triamterene at some point (if not from the start) to avoid the hyperkalemia.

Prazosin (b), a selective α_1-adrenergic blocker, is not at all likely to have elicited the hyperkalemia. Diltiazem (a) and verapamil (e), both nondihydropyridine calcium channel blockers, are not likely to affect serum potassium levels in a measurable way. (β-adrenergic blockers (e.g., propranolol, c) have been reported to lower serum potassium levels, presumably by enhancing K^+ uptake into skeletal muscle. These drugs are not, therefore, a likely cause of the hypokalemia, even when used in combination with the diuretics.

252. The answer is c. (*Brunton, pp 242, 254, 263–264; Craig, pp 100–102; Katzung, pp 133–134, 136–138, 148.*) Phenylephrine is the prototypic α-adrenergic agonist. It terminated the arrhythmia reflexly, via the baroreceptors, in response to a vasopressor effect. (Raising blood pressure quickly and markedly is a risky way of terminating this tachycardia, of course, due to such risks as causing a hemorrhagic stroke.) All the other drugs would also terminate the arrhythmia, but by actions in the heart. Edrophonium (a) is an ACh esterase inhibitor with a fast onset of action and a brief duration. It would slow heart rate by increasing the effects of ACh on the SA node, slowing the spontaneous rate of phase 4 depolarization. Esmolol is a β blocker (nonselective) that also has a fast onset and short duration of action. It and propranolol (d) would slow heart rate via the direct β-blocking effects on the SA node. Verapamil (e) will do the same by blocking AV nodal calcium channels.

253. The answer is b. *(Brunton, pp 912, 921–922; Craig, pp 152–154, 192; Katzung, pp 206–208.)* Answering this question, of course, requires that you not only know the expected effects of digoxin, but also that you can "translate" those effects into interpretations of findings from a most useful diagnostic tool, the electrocardiogram.

An expected and important effect of digoxin is slowed atrioventricular nodal conduction velocity, manifest as prolongation of the P-R interval. The effect, which can lead to increasing degrees of heart block, depends on the serum concentration of digoxin and on serum concentrations of several ions, potassium arguably the most important.

Digoxin tends to speed electrical impulse velocity through the atrial myocardium, and so widening of P waves (a) would be the opposite of the expected response. There is no good reason to expect increased P-wave amplitude due to the digoxin. (Atrial enlargement, a result of the heart failure and not the drug, is likely.)

Digoxin also speeds electrical impulse conduction velocity through the ventricles (e.g., the His-Purkinje system), and so widened QRS complexes, compared with baseline, would be counter to the expected effect.

R-R intervals essentially reflect ventricular rate. Before treatment of heart failure there are varying degrees of compensatory "sympathetic drive" over the heart, leading to tachycardia and shortened R-R intervals (d). Once digoxin starts increasing cardiac output, there is a lessening of sympathetic drive (and the physiologic need for it). Thus, compared with baseline heart rate, posttreatment heart rate is slower; this is manifest as a longer R-R interval compared with baseline.

S-T segment changes are among the manifestations of acute coronary syndrome and regional myocardial ischemia. Based on the description of the patient, who appears to have normal blood profiles and no evidence of acute ischemia, S-T elevation (e) is not a reasonable answer.

254. The answer is a. *(Brunton, pp 308–311; Katzung, pp 276–278.)* Although ergotamine and the ergot alkaloids in general, may not be considered typical cardiovascular drugs, they clearly can cause significant, cumulative, and sometimes dangerous cardiovascular effects. Ergotamine can cause intense and prolonged vasoconstriction in both the peripheral and coronary vasculatures. Thus, of the answer choices given myocardial ischemia and ischemia of, for example, one or more extremities are the most likely outcomes. These vascular responses pose particular problems for patients with ischemic heart disease, especially those who have vasospastic, or variant, angina; or patients with peripheral vascular disease. (One ergot alkaloid, ergonovine, is such a powerful coronary vasoconstrictor that it is sometimes used in angiographic studies of the heart to diagnose vasospastic angina.) The coronary effects may be rapidly fatal; limb ischemia may be sufficiently intense and prolonged to induce gangrene and require amputation of the affected limb(s). Rhabdomyolysis, with or without renal failure (b) is unlikely, at least as a direct consequence of ergotamine, as the ergot compounds in general have no appreciable effects on skeletal muscle structure or function. There are no direct effects on platelet activation or aggregation that would lead to spontaneous bleeding (c); however, platelet activation and thrombotic events certainly may occur secondary to stasis in vascular beds that have been intensely constricted by the drug. Hypertension, not hypotension with or without syncope (d), is a likely consequence of peripheral vasoconstriction. Sudden rises in blood pressure are likely to cause bradycardia (not tachycardia, e) *via* baroreceptor reflex activation. Members of the ergot alkaloid class (e.g., ergotamine, ergonovine) have variable agonist or antagonist effects (direct or indirect) on α-adrenergic, dopaminergic, and serotoninergic receptors), but not on β-adrenergic receptors.

(For study purposes in other areas of pharmacology you may want to recall the following: (1) Triptans [e.g., sumatriptan] or methysergide tend to be used more than ergotamine or similar drugs for migraine. (2) Ergonovine is sometimes used as an alternative or back-up to oxytocin for controlling postpartum uterine bleeding or hemorrhage: it causes intense and prolonged uterine smooth muscle contraction, and relatively slight cardiovascular effects. (3) Another ergot drug, bromocriptine, is used to manage hyperprolactinemia [due to its strong dopaminergic effects] such as that which may occur with pituitary tumors, and is also sometimes used for managing Parkinson's disease.)

255. The answer is e. (*Brunton, pp 143t, 164, 269–270; Craig, p 232; Katzung, pp 146–147, 147i.*) Pheochromocytomas are epinephrine-secreting tumors, and so the worrisome and dangerous consequences are due to excessive vasoconstriction (α-mediated) and cardiac chronotropic and inotropic responses (β_1). A β-adrenergic blocker is an essential component of pharmacotherapy. It must be administered along with another drug that blocks α-adrenergic receptors, but should not be given before the α-adrenergic blocker is given. Activation of β_2 adrenergic receptors in the peripheral vasculature plays a small but important role in blood pressure control (since β_2 activation in some vascular beds causes vasodilation). Block that effect in a patient with epinephrine excess—a pheochromocytoma—and any potentially blood pressure-lowering effects are lost. Blood pressure will, therefore, either rise or stay the same in terms of peripheral vascular effects.

In the face of this still high blood pressure and total peripheral resistance the β blocker will reduce both heart rate and contractility, and so cardiac output will fall (recall that $CO = HR \times SV$). The outcome may be not merely a fall of cardiac output, but a considerable fall in a very short time that might well put the patient into acute heart failure.

Blood pressure is not at all likely to fall promptly due to any peripheral vasodilator effects; if it did (and it won't), the β blocker would prevent reflex tachycardia (a) via direct actions on cardiac β_1 receptors. The β blockers do not inhibit catecholamine release (b), whether from a catecholamine-secreting tumor or from a normal sympathetic nervous system. A β blocker will not trigger catecholamine release from a pheochromocytoma (c), nor will it normalize cardiovascular status in any other way if given without an α blocker. A β blocker alone, in this situation, will raise left ventricular afterload, and reduce cardiac output by effects on both heart rate and stroke volume. Thus, answer e is wrong.

256. The answer is d. (*Brunton, pp 830–832; Craig, pp 197–199; Katzung, pp 186–190.*) Nitroglycerin and other nitrovasodilators provide immediate symptom relief in most patients with an acute coronary syndrome or MI. However, there is no evidence that these drugs provide long-term preventative effects against sudden death from an acute MI. In contrast, aspirin (a; antiplatelet drug), a lipid-lowering drug such as atorvastatin (b), ACE inhibitors such as captopril (c), and β blockers such as propranolol (e), have documented protective effects to reduce the risk of death from a subsequent MI.

257. The answer is a. (*Brunton, pp 250–251, 889–894; Craig, pp 105, 108; Katzung, pp 133–135, 209.*) Intravenous infusion of dobutamine, a β_1 agonist, was the most likely cause of the increased heart rate. Blood pressure probably rose secondary to a positive inotropic effect of the drug, rather than by any direct peripheral vasoconstrictor activity. Esmolol (b) is a nonselective β blocker with a rapid onset of action, and a brief duration of action (due to rapid hydrolysis by plasma esterases. Being a β blocker, neither it nor propranolol (d) would raise heart rate or blood pressure. Neostigmine (c) is an ACh esterase inhibitor. It and verapamil (e), a nondihydropyridine calcium channel blocker, would be expected to reduce heart rate. Verapamil would also tend to lower, not raise, blood pressure by virtue of its peripheral vasodilator action.

258. The answer is b. (*Brunton, pp 655, 657–658, 660, 1470, 1482; Craig, pp 262–263, 425–428; Katzung, pp 554–555, 580, 581t.*) At the usual low cardioprotective doses of aspirin, the main effect of the drug is rather selective inhibition of thromboxane A2 (TXA$_2$) synthesis via the COX-1 pathway. Recall that TXA$_2$ is a major—but not the only—trigger of platelet activation, amplification, and aggregation. However, at high(er) doses, aspirin also inhibits synthesis of other eicosanoids, of which PGI$_2$ (prostacyclin), synthesized in the vascular endothelium, is of most importance here. Endothelial prostacyclin synthesis helps prevent platelets from adhering to the vascular wall. Suppress PGI$_2$ in the endothelium, and platelet adherence is increased, despite the fact that platelet TXA$_2$ synthesis has already been blocked. It's important to remember here that aspirin does nothing to inhibit platelet activation by such other agonists as collagen or ADP. By lowering endothelial PGI$_2$ levels we've increased the likelihood that platelets activated by eicosanoid-independent agonists will adhere to the lining of blood vessels, and potentially occlude them.

Aspirin has no effect on Gp IIb/IIIa receptors (a); it does not rupture or otherwise damage vascular plaques (c) to expose collagen; inhibit synthesis of any liver-based clotting factors (d); or amplify or otherwise enhance the effects of ADP (e) or of other platelet activators.

259. The answer is d. (*Brunton, pp 264–269, 851–852; Craig, pp 111–112, 231; Katzung, pp 145, 172–173.*) Prazosin causes competitive α blockade. This is in stark contrast with phenoxybenzamine, which causes insurmountable (noncompetitive) and long-lasting blockade of α receptors by alkylating them. Phenoxybenzamine is chemically classified as a haloalkylamine. You probably don't need to remember that, but perhaps it will help you realize that the drug alkylates the α-adrenergic receptors. This covalent interaction, in comparison with typical weak ionic interactions between most drugs and their receptors, accounts for phenoxybenzamine's long-lasting (not shorter-acting; a) and noncompetitive blockade. As a result of altering receptor confirmation, not merely occupying them as prazosin and most other α blockers do, phenoxybenzamine renders largely ineffective α agonists that ordinarily would be used to counteract effects of excessive receptor blockade. Thus, if the patient became hypotensive in response to phenoxybenzamine, raising pressure with typical and usually effective drugs may not succeed. Neither drug has intrinsic β-blocking activity (b), and so regardless of which of these drugs we use for the pheochromocytoma patient, a β blocker will need to be used adjunctively to control (primarily) heart rate and contractility. Neither drug suppresses epinephrine release from the adrenal/suprarenal medulla (c); both tend to cause orthostatic hypotension by blocking peripheral α-mediated vasoconstriction that occurs upon standing up suddenly.

260. The answer is e. (*Brunton, pp 272–275, 864; Craig, pp 230–231; Katzung, p 175.*) Nitroprusside is likely to elicit baroreceptor reflex-mediated rises of heart rate and contractility. It may be significant and dangerous for any patient, more so for patients with ischemic heart disease, and potentially deadly for patients with aneurysms, such as our patient. For aortic aneurysm patients, the problem is not the rise of heart rate, but rather of left ventricular contractility (left ventricular dP/dt). The bounding aortic pressure pulse with each systole favors rupture of the aneurysm, and use of a β blocker such as propranolol is an effective and common way to minimize the risk (and, of course, reflex cardiac stimulation overall). Atropine (a) is an illogical choice. It will increase heart rate (and, indirectly, contractility) further by removing parasympathetic tone on the SA node. Diazoxide (b) is a rapidly acting antihypertensive/vasodilator, given as an IV bolus in situations where safe nitroprusside use (and the invasive monitoring it normally requires) is not practical. Diazoxide, like nitroprusside, triggers reflex cardiac stimulation as blood pressure falls. The drug also has some direct cardiac-stimulating effects (not involving antimuscarinic or adrenergic-agonist effects). Diazoxide also tends to cause hyperglycemia (an oral dosage form of the drug is sometimes prescribed to manage blood glucose levels in patients prone to developing hypoglycemia.) Furosemide (c) is a loop diuretic that is an important adjunct in such conditions as hypertensive crisis due to volume overload, heart failure, and acute pulmonary edema. However, the volume depletion and hypotension it would cause would exacerbate the clinical situation we have described. The prompt diuresis and fall of blood pressure may also trigger unwanted baroreceptor-mediated cardiac stimulation. Phentolamine (d), an α-adrenergic blocker, would be irrational. It is a powerful vasodilator (indeed, it is often used for vasoconstrictor drug-induced hypertensive emergencies) that would add to—unfavorably—nitroprusside's prompt antihypertensive effect and the reflex cardiac stimulation that is so dangerous for our patient.

The Renal System and Diuretics

Carbonic anhydrase inhibitors
Loop ("high-ceiling") diuretics
Osmotic diuretics

Potassium (K^+)-sparing diuretics
Thiazide diuretics (benzothiadiazides)

Questions

DIRECTIONS: Each item contains a question or incomplete statement that is followed by several responses. Select the **one best** response to each question.

261. Diuretic-induced hypokalemia can have clinically significant consequences, and so it's important to know which diuretics are potassium-wasting and which spare (reduce net renal excretion of) potassium, because potassium-sparing diuretics play an important role in preventing hypokalemia or treating asymptomatic deficiencies of this cation. Which of the following is classified as potassium-sparing?

a. Amiloride
b. Bumetanide
c. Hydrochlorothiazide
d. Metolazone
e. Torsemide

262. We have a patient with heart failure, unacceptably low cardiac output, and intense reflex-mediated sympathetic activation of the peripheral vasculature that is attempting to keep vital organ perfusion pressure sufficiently high. The patient is edematous, and has ascites, because of the poor cardiac function and renal compensations for it. Which one of the following drugs should be *avoided* in this patient because it is most likely to compromise function of the already failing heart and the circulatory system overall?

a. Amiloride
b. Ethacrynic acid
c. Hydrochlorothiazide
d. Mannitol
e. Spironolactone

263. One of your clinic patients is being treated with spironolactone. Which of the following statements best describes a property of this drug?

a. Contraindicated in heart failure, especially if severe
b. Inhibits Na^+ reabsorption in the proximal renal tubule of the nephron
c. Interferes with aldosterone synthesis
d. Is a rational choice for a patient with an adrenal cortical tumor
e. Is more efficacious than hydrochlorothiazide in all patients who receive the drug

264. A patient taking an oral diuretic for about 6 months presents with elevated fasting and postprandial blood glucose levels. You check the patient's HbA_{1c} and find it is elevated compared with normal baseline values obtained 6 months ago. You suspect the glycemic problems are diuretic-induced. Which of the following was the most likely cause?

a. Acetazolamide
b. Amiloride
c. Chlorothiazide
d. Spironolactone
e. Triamterene

265. Chlorthalidone and torsemide are members of different diuretic classes, in terms of mechanisms of action, but they share the ability to cause hypokalemia. Which of the following statements best describes the general mechanism by which these drugs cause their effects that lead to net renal loss of potassium?

a. Act as aldosterone receptor agonists, thereby favoring K^+ loss
b. Block proximal tubular ATP-dependent secretory pumps for K^+
c. Increase delivery of Na^+ to principal cells in the distal nephron, where tubular Na^+ is transported into the cells via a sodium channel in exchange for K^+, which gets eliminated in the urine
d. Inhibit a proximal tubular Na,K-ATPase such that K^+ is actively pumped into the urine
e. Lower distal tubular urine osmolality, thereby favoring passive diffusion of K^+ into the urine

266. A patient was in a recumbent position for a 45-minute dental procedure. When the procedure was completed she stood up quickly and promptly got light-headed and fainted. The cause was hypotension due to hypovolemia from excessive diuresis, attributed to a drug prescribed by her physician and taken for several months. Which of the following was the *most likely* cause?

a. Acetazolamide
b. Furosemide
c. Hydrochlorothiazide
d. Spironolactone
e. Triamterene

267. A 52-year-old man presents to your clinic for his first visit with you, after moving from a distant town. His only medications are a statin, aspirin (81 mg/day) and metolazone. The pharmacist who filled his prescriptions told the gentleman why he was taking the aspirin and the statin, but unfortunately referred to the metolazone as a "water pill." Thus, you're asked about it. Assuming proper prescribing, which of the following is the most likely reason why the metolazone was prescribed?

a. Adjunctive management of an adrenal cortical tumor
b. Adjunctive management of hepatic cirrhosis from years of excessive alcohol consumption
c. Hypertension accompanied by a history of gout and diabetes
d. Treatment of essential hypertension
e. Treatment of edema and ascites from heart failure

268. Urinary potassium concentrations are measured before and after several weeks of administering a loop diuretic (typical daily dosages). We find that posttreatment urine K^+ concentrations are substantially lower than those measured at baseline. Which of the following is the most likely explanation for this observation?

a. An expected response to the drug
b. Loop diuretics cause potassium-wasting only in *in vitro* experimental models
c. Measurements of posttreatment urine K^+ concentrations were erroneous
d. The patient has hypoaldosteronism from bilateral adrenalectomy
e. The patient has significantly impaired renal function

269. A patient has very high serum uric acid levels, has had two acute gout attacks, and is at imminent risk of developing acute uric acid nephropathy. We will treat the patient with proper anti-inflammatory drugs and other agents, but feel that reducing solubility of uric acid in the urine, by raising urine pH, might help stave-off the development of renal problems. Which of the following drugs produce this desired renal effect without appreciably increasing systemic risks of the hyperuricemia?

a. Acetazolamide
b. Antidiuretic hormone (ADH) (vasopressin [VP])
c. Ethacrynic acid
d. Furosemide
e. Hydrochlorothiazide

270. A 58-year-old man with a history of hypertension and hypercholesterolemia is diagnosed with heart failure. We start therapy with a loop diuretic. Which of the following would you expect to occur along with the increased urine volume caused by the diuretic?

a. Dilute (hypotonic) urine because normal urine concentrating mechanisms are impaired
b. Hypercalcemia due to impaired renal Ca^{2+} excretion
c. Reduced net excretion of Cl^-
d. Metabolic acidosis due to increased renal bicarbonate excretion
e. Reduced serum uric acid (urate) concentrations because of increased urate excretion

271. A patient with mild heart failure and edema fails to respond adequately to maximum recommended dosages of chlorthalidone. Which of the following is the most likely appropriate and most fruitful next step in terms of restoring the diuretic response?

a. Add hydrochlorothiazide
b. Add metolazone
c. Replace chlorthalidone with furosemide
d. Replace chlorthalidone with hydrochlorothiazide
e. Try increasing the chlorthalidone dose anyway

272. A hypertensive patient has been on long-term therapy with lisinopril for hypertension. The drug isn't controlling pressure as well as wanted, so the physician decides to add triamterene as the (only) second drug. Which of the following is the most likely outcome of adding this diuretic to the ACE inhibitor regimen?

a. Blood pressure would rise abruptly
b. Better BP control, but with a risk of hyperkalemia
c. Cardiac depression, because both drugs directly depress the heart
d. Cough that may be severe, even though there was no cough with lisinopril alone
e. Hypernatremia, because ACE inhibitors counteract triamterene's natriuretic effect

273. Package inserts for a drug caution against administering the medication concurrent with any other drug that can raise or lower serum sodium concentrations. The risks are inadequate or excessive effects of the drug, depending on the direction in which serum sodium concentrations change. This, of course, requires cautious use or avoidance (if possible) of the common diuretics. To which of the following drugs does this caution or warning most likely apply?

a. Cholestyramine
b. Lithium
c. Nifedipine
d. Phenylephrine
e. Statin-type cholesterol-lowering drugs

274. Your patient, who lives in Death Valley, California (altitude 240 feet below sea level), is planning a vacation that includes a short hike to the top of Mount Everest (altitude approx. 29,000 feet above sea level). You're concerned about "altitude sickness." He has no other significant medical conditions, and takes no other drugs that would interact with the drug you will prescribe for his trip. Which of the following drugs would you recommend that this adventurer start taking before his trek, and continue until he returns to an altitude much closer to sea level?

a. Acetazolamide
b. Amiloride
c. Bumetanide
d. Furosemide
e. Spironolactone
f. Triamterene

275. A patient with heart failure has been managed with digoxin and furosemide and is doing well by all measures, for 3 years. He develops acute rheumatoid arthritis and is placed on rather large doses of a very efficacious nonsteroidal anti-inflammatory drug—one that inhibits both cyclooxygenase pathways (COX-1 and -2). Which of the following is the most likely outcome of adding the NSAID?

a. Hyperchloremic acidosis indicative of acute diuretic toxicity
b. Dramatic increase of furosemide's potassium-sparing effects
c. Edema, weight gain, and other signs/symptoms indicative of reduced diuresis
d. Increased digoxin excretion
e. Reduced digoxin effects because the NSAID competes with digoxin for myocyte receptor-binding sites

276. A patient presents with chronic open angle glaucoma. Which of the following "renal" drugs might be prescribed as an adjunct to lower intraocular pressure and help manage his condition?

a. Acetazolamide
b. Amiloride
c. Furosemide
d. Spironolactone
e. Triamterene

277. Furosemide's main mechanism of action involves inhibition of a Na^+, K^+, $2Cl^-$ cotransporter. In which part of the nephron is this cotransporter located?

a. Ascending limb, loop of Henle
b. Collecting duct
c. Descending limb, loop of Henle
d. Distal convoluted tubule
e. Proximal tubule

278. A patient with severe infectious disease is being treated with an aminoglycoside antibiotic. Which of the following diuretics should be avoided, if possible, for this patient, because of the risk of a serious common and additive adverse effect?

a. Acetazolamide
b. Furosemide
c. Metolazone
d. Spironolactone
e. Triamterene

279. We have a patient with a recently diagnosed adrenal cortical adenoma. Among the pertinent cushingoid signs and symptoms are hypertension and weight gain from fluid retention, and hypernatremia and hypokalemia. Which of the following drugs would be the most rational to prescribe, alone or adjunctively, to specifically antagonize both the renal and the systemic effects of the hormone excess?

a. Acetazolamide
b. Amiloride
c. Furosemide
d. Metolazone
e. Spironolactone

280. A patient has been referred to your academic medical center because of recent-onset ventricular ectopy, second degree AV nodal block, chromatopsia, and other extracardiac signs and symptoms of digoxin intoxication. His family doctor, who has been treating him for a host of common medical problems over the last 30 years, had prescribed furosemide and digoxin for this gentleman's heart failure. Blood tests show that serum digoxin levels are well within a normal range. We believe the problems are diuretic-induced. Which of the following does the diuretic most likely do to account for the digoxin toxicity?

a. Caused hypercalcemia
b. Caused hypokalemia
c. Caused hyponatremia
d. Displaced digoxin from tissue binding sites
e. Inhibited digoxin's metabolic elimination

281. A 48-year-old man develops acute heart failure as one consequence of septicemia. His medical history is well documented. Among other things, it reveals poorly controlled Type I diabetes mellitus, and a near-fatal allergic response, 10 years ago, to a sulfonamide antibiotic. The patient has now developed significant edema and ascites, among other important clinical findings, due to sepsis. We will administer appropriate antibiotics and cardiac inotropes, but also need to administer a diuretic to promptly reduce circulating fluid volume and hemodynamically "unload" the failing heart.

Which of the following diuretics would be most appropriate in terms of managing the hemodynamic problems and posing the lowest risk of altering blood glucose levels or eliciting a sulfonamide-related allergic reaction?

a. Ethacrynic acid
b. Furosemide
c. Hydrochlorothiazide
d. Mannitol
e. Metolazone

282. Amiloride is a useful drug for managing hypokalemia caused by other drugs. Which of the following statements best describes the mechanism by which amiloride causes its potassium-sparing effects?

a. Blocks the agonist effects of aldosterone with its renal tubular receptors
b. Blocks distal tubular sodium channels and, ultimately, Na^+-K^+ exchange
c. Hastens metabolic inactivation of aldosterone
d. Stimulates a proximal tubular Na,K-ATPase
e. Suppresses cortisol and aldosterone synthesis and release in the adrenal cortex

283. A patient with severe heart failure is in the ICU. His urine output is dangerously low. We begin an intravenous infusion of dopamine at a usual therapeutic dose and urine output rises quickly and dramatically. Which of the following is the most likely mechanism by which the dopamine causes this effect?

a. Blocked β-adrenergic receptors in the juxtaglomerular apparatus, thereby inhibiting renin release and susequent angiotensin-mediated aldosterone release from the adrenal cortex.
b. Directly inhibited a renal Na^+-K^+-$2Cl^-$ cotransporter in the loop of Henle.
c. Improved renal blood flow and glomerular filtration
d. Lowered the medullary-to-cortical osmotic gradient, such that normal urine concentrating mechanisms were impaired
e. Reduced the permeability of the ascendng limb, loop of Henle, and of the collecting ducts, to water

284. A patient has had recurrent episodes of symptomatic hyponatremia, and is at great risk of recurrences. He now requires administration of a diuretic. Which of the following diuretics is most likely to precipitate another recurrence of the hyponatremia, and so should be avoided for that reason?

a. Bumetanide
b. Ethacrynic acid
c. Furosemide
d. Hydrochlorothiazide
e. Torsemide

285. We have a patient with essential hypertension. He is being treated with hydrochlorothiazide and a calcium channel blocker, and is doing well. He also takes atorvastatin for hypercholesterolemia, and aspirin for pro-phylaxis of MI due to thrombosis.

He is now diagnosed with a seizure disorder. We begin therapy with one of the suitable anticonvulsants that, fortunately, does not alter the metabolism of any of the medications prescribed for his cardiovascular problems. We've also read that systemic administration of acetazolamide may prove to be a useful adjunct to the anticonvulsant therapy: the meta-bolic acidosis it causes may help suppress seizure development or spread. So, we start acetazolamide therapy too. Which of the following is the most likely outcome of adding the acetazolamide?

a. Excessive rises of serum sodium concentrations
b. Hypertensive crisis (antagonism of both antihypertensive drugs)
c. Hypokalemia via synergistic actions with the thiazide
d. Spontaneous bleeding (potentiation of aspirin's actions)
e. Sudden circulating volume expansion, onset of heart failure

286. The table shows the urinary electrolyte excretion patterns typical of various prototype diuretics. These are qualitative changes, and do not reflect the magnitude of the changes. They show whether excretion of an electrolyte (*net amount*) is increased or decreased; they do not reflect changes in urine *concentrations* of these substances.

Drug	Na⁺	K⁺	Ca²⁺	Mg²⁺	Cl⁻	HCO₃⁻
1.	↑	↑	↓	↑	↑	0/↑
2.	↑	↑	↑	↑	↑	0
3.	↑	↓	0	0	↑	↑
4.	↑	↑	0	0	↓	↑

↑, increased net loss into urine; ↓, decreased loss into urine; 0, no change; +/−, increased or decreased, largely dependent on dose.

Which of the following drugs causes effects most similar, if not identical, to unknown Drug 2?

a. Acetazolamide
b. Amiloride
c. Chlorthalidone
d. Furosemide
e. Hydrochlorothiazide

The Renal System and Diuretics

Answers

261. The answer is a. (*Brunton, 744t, 751, 755–756, 758–759, 761–763; Craig, pp 247–249; Katzung, pp 256–257.*) Amiloride is potassium-sparing. Its mechanism of action is largely similar to that of triamterene, and is aldosterone-independent. The other main potassium-sparing diuretic, spironolactone, causes natriuresis and potassium loss by blocking aldosterone receptors. All the others are potassium-wasting. Bumetanide (b) and torsemide (e) are loop diuretics. Hydrochlorothiazide (c) can be considered the prototype of the thiazides (benzothiadiazides); metolazone (d) is not, chemically, a thiazide, but it is thiazide-like in terms of its main actions and uses.

262. The answer is d. (*Brunton, pp 747–748; Craig, pp 250–251; Katzung, pp 252–253.*) Mannitol is an osmotic diuretic, the prototype of that small class of drugs (glycerin/glycerol is another somewhat noteworthy member of the group) with indications and potential side effects that are quite different from those of "typical" diuretics like the thiazides or loop agents. What happens when you inject (intravenously) this nonmetabolizable sugar, which has a structure similar to that of glucose and the same molecular weight? Initially, and until it is excreted by glomerular filtration, mannitol increases plasma osmolality. That, in turn, osmotically withdraws water from the extracellular space and, ultimately, from the parenchymal cells, and into the blood. If the patient has good renal function, renal blood flow and GFR rise, and the drug is eventually excreted. If he or she has adequate cardiac function, circulating that extra volume (up to a limit) is not a problem.

However, if the patient has a sufficiently low cardiac output to begin with, or renal perfusion is compromised, the increased blood volume and pressure may be such that the heart simply cannot handle the added work load. Indeed, in a futile attempt to circulate that additional volume and eject it against a higher afterload, the heart may fail acutely.

Amiloride (a), a potassium-wasting diuretic with relatively low efficacy in terms of its ability to increase urine volume, should have no adverse effects in this patient. The same applies to hydrochlorothiazide (c), which is potassium-wasting. Ethacrynic acid (b) is a loop diuretic. It is one of several loop agents we might choose to help "unload" this patient's ventricles, provided the patient isn't hypovolemic already. Spironolactone (e), a potassium-sparing aldosterone antagonist, might ultimately be prescribed for this patient, particularly if his heart failure worsens. Nonetheless, at this time it is not a drug we should avoid.

263. The answer is d. (*Brunton, pp 759–762; Craig, pp 247–248; Katzung, pp 250–252.*) Spironolactone is a potassium-sparing diuretic. Its active metabolite displaces aldosterone from aldosterone receptors in the collecting ducts. The drug is ineffective in the absence of aldosterone. (Recall that aldosterone normally causes renal Na^+ retention and K^+ loss. The effects of aldosterone are qualitatively the opposite: Na^+ loss, K^+ retention.)

Owing to the ability of spironolactone to counteract the effects of aldosterone, it is particularly suited for patients with primary or secondary hyperaldosteronism (e.g., adrenal cortical tumor or hepatic dysfunction, as might occur with long-term/high-dose alcohol consumption, respectively). There is abundant data that the drug is beneficial in heart failure and probably reduces morbidity in severe heart failure.

In addition to the potential for causing hyperkalemia (especially if combined with oral potassium supplements, which should not be done) and hyponatremia (overall risk is low), spironolactone may cause several other side effects. CNS side effects include lethargy, headache, drowsiness, and mental confusion. Other side effects that are fairly common arise from the drug's androgen receptor–blocking actions: gynecomastia (in men and women) and erectile dysfunction. It may also cause seborrhea, acne, and coarsening of body hair. (Paradoxically, the drug can cause hirsutism in some patients, but it is also used to manage hirsutism in others.)

264. The answer is c. (*Brunton, p 756; Craig, p 246; Katzung, p 250.*) Thiazides and thiazide-like diuretics (e.g., chlorthalidone, metolazone) may elevate blood glucose levels, impair glucose tolerance, and cause frank hyperglycemia. The loop diuretics may do the same.

Several mechanisms have been proposed to explain the effect: decreased release of insulin from the pancreas; increased glycogenolysis and decreased glucogenesis; a reduction in the conversion of proinsulin to insulin; and a reduced responsiveness of adipocyte and skeletal myocyte insulin receptor response to the hormone.

(You might recall that diazoxide [mainly used as a parenteral drug for prompt lowering of blood pressure] can be used in its oral dosage form to raise blood glucose levels in some hypoglycemic states. It is, chemically, a thiazide, but is not used as a diuretic.)

265. The answer is c. *(Brunton, pp 742, 749–751, 755; Craig, pp 241, 243–244; Katzung, p 244.)* Thiazides (and thiazide-like agents such as chlorthalidone and metolazone) and loop diuretics (furosemide, bumetanide, torsemide, ethacrynic acid) increase delivery of Na^+ to the distal nephron because they inhibit reabsorption of Na^+ at more proximal sites. This extra Na^+ reaches the principal cells in the distal nephron, and some of it is taken from the tubular fluid *via* sodium channels. This reclamation of Na^+ leads to exchange of K^+, which is lost into the urine (i.e., potassium "wasting"). In essence, the more Na^+ delivered (and recovered) distally, the more K^+ that is eliminated in exchange. No diuretic acts as an aldosterone receptor agonist; spironolactone (not listed here) exerts its natriuretic and potassium-*sparing* effects by *blocking* aldosterone receptors.

266. The answer is b. *(Brunton, pp 752–753; Craig, pp 249–250, 253–254; Katzung, pp 247–248.)* One way to simplify answering this question involves merely asking "which diuretic has the greatest ability to cause hypovolemia?" That narrows the choice to furosemide or the other loop diuretics (bumetanide, torsemide, ethacrynic acid). In terms of extra free water loss (and the concomitant risk of hypovolemia) the maximal efficacy of acetazolamide (carbonic anhydrase inhibitor; a) is modest at best, and self-limiting to boot. Hydrochlorothiazide (c) and the two potassium-sparing diuretics listed (spironolactone and triamterene; d, e) also have modest efficacy in terms of the peak diuretic effect, even if unusually large doses were to be given.

Note: Hyponatremia reduces the responsiveness of the peripheral vasculature to vasoconstrictors (e.g., EPI, NE, and angiotensin II). If we stated that the patient's hypotension were due to diuretic-induced hyponatremia, then the best answer would be hydrochlorothiazide or another thiazide or thiazide-like diuretic (e.g., metolazone); of all the diuretics classes (and most other classes of drugs), they are the most common cause of hyponatremia.

267. The answer is d. (*Brunton, pp 756–757, 764–765; Craig, pp 245–246, 251–253; Katzung, pp 248–250.*) Metolazone, although not a thiazide (benzothiadiazide) in the chemical sense, is largely (hydrochloro) thiazide-like in terms of its pharmacologic properties and uses, although it has a much longer duration of action than the prototype, hydrochlorothiazide. As far as the "main use" of thiazides goes, that would be essential hypertension (assuming no contraindications), with lesser uses being "mild" and especially transient edema, management of idiopathic hypercalciuria, adjunctive management of nephrogenic diabetes insipidus, and perhaps management of Meniere's disease. Thiazides (or such thiazide-like drugs as metolazone) would not be rational, nor very efficacious, for drug therapy of an adrenal cortical tumor (a). In that instance, if we are considering only diuretics, the proper drug would be spironolactone, the aldosterone receptor blocker. Likewise, since thiazides can raise serum urate and glucose levels, they would not be good choices for the patient with hepatic cirrhosis or other diseases characterized by poor liver function (b; here too spironolactone would be the best choice) or gout or diabetes (e). If our goal were to manage severe edema (e) with or without ascites (as in a patient with heart failure), our best choice would be a loop diuretic.

268. The answer is a. (*Brunton, pp 751–753; Craig, pp 249–250; Katzung, p 247.*) One expected response to therapeutic doses of loop diuretics, which are clearly and correctly classified as potassium-wasting, is a reduction of urinary potassium *concentrations*. How can this be? Note that the term concentration reflects the amount of a substance (here, potassium) per unit volume. The loop diuretics do increase K^+ excretion in exchange for an added load of Na^+ delivered to the distal nephron. They also impair the ability of the kidneys to form a concentrated urine—that is, they promote formation of a large volume of more dilute urine. The net loss of K^+ (say, on a 24-h basis) is increased, but it's accompanied by a disproportionate increase in free water loss such that urine K^+ concentration (but not total amount) is decreased.

269. The answer is a. (*Brunton, pp 743–747; Craig, pp 244–245, 442, 445; Katzung, pp 248, 250, 596, 599.*) Here we asked about reducing the risk of urate nephropathy acutely by increasing uric acid solubility, through urinary alkalinization. One key to answering this question correctly is to realize that uric acid becomes more soluble (less likely to precipitate or crystallize) as local pH rises. (Yes, we have asked a question in the renal drugs chapter that requires your knowledge of other areas of pathophysiology and pharmacology.) Recall that normal urine is acidic. We want to alkalinize the urine, and that is precisely what acetazolamide does, by inhibiting carbonic anhydrase in the proximal nephron. Note that acetazolamide is only an adjunct, and in addition to (or instead of) using it, we might also administer sodium bicarbonate, which will alkalinize the urine; and keep the patient well hydrated to help form large amounts of a dilute urine. Acetazolamide does cause a metabolic acidosis, which would seemingly favor reductions of uric acid solubility in the blood. However, we are keeping our patient well hydrated (helps reduce precipitation), and the volume of blood is far greater than urine volume at any given time, and given the great size of the "blood pool" we have little to worry about in terms of urate precipitation systemically.

Antidiuretic hormone (b) would be illogical. It would reduce urine volume and concentrate solutes (such as uric acid) in it. Ethacrynic acid (c) and furosemide (d) lead to the formation of copious volumes of dilute urine. In terms of renal problems, that may be beneficial. However, the loop diuretics tend to cause such large amounts of fluid loss via the urine that the concentration of solutes (including uric acid) in the blood may go up.

Hydrochlorothiazide (e) and related drugs tend to form a very concentrated urine by interfering with normal urine-diluting mechanisms in the kidneys. While some of these drugs have carbonic anhydrase activity, and alkalinize the urine, these effects are weak in comparison with acetazolamide. The most likely predominant renal effect is the unwanted one: increased risk of urate nephropathy. In addition, thiazides tend to elevate serum urate levels (by interfering with tubular secretion of urate), and so these drugs are likely to pose additional systemic problems.

270. The answer is a. (*Brunton, p 751; Craig, pp 249–250; Katzung, pp 247–248.*) Recall one of the main mechanisms by which a concentrated urine is formed: a hypertonic milieu in the renal medulla—and a medullary-to-cortical osmotic gradient—osmotically withdraws water (but not solute) from the tubular fluid as it passes through the collecting ducts. What creates that hypertonic medullary-to-cortical gradient? Reabsorption of Na^+ and Cl^- as tubular fluid ascends the loop of Henle, which ultimately increases interstitial osmolality. However, that process of ion resorption is impaired by loop diuretics. That reduces osmolality in the medullary interstitium, thereby dramatically reducing the osmotic gradient that enables the tubular fluid to become hypertonic as water is lost in the distal nephron. Thus, in the presence of a loop diuretic the urine remains dilute and hypotonic.

Hypercalcemia (b) is not an expected accompaniment. Loop diuretics (in contrast with thiazides) increase renal Ca^{+2} elimination.

Recall that the main anion excreted (along with Na^+, K^+, etc.) in response to a loop diuretic is chloride, and so net Cl^- excretion goes up (not down; c). Metabolic acidosis from increased bicarbonate excretion (d) doesn't occur. Bicarbonate tends to be reabsorbed, therefore. You should recall that hypochloremic alkalosis (also called contraction alkalosis, because blood volume contracts as the result of excessive fluid loss in the urine) is one potential and quite dangerous adverse responses caused by loop diuretics.

Loop diuretics do not lower serum urate concentrations (e). Rather, urate levels tend to rise, in part, because of reduced urate excretion combined with a "concentration" of urate in the blood owing to increased free water loss via urine. Serum uric acid concentration tends to rise. The loop diuretics reduce urate excretion through a direct renal tubular action. More important, perhaps, the proportionally large extra free water loss shrinks blood volume and tends to increase solute concentration, independent of any renal tubular effects on urate elimination.

271. The answer is c. (*Brunton, pp 753, 756–757, 764–765; Craig, p 253; Katzung, pp 249–250, 254–256.*) Chlorthalidone is a thiazide-like diuretic. If maximum dosages don't yield the desired effects, there is probably little to be gained by switching (c) to another thiazide or thiazide-like agent (e.g., hydrochlorothiazide, metolazone, many others) will do better. Likewise, and given the relatively "flat" dose-response relationship for these drugs, nothing good is likely to be gained by adding (a, b) "yet another" agent that works in precisely the same way as the drug that has already proven inadequate. If a maximum recommended dose isn't adequate, giving more of the same or a similar drug won't be better (e). So, in situations such as this, it's time to switch to a drug that is intrinsically more efficacious and works via a different mechanism: a loop diuretic. There is a more prescient question to ask: If our patient had edema and heart failure, why didn't we initiate therapy with a loop diuretic in the first place?

272. The answer is b. *(Brunton, pp 757–759, 848–850, 858–859, 866–867; Craig, p 249; Katzung, pp 178–180, 252–256.)* The combined use of an ACE inhibitor and a diuretic is quite common, because the combination often provides better blood pressure control than can either agent alone. However, this combination usually involves a thiazide, not triamterene or another K-sparing diuretic because of the risk of hyperkalemia. Recall that one ultimate effect of any ACE inhibitor is potassium retention (and, of course, renal Na^+ loss); add to this the K-sparing effects of triamterene, amiloride, or spironolactone; and there's a definite risk of causing hyperkalemia that can be more of a problem than the prior issues with blood pressure control.

You should also recall that although it is common to use both an ACE inhibitor and a thiazide, adding the thiazide is often associated with an excessive (but, fortunately, transient) fall of blood pressure that may lead to symptoms of hypotension. So, caution is required.

There is no known interaction involving a rise of blood pressure (a) when adding a diuretic (triamterene or other) to an ACE inhibitor regimen. The more likely approach would be a fall. Neither the ACE inhibitor nor the triamterene has cardiac-depressant activity (c). Cough from an ACE inhibitor—not uncommon, and for some patients severe—apparently involves inhibition of bradykinin metabolism by bradykininase, an enzyme that is, for all practical purposes, identical to angiotensin-converting enzyme. Diuretics do not potentiate or cause that effect (d).

Hypernatremia (e) is not a reasonable answer. Note that through different mechanisms both ACE inhibitors and diuretics (all) increase renal sodium loss. If anything, there would be a risk of hyponatremia.

273. The answer is b. *(Brunton, pp 429, 485–490, 753; Craig, pp 393–395; Katzung, p 478.)* In essence, the intensity of effects from any given serum level of lithium are inversely related to serum sodium concentrations. When serum sodium concentration falls, the effects of lithium can be intensified to the point of causing toxicity. Via their actions to increase renal sodium loss, virtually all the common diuretics also reduce renal lithium excretion. It is probably of greatest concern with thiazides or thiazide-like diuretics, which have the greatest potential of all the common diuretics to cause hyponatremia. Cholestyramine (a) is a cholesterol-binding resin. Given concomitantly with an oral diuretic, the most likely outcome would be reduced bioavailability of the diuretic, not increased or decreased cholestyramine effects. Nifedipine (c), a dihydropyridine calcium channel blocker, may cause excessive antihypertensive effects when administered with any diuretic (although combined administration is common and usually problem-free). If excessive effects of nifedipine occur in conjunction with a diuretic, they are most likely blood volume-related, not specifically due to changes of serum sodium concentrations. Phenylephrine's (d) vasoconstrictor effects are not likely to be altered appreciably in the presence of a diuretic. The same lack of a clinically significant interaction applies to the statins (e; HMG CoA reductase inhibitors, e.g., atorvastatin).

274. The answer is a. (*Brunton, pp 391, 743–747; Craig, pp 244–245; Katzung, p 246.*) The signs and symptoms of altitude sickness are related to the development of respiratory alkalosis: ventilatory rate is increased in response to breathing the rarefied air, which increases net ventilatory loss of CO_2. Blood pH rises. Acetazolamide effectively inhibits carbonic anhydrase and so increases bicarbonate loss. This, in turn, causes a metabolic acidosis that counteracts the ventilatory-induced rise of blood pH. It is the drug of choice for prophylaxis or management of altitude sickness. It is true that some of the thiazide or thiazide-like diuretics inhibit carbonic anhydrase, but the effect is very weak in comparison to that of acetazolamide. None of the other drugs listed would be suitable for this patient and the altitude sickness he is likely to experience.

275. The answer is c. (*Brunton, pp 685–686, 752–753; Craig, pp 249–250, 428; Katzung, p 247.*) An important element in the renal responses to furosemide is maintenance of adequate renal blood flow. That is, to a degree, prostaglandin-mediated. The NSAIDs, such as the hypothetical one described here, inhibit prostaglandin synthesis. That, in turn, antagonizes the desired effects of the loop diuretic, leading to less fluid and salt elimination: edema, weight gain, and other markers of heart failure are likely to develop as a result. Hyperchloremic alkalosis (a) is incorrect, in part, because chronic or acute excessive effects of loop diuretics are characterized by hypochloremic metabolic alkalosis. Regardless, NSAIDs are not likely to potentiate the effects of these diuretics. "Dramatic increases of furosemide's K-sparing effects (b)" is incorrect. Recall that loop diuretics are K-wasting. Digoxin is eliminated by renal excretion. If we accept the notion that loop diuretics may increase excretion of digoxin, then we should accept the likely possibility that NSAID-induced reductions of diuretic action should reduce the glycoside's renal loss, not increase it (d). The NSAIDs do not bind to and inhibit the myocyte Na^+,K^+-ATPase, which is digoxin's cellular receptor (e). Do remember that furosemides (and thiazides) are apt to increase the risk or severity of digoxin toxicity. The mechanism mainly involves diuretic-induced hypokalemia, not changes in circulating fluid volume or urine volume *per se*.

276. The answer is a. *(Brunton, pp 743–747, 1709–1711, 1723; Craig, p 245; Katzung, pp 245–246.)* Aqueous humor formation (as well as that of cerebrospinal fluid) involves carbonic anhydrase activity. Reduce aqueous humor synthesis and, all other factors being equal, intraocular pressure goes down. Acetazolamide is, of course, "the" carbonic anhydrase-inhibiting diuretic.

Note that when a carbonic anhydrase inhibitor is used to manage glaucoma, the drug's renal/diuretic effects, which certainly occur if the drug is given systemically, have nothing to do with the beneficial effects that are due to an ocular (ciliary body) site of action. If fact, those extraocular effects aren't needed for glaucoma control. That is why, when we prescribe a carbonic anhydrase inhibitor for glaucoma, we usually choose a topical ophthalmic agent (e.g., dorzolamide or methazolamide).

277. The answer is a. *(Brunton, pp 738f, 749–751, 763f; Craig, p 249; Katzung, p 247.)* As soon as you realize (it should be instantaneous) that furosemide (and bumetanide, torsemide, and ethacrynic acid) is a loop diuretic, you're half-way toward picking the right answer. These agents inhibit a Na^+, K^+, $2Cl^-$ cotransporter in the *ascending* limb. Recall that unimpaired Na^+ and Cl^- reabsorption in the ascending limb is what is responsible and necessary for making the medullary milieu hypertonic, thereby providing the osmotic force necessary for withdrawing water (i.e., concentrating the urine) as urine passes through the collecting ducts—the "countercurrent multiplier." You may also recall that the ability of loop agents to increase Ca^{2+} and Mg^{2+} excretion also involves actions in the ascending limb.

278. The answer is b. *(Brunton, pp 753, 1162–1163; Craig, p 250; Katzung, pp 248, 767–768.)* Both the loop diuretics and the aminoglycosides (tobramycin, streptomycin, gentamicin, others) are ototoxic—capable of causing vestibular damage (e.g., balance problems) or cochlear damage (tinnitus or sensorineural hearing loss). The ototoxic effects of each drug is enhanced (often significantly) by the other's, and so it is best to avoid use of both these drugs (or other ototoxins) unless the benefits clearly outweigh the risk of perhaps permanent and total hearing loss. Of course, there are instances in which it's impossible to avoid such combinations. There's strong evidence that of all the loop diuretics, the risk of ototoxicity is highest with ethacrynic acid (and its parenteral formulation, sodium ethacrynate). Nonetheless, all the other loop diuretics—bumetanide, furosemide, and torsemide—are definitely on the short list of ototoxic drugs.

279. The answer is e. (*Brunton, p 762; Craig, pp 246–248; Katzung, pp 250–252, 256.*) The most rational choice for specifically antagonizing the consequences of hormone excess—aldosterone being the hormone of most importance in terms of the renal, hemodynamic, and electrolyte problems here—is spironolactone. Its primary mechanism of action is blockade of aldosterone receptors. Remember that the main renal effects of aldosterone are sodium (and water) retention, and increased renal loss of potassium.

Acetazolamide (a), the carbonic anhydrase inhibitor, exerts weak and self-limiting diuretic and natriuretic effects. It is also potassium-wasting, and increased excretion of potassium is what we do not want to do in situations of preexisting hypokalemia. Amiloride (b) would help increase sodium excretion and help normalize serum potassium levels too. However, it does not provide the "rational" approach to hyperaldosteronism because it does not block aldosterone receptors. Furosemide (c) or another loop diuretic might prove effective in terms of increasing excretion of sodium and reducing that of potassium. Indeed, if the hyperaldosteronism is sufficiently great to cause dangerous degrees of fluid retention (hypervolemia) and heart failure we may need to administer it. Nonetheless, spironolactone would be a reasonable, rational, and probably necessary element of management. Metolazone (d), a thiazide-like diuretic, would desirably help increase renal sodium excretion and lower blood pressure. Having relatively low efficacy in terms of increased urine production, it may not do much to manage the hypervolemia and the resulting weight gain. More important, metolazone is likely to aggravate the preexisting hypokalemia because it is, of course, a potassium-wasting diuretic.

280. The answer is b. (*Brunton, pp 751, 763, 765–766, 886–889; Craig, pp 249–251, 154–155; Katzung, pp 211–212.*) While many ionic and other factors can predispose a patient to digoxin toxicity, hypokalemia, as can be caused by a loop diuretic (usually used for edema and/or ascites, including that associated with heart failure) or thiazide diuretic (mainly used for treating essential hypertension), is arguably the most important, if not the most common. There is a competition between extracellular K^+ and digoxin for binding to digoxin's cellular receptor, the Na^+,K^+-ATPase on the sarcolemma. When serum K^+ levels are reduced (i.e., when hypokalemia develops), the binding of digoxin is enhanced and so its effects are increased, even without a rise of serum digoxin concentrations, and usually those increased effects are deleterious, as described here. Hypercalcemia can increase the risk or severity of digoxin toxicity. However, loop diuretics increase renal Ca^{2+} loss, and so hypercalcemia (a) is not a likely explanation. Hyponatremia (c) is not likely to have occurred with a loop diuretic, which tends to increase both renal Na^+ and H_2O loss proportionally, such that hyponatremia is not likely to occur as it may with a thiazide. Loop diuretics do not displace digoxin from tissue binding sites (d) or inhibit digoxin's elimination (which involves renal excretion, not metabolism).

Note that in the scenario we described the patient as having been treated by "his family doctor who has been treating him . . . for the last 30 years." This is not at all meant to impugn family doctors or general practitioners. The point is that nowadays, and for a variety of reasons (toxicity being one), digoxin is no longer considered an appropriate drug for managing heart failure, with or without signs or symptoms of congestive failure, until all other reasonable and more suitable options have been tried and the patient's condition has deteriorated to the point that inotropes (digoxin or parenteral agents) are warranted. Recall that our preferred approach for initial therapy of failure involves ACE inhibitors, a β blocker, and perhaps a loop diuretic. Nonetheless, and unfortunately, some physicians still use the "old way," involving digoxin. It is these patients who are likely to be seen in the hospital when the almost inevitable problems due to digoxin develop.

281. The answer is a. (*Brunton, pp 749–753; Craig, pp 249–250; Katzung, pp 252–254.*) This patient needs a diuretic that can be administered in such a way that its actions develop promptly, and has properties that can increase considerably the renal excretion of sodium free water to unload hemodynamically the heart. This should narrow the answer choice to ethacrynic acid and furosemide. Thiazides and thiazide-like diuretics (e.g., metolazone) would not be suitable; their efficacies are low in terms of managing edema; they impair glycemic control in diabetic patients; and they have sulfonamide-like structures and so pose a risk of allergic reactions in the patient we described.

However, we must consider significant patient-related issues that should lead us to decide which loop diuretic we will use for this particular patient. The patient has a documented history of allergic reactions to sulfonamides. Furosemide (and the related drugs bumetanide and torsemide) has a sulfonamide structure, and so may elicit an allergic response in this patient). Ethacrynic acid does not (it is a phenoxyacetic acid derivative...a point you probably should not commit to memory). Furosemide and most of the other common diuretics (thiazides, thiazide-like agents such as metolazone and chlorthalidone; and the other loop diuretics) also tend to elevate blood glucose in one way or another. Ethacrynic acid does not. One other noteworthy point: although all the loop diuretics are quite similar in terms of their clinical uses, and in terms of their likely adverse effects, ethacrynic acid differs not only in the ways noted above but also because it seems to have the greatest potential for causing ototoxicity—a point you should always associate with all the loop diuretics.

282. The answer is b. (*Brunton, pp 758–759; Craig, p 248; Katzung, p 251.*) Amiloride and triamterene block distal tubular Na^+ channels that provide for Na^+ reabsorption in exchange for K^+, which is lost into the urine. This sodium channel, which is the main site of action of amiloride, is on the luminal side of the principal cell membranes. (Principal cells in the nephron are located in the late distal tubule and collecting ducts.) There is an ATPase on the interstitial face of the principal cells (again, these are in the distal nephron, not proximal; d). The ATPase is responsible for the extrusion of potassium into the urine in exchange for extra sodium taken up by the luminal sodium channels, and so it is essential in the overall actions of potassium-sparing diuretics. Nonetheless, the ATPase is not inhibited (or stimulated; d) directly by amiloride.

Amiloride has no direct effects on aldosterone synthesis or metabolism (c), or on aldosterone receptors (a; those receptors are blocked by spironolactone).

283. The answer is c. (*Brunton, pp 248–249; Craig, pp 103–104; Katzung, pp 133, 137, 212–213.*) The often dramatic increase in urine output caused by therapeutic doses of dopamine (so-called "renal doses") is mainly due to improved hemodynamics. The drug, under these conditions, not only improves cardiac contractility and cardiac output (which, in turn, improves renal perfusion), but also dilates the renal arterioles; these effects lead to improved glomerular filtration, and the increased urine volume Improved hemodynamics will suppress the renin-angiotensin-aldosterone system, which was activated in response to poor renal perfusion. Weak β_1 receptor activation also contributes to this effect (particularly with such drugs as dobutamine). However, dopamine does not block (a) any of the adrenergic receptors.

Dopamine also has renal tubular effects, much like traditional diuretics do, although we often overlook them (perhaps because they are less important than the effects described here). The drug, *via* its D_1 receptor agonist actions, increases c-AMP formation in the proximal tubules and also in the thick ascending limb of the loop of Henle. At the latter site the result is inhibition of both the Na^+-H^+ exchange mechanism and the Na^+, K^+-ATPase, but not of water (e; recall that the thick ascending limb of the loop of Henle is impermeable to water.) Taken together, the renal hemodynamic and tubular actions of dopamine make it particularly useful for managing heart failure that is accompanied by reduced renal function.

Higher dose causes positive inotropy via β_1 receptor activation, and causes neuronal NE release. High doses activate α_1 receptors in various vascular beds, including the renal, leading to vasoconstriction that can raise blood pressure and total peripheral resistance, and can reduce renal blood flow, thereby reducing renal excretory function.

284. The correct answer is d. *(Brunton, pp 752, 756; Craig, pp 245–246; Katzung, pp 249–250.)* Thiazide and thiazide-like diuretics should be high (highest?) on your list of drugs that are likely to cause hyponatremia, and in some cases the outcome has been fatal. Was it easy to select hydrochlorothiazide as the correct answer because it was the only drug listed that was not a loop diuretic? Were you puzzled because you knew that furosemide is the prototype loop agent, and weren't sure about the classification bumetanide, ethacrynic acid, or torsemide. Or did you not select the thiazide because you considered its diuretic effects to be mild, or modest, and therefore least likely to cause hyponatremia?

In absolute or relative terms the natriuretic (sodium-wasting) effects can be considered weak (especially in comparison with loop diuretics).

They cause relatively slight increases in free water loss in the urine (compared with normal), interfere with normal urine-diluting mechanisms and lead to the formation of a concentrated (in terms of such solutes as sodium) urine. That is, the amount of extra sodium lost is disproportionate to the extra volume lost. This is reflected, in the blood, as not much extra volume loss coupled with proportionally greater declines in the amount of sodium. Remember that hyponatremia means excessively reduced serum sodium *concentration*, and concentration is a function of amount per unit volume. The thiazides have caused "dilutional hyponatremia." Contrast this with the typical response to a loop diuretic. They do cause appreciable extra renal sodium loss, but they simultaneously impair normal renal urine concentrating mechanisms. That leads to the formation of large volumes of urine that is dilute in terms of solute concentration. We can lose much extra sodium in response to a loop diuretic, but the concomitant and large(r) decrease of circulating fluid volume counteracts the tendency to reduce serum concentrations of sodium. This rather unusual effect of loop diuretics accounts for why they may be used adjunctively to treat hyponatremia, including that which was caused by a thiazide.

285. The answer is c. (*Brunton, pp 743–746; Craig, p 245; Katzung, p 246.*) We seldom administer acetazolamide as a diuretic, because its effects are "mild;" associated with significant changes of both urine pH (up) and blood pH (down); and self-limiting (once sufficient bicarbonate has been lost from the blood, into the urine, refractoriness to further diuresis occurs). More often we administer acetazolamide and other carbonic anhydrase inhibitors for nonrenal/noncardiovascular problems, such as an adjunct to anticonvulsant therapy as described here. As a result, we may forget that these systemically administered drugs *are* diuretics, one common property of all the diuretics being increased renal sodium loss (thus, answer a is not correct). We may even forget that carbonic anhydrase inhibitors, given systemically, are potassium-wasting diuretics.

In this scenario we have a patient taking a thiazide, which is obviously potassium-wasting and has the potential in its own right to cause hypokalemia. Add a carbonic anhydrase to the regimen and the risks of hypokalemia increase. Acetazolamide does not antagonize the antihypertensive effects of thiazides or calcium channel blockers, nor provoke hypertension or a hypertensive crisis (b). If there were any interactions between the acetazolamide and the aspirin, it would be antagonism, not potentiation (d) of aspirin's antiplatelet effects. Aspirin undergoes renal tubular reabsorption, and that is a pH-dependent effect. Aspirin's reabsorption is reduced in the presence of an alkaline urine, which is precisely what occurs with acetazolamide. (You should recall that alkalinizing the urine is one of the important adjunctive measures in treating severe salicylate poisoning, and it is beneficial in part because salicylate reabsorption is reduced.)

There is no reason to suspect sudden rises of blood volume, with or without concomitant heart failure from that (e). Indeed, the added diuresis from the acetazolamide may, at least transiently, potentiate the effects of the thiazide on urine volume, blood pressure, or both.

286. The answer is d. (*Brunton, p 744t; Craig, p 244; Katzung, p 254.*) And so the other drugs? Acetazolamide has a profile that best matches Drug 4 (note the increased bicarbonate loss and decreased chloride loss). Amiloride's profile fits that of Drug 3 (note the reduced renal potassium loss). Chlorthalidone and hydrochlorothiazide would produce profiles like Drug 1 (more potassium loss, a decrease in the excretion of calcium, and variable effects on bicarbonate loss due to variable effects on carbonic anhydrase).

Rather than rehashing the sites and mechanisms by which the "main" diuretics cause their effects—that's largely all been addressed above—what follows are some tips for arriving at the correct answer more or less easily. We'll add some additional comments that may not have been emphasized before.

Note that all the profiles show an increased (qualitative) renal excretion of Na. The essence of this is that it reflects the fact that all the common diuretics do that. Indeed, this natriuretic effect is part of the "definition" of "diuretic."

The next step is to identify which agents increase renal K excretion and which do the opposite, because the main diuretics are either K-sparing or K-wasting. That will narrow your choices nicely. You should be able to place a drug in the proper K-related class instantaneously (with the possible exception of acetazolamide, a K-wasting drug, because we tend to emphasize its carbonic acid–inhibitory effects and overload other important properties; see the answer to Question 285).

Finally, once you see that a drug's profile involves increased K elimination, you have narrowed your choices to a thiazide or thiazide-like agent (hydrochlorothiazide, chlorthalidone, metolazone, many others), a loop agent, or a carbonic anhydrase inhibitor.

Look now at what happens to urinary Ca^{2+} excretion. If it's reduced, it's a thiazide or a related agent (recall we can use these drugs for idiopathic hypercalciuria, an effect that capitalizes on reduced presence of Ca^{2+} in the urine). If Ca^{2+} excretion is increased, it's a loop diuretic.

Now how do you identify which agent is a carbonic anhydrase inhibitor (i.e., acetazolamide)? In addition to looking at Na^+ and K^+, note what happens to HCO_3^- and Cl^-. Acetazolamide causes profound urinary alkalinization from the HCO_3^- loss; so much so that the blood's other major anion, Cl^-, is retained. Just looking at the table you would probably rule out a thiazide (e) or chlorthalidone (c) because we indicate that the effect on that anion is variable (+/−).

How could you rule out triamterene, because we showed increased HCO_3^- loss with it? (It's a slight effect, by the way, and carbonic anhydrase inhibition is not its main nor an important mechanism or outcome, but you can't tell from the table.) Look at the Cl^- profile and you will see that acetazolamide is the only diuretic that lowers Cl^- excretion. That's because one of the blood's major anions, HCO_3^-, is lost to such a great degree that the other main anion, Cl^-, is conserved.

The Respiratory System: Asthma and COPD

Adrenergic agonists
Antimuscarinics
Methylxanthines
Leukotriene synthesis inhibitors
and receptor blockers

Mast cell "stabilizers"
Mucolytics
Antitussives
Histamine receptor (H_1) blockers

Questions

DIRECTIONS: Each item contains a question or incomplete statement that is followed by several responses. Select the **one best** response to each question.

287. Adrenergic agonists clearly play a role in managing some patients with asthma, whether for prophylaxis (control medication) or for rescue therapy. Which of the following drugs is classified as an adrenergic agonist, but has no physiologically relevant or clinically useful effects on airway smooth muscle tone?

a. Albuterol
b. Epinephrine
c. Norepinephrine
d. Salmeterol
e. Terbutaline
f. Theophylline

288. A patient with asthma has moderate bronchospasm and wheezing about twice a week. Current medications are inhaled albuterol, used for both prophylaxis and to abort ongoing attacks (rescue therapy), and inhaled beclomethasone. If the physician chooses to use salmeterol, which of the following states best the way it should be used in this patient's management?

a.   A replacement for the albuterol
b.   A replacement for the corticosteroid
c.   An add-on to current medications for additional prophylactic benefits
d.   Primary (sole) therapy, replacing both albuterol and the steroid
e.   The preferred agent for acute symptom control (rescue therapy)

289. A 22-year-old patient moves from a small town to your city, and is now under your care. They have a history of asthma, and their previous primary care physician was managing it with oral theophylline. Which of the following best summarizes the efficacy or current status of this drug in such patients as the one we described?

a.   Dosing is simple and convenient, rarely needs to be adjusted
b.   Excellent alternative to an inhaled steroid for "rescue" therapy
c.   Is, at best, a second or third-line agent for long-term asthma control
d.   Possesses strong and clinically useful anti-inflammatory activity
e.   Sedation is a major side effect, even with therapeutic doses or blood levels

290. An elderly man with COPD is being managed with several drugs, one of which is inhaled ipratropium. Which of the following is the main mechanism that accounts for the beneficial effects of this drug?

a.   Blocks of an endogenous bronchoconstrictor mediator
b.   Enhances release of epinephrine from the adrenal medulla
c.   Inhibits cAMP breakdown via phosphodiesterase inhibition
d.   Prevents antigen-antibody reactions that lead to mast cell mediator release
e.   Stimulates ventilatory rates (CNS effect in brain's medulla)
f.   Suppresses synthesis and release of inflammatory mediators

291. A 16-year-old girl treated for asthma develops skeletal muscle tremors that are drug-induced. Which of the following was the most likely cause?

a. Albuterol
b. Beclomethasone
c. Cromolyn
d. Ipratropium
e. Montelukast

292. A 26-year-old patient with asthma is being treated with montelukast. Which of the following is the main mechanism by which this drug works?

a. Blocks the proinflammatory effects of certain arachidonic acid metabolites
b. Enhances release of epinephrine from the adrenal (suprarenal) medulla
c. Increases airway β-adrenergic receptor responsiveness to endogenous norepinephrine
d. Inhibits cAMP breakdown via phosphodiesterase inhibition
e. Prevents antigen-antibody reactions that lead to mast cell mediator release
f. Stimulates ventilatory rates (CNS effect in brain's medulla)

293. An elderly man, in obvious respiratory distress due to exacerbation of his emphysema and chronic bronchitis, presents in the emergency department. One drug ordered by the physician, to be administered by the respiratory therapist, is N-acetylcysteine. Which of the following is the main action or purpose of this drug?

a. Block receptors for the cysteinyl leukotrienes
b. Inhibit metabolic inactivation of epinephrine or β_2 agonists that were administered
c. Inhibit leukotriene synthesis
d. Promptly suppress airway inflammation
e. Reverse ACh-mediated bronchoconstriction
f. Thin airway mucus secretions for easier removal by suctioning or postural drainage

294. A 23-year-old woman with asthma has what is described as "aspirin (hyper)sensitivity" and experiences severe bronchospasm in response to even small doses of the drug. Which of the following is the most likely mechanism by which the aspirin provokes her pulmonary problems?

a. Blocks synthesis of endogenous prostaglandins that have bronchodilator activity
b. Induces formation of antibodies directed against the salicylate on airway mast cells
c. Induces hypersensitivity of H_1 receptors on airway smooth muscles
d. Induces hypersensitivity of muscarinic receptors on airway smooth muscles
e. Prevents or reduces epinephrine binding to β_2-adrenergic receptors (airways and elsewhere)

295. A young boy is diagnosed with asthma. His primary symptom is frequent cough, not bronchospasm or wheezing. Other asthma medications are started, but until their effects develop fully we wish to suppress the cough without running a risk of suppressing ventilatory drive or causing sedation or other unwanted effects. Which of the following would best meet these needs?

a. Codeine
b. Dextromethorphan
c. Diphenhydramine
d. Hydrocodone
e. Promethazine

296. A mother brings her 10-year-old son, who has a long-standing history of poorly controlled asthma, to the emergency department (ED). He is in a relatively early stage of what will prove to be a severe asthma attack. Arterial blood gases have not been analyzed yet, but it is obvious that the lad is in great distress. He is panting with great effort at a rate of about 160/min.

Given the boy's history and the likely diagnosis, the health care team administers all the drugs listed by the stated routes, and with the expected purposes noted. The child's condition quickly improves, and the team leaves the boy with his mother while they go to care for other ED patients. Within a couple of minutes the mother comes out of her son's cubicle frantically screaming "he's stopped breathing!" Which of the listed drugs most likely caused the ventilatory arrest?

a. Albuterol, inhaled, given by nebulizer for prompt bronchodilation
b. Atropine, inhaled, given with the albuterol
c. Midazolam, IV, to normalize ventilatory rate and allay anxiety
d. Methylprednisolone (glucocorticosteroid), IV, for prompt suppression of airway inflammation
e. Normal saline, inhaled, to hydrate the airway mucosae

297. We prescribe an orally inhaled corticosteroid for a patient with asthma. Previously they were using only a rapidly acting adrenergic bronchodilator for both prophylaxis and for treatment of acute attacks. They use the steroid as directed for 5 days, then stop taking it. Which of the following is the most likely reason why the patient quit using the drug?

a. Disturbing tachycardia and palpitations occurred
b. Relentless diarrhea developed after just one day of using the steroid
c. She experienced little or no obvious improvement in breathing
d. The drug caused extreme drowsiness that interfered with daytime activities
e. The drug caused him to retain fluid and gain weight

298. A patient consumes an excessive dose of theophylline and develops toxicity in response to the drug. Which of the following is the most likely consequence of this?

a. Bradycardia
b. Drowsiness progressing to sleep and then coma
c. Hepatotoxicity
d. Paradoxical bronchospasm
e. Seizures

299. Acetylcholine esterase inhibitors, muscarinic agonists such as pilocarpine, and β blockers, are among the drugs used to manage many patients with glaucoma. They also share properties that are particularly relevant to patients with asthma. Which of the following statements summarizes best what that relevance is?

a. Contraindicated, or pose great risks, for people with asthma
b. Degranulate mast cells, cause bronchoconstriction
c. Tend to raise intraocular pressure in patients who have both glaucoma and asthma
d. Trigger bronchoconstriction by directly activating H_1 histamine receptors on airway smooth muscle cells
e. Useful for acute asthma, not for ambulatory patients

300. A patient suffering status asthmaticus presents in the emergency department. Blood gases reveal severe respiratory acidosis and hypoxia. Even large parenteral doses of a selective β_2 agonist fail to dilate the airways adequately; rather, they cause dangerous degrees of tachycardia. Which of the following pharmacologic interventions or approaches is most likely to control the acute symptoms and restore the bronchodilator efficacy of the adrenergic drug?

a. Add inhaled cromolyn
b. Give a parenteral corticosteroid
c. Give parenteral diphenhydramine
d. Switch to epinephrine
e. Switch to isoproterenol (β_1/β_2 agonist)

The Respiratory System: Asthma and COPD

Answers

287. The answer is c. *(Brunton, pp 144–145, 127–238, 248; Craig, pp 93, 101; Katzung, p 86.)* By way of a brief but essential review of autonomic pharmacology, recall that "adrenergic bronchodilation" requires activation of β_2-adrenergic receptors on airway smooth muscle cells. Norepinephrine is an α and β_1 agonist, with no ability to activate β_2s, and so it has no bronchodilator activity. Albuterol (a), a β_2 agonist, can be considered the prototype of adrenergic bronchodilators used for asthma (prophylaxis/control, but mainly rescue therapy). Epinephrine (b) is a very efficacious bronchodilator, but its use for routine management of asthma is considerably limited due to its ability to cause vasoconstriction (α-agonist activity) and cardiac stimulation (β_1 agonist activity). In terms of pulmonary problems, it is reserved mainly for managing anaphylaxis or status asthmaticus, but it indeed causes bronchodilation well and promptly. Salmeterol (d) is a β agonist also. Given by inhalation, its bronchodilator effects are slow in onset, but it has a long duration compared with similarly classified drugs such as albuterol. Thus, salmeterol is an efficacious bronchodilator, but not suitable for prompt effects (rescue therapy). Terbutaline (e) is classified similar to albuterol (and salmeterol) and is not an adrenergic drug in any respect. Theophylline (f) has reasonable bronchodilator activity, but it is not an adrenergic agonist. It may inhibit phosphodiesterase, and so catabolism of cAMP (the second messenger formed by adrenergic bronchodilators in airway smooth muscle), but it has no direct effects on the adrenergic receptors.

288. The answer is c. *(Brunton, pp 253, 720–721; Craig, p 462; Katzung, pp 324–325, 332.)* If we were to decide to use salmeterol in this situation it would be best to consider it as an add-on. Recall that salmeterol, like albuterol, is mainly a β_2 agonist, but salmeterol's onset of action is much slower, its duration of action much longer. The slow onset of salmeterol makes it a useful prophylactic agent for some patients, but renders it completely inappropriate for rescue therapy (a, e). It can be administered separately, or the physician might prescribe one of the proprietary fixed-dose combination products that contain both salmeterol and a steroid (given by oral inhalation). One could reasonably argue that salmeterol is also dangerous if used as the sole intervention for rescue, because serious ventilatory compromise can develop before its bronchodilator effects develop. The patient described needs a corticosteroid. We might increase the dose of the inhaled steroid as a start, or perhaps try a burst of an oral steroid (e.g., prednisone) for a while. Regardless, using salmeterol as a replacement for any corticosteroid (b) or for all the other current medications (d) is likely to provoke more and more severe asthma attacks; it's simply bad management. Remember: the key to success in asthma therapy long-term requires controlling airway inflammation, and corticosteroids are the key drugs for doing just that.

289. The answer is c. (*Brunton, pp 727–730; Craig, pp 349, 351, 463; Katzung, pp 325–327.*) Theophylline, the prototype methylxanthine, is an oral bronchodilator that has some beneficial pulmonary effects in patients with asthma or COPD. We don't know precisely how it exerts its bronchodilator activity, at least at concentrations found in human beings (*in vitro* it inhibits phosphodiesterase, preserving cAMP levels; it also blocks receptors for adenosine, which has bronchoconstrictor activity).

However, there are serious problems with this old drug that relegate it to second or third status in therapy; that render it a drug that should be prescribed only by pulmonologists who are quite familiar with the limitations, side effects, and toxicity; and that make its use as primary therapy for asthma usually inappropriate (at best).

Theophylline (and other methylxanthines) have a very low therapeutic index: it is all too easy (whether because of drug-drug interactions, or simply improper dosing) to have blood levels rise into a range that can cause toxicity (mainly excessive cardiac and CNS stimulation, with the potential for arrhythmias or seizures). Moreover, and because of the problems stated here, frequent blood testing is necessary in order to get, and keep, serum levels within an acceptable therapeutic range and hopefully avoid subtherapeutic or toxic blood levels. The drug depends on hepatic P450 status for its elimination, and that makes elimination very easily influenced by liver dysfunction or other interacting drugs that can either induce or inhibit its metabolism.

Most important is the fact that theophylline has no anti-inflammatory activity; as we said, if we are treating asthma long-term, the "secret to success" is controlling airway inflammation. For our foundation we use corticosteroids to suppress inflammation.

And if we are dealing with COPD and the goal is bronchodilation, such drugs as ipratropium (inhaled antimuscarinic) are not only more efficacious, but also associated with fewer dosing problems, monitoring needs, and side effects.

290. The answer is a. *(Brunton, pp 189–190, 194–196, 730–732; Craig, pp 137–138, 463–464; Katzung, pp 327–328, 332.)* You should be able to deduce quickly (if not simply know outright) that ipratropium is an atropine-like drug—an antimuscarinic that blocks the bronchoconstrictor effect of ACh on airway smooth muscle. It is a quaternary, inhaled antimuscarinic: that is, it acts locally in the airways, and very little of the "always charged" molecule diffuses into the circulation to cause systemic effects. Ipratropium has no effects on the adrenal medulla, on mast cells or other elements of the inflammatory response, or in the CNS. Ipratropium is approved for managing COPD, but is often used for some asthma patients. The drug has a rapid onset of action. However, some studies indicate that it is not as efficacious a bronchodilator as β_2 agonists, and so it is not a suitable agent for rescue therapy. Finally, the bronchodilator effects of ipratropium and β agonists are synergistic (same effect, different mechanisms), and so there's some logic to using them both.

291. The answer is a. *(Brunton, pp 719–721, 252–253; Craig, p 462; Katzung, p 325.)* Of the drugs listed in the question, skeletal muscle tremor is a side effect most often associated with β_2-adrenergic agonists—albuterol and others. It is almost always a dose-dependent phenomenon. (Note: Some physicians titrate the dose of adrenergic bronchodilators upward, stopping when tremors develop and equating the blood level associated with that dose as being therapeutic with respect to controlling the pulmonary disease. The wisdom of that is questionable; proper dosage adjustments or other therapy changes should be based on pulmonary symptom relief [subjective assessment] in general and, ideally, quantitative pulmonary function tests.) None of the other drugs listed is associated with skeletal muscle tremor. Beclomethasone (b) is an inhaled corticosteroid; cromolyn (c), also inhaled for asthma, reduces mast cell degranulation;

ipratropium (d) is an inhaled antimuscarinic indicated for COPD; montelukast (e) is a leukotriene receptor blocker that is also indicated for asthma prophylaxis.

292. The answer is a. (*Brunton, pp 722–724; Craig, pp 465–466; Katzung, pp 330–331.*) Montelukast (and a related drug, zafirlukast) block receptors for leukotrienes (LTs). (When you see "leuk" or "luk" as part of these drugs' generic names, think leukotrienes or leukotriene modifiers, and think of drugs for asthma.)

Recall that the LTs are proinflammatory and bronchoconstrictor mediators formed as part of normal arachidonic acid metabolism via the 5'-lipoxygenase pathway. (The other main part of arachidonic acid metabolism, involving cyclooxygenases, forms various prostaglandins and thromboxane A_2.) A somewhat related drug, zileuton, inhibits 5'-lipoxygenase directly, thereby mainly blocking LT synthesis rather than mainly blocking LT receptors.

These leukotrienes receptor blockers are indicated for prophylaxis (control therapy) only, and should not be used in lieu of corticosteroids (oral or orally inhaled) when corticosteroids are suitable which is most of the time. They will do virtually no good in a short enough time if they were administered to suppress ongoing bronchoconstriction (e.g., for rescue therapy), mainly because they are too slow-acting. And, although this class of drugs is among the newest approved for asthma in many years, they are not panaceas for all asthma patients, and for some patients their efficacy appears to be no better than placebo.

Note: Montelukast has at least two advantages over zafirlukast. It does not inhibit the hepatic P450 system to cause drug-drug interactions, particularly with such other drugs as theophylline or warfarin. The risk of hepatotoxicity also seems substantially lower with montelukast.

Another "leukotrienes modifier" is zileuton; it inhibits lipoxygenase, thereby inhibiting leukotriene synthesis. Although this oral prophylactic drug is relatively new, it is falling into disuse because of the risks of hepatotoxicity that requires frequent monitoring of liver enzymes (e.g., ALT); its dependence on hepatic metabolism by the P450 system to the extent that is significantly inhibits the metabolism of such drugs as propranolol, theophylline, warfarin, and many others; and the inconvenience of four times a day dosing.

The leukotrienes modifiers do not enhance epinephrine release from the adrenal medulla (suprarenal medulla; b); increase β-adrenergic receptor responsiveness (c; note that norepinephrine, mentioned in the question, has no bronchodilator/β$_2$ activity); inhibit phosphodiesterase (d); or interfere with mast cell function or mast cell responsiveness to antigens (e).

293. The answer is f. (*Katzung, p 333.*) You should know *N*-acetylcysteine as an antidote for acetaminophen poisoning. When used for that purpose, it is given orally or intravenously. The sulfhydryl groups that are part of the molecule are important, as they react with the toxic acetaminophen metabolite and spare glutathione-depleted hepatocytes from oxidative attack. N-acetylcysteine is also a mucolytic (mucus-thinning) drug, given by inhalation in a nebulized solution or by intratracheal instillation, to reduce the viscosity of airway mucus that can then be removed easier by coughing, postural drainage and chest percussion, or by airway suctioning. Here, too, the mechanism is based on its—SH rich composition. N-acetylcysteine lacks other airway effects such as bronchodilation or suppression or inflammation.

294. The answer is a. (*Brunton, pp 683–689; Craig, pp 313, 426–427; Katzung, pp 319–321, 581.*) Aspirin, the prototype of the nonsteroidal anti-inflammatory drugs (NSAIDs), inhibits cyclooxygenases (COX-1 and -2) and the "arachidonic acid cascade." One outcome of that is inhibited synthesis of PGE$_2$. The PGE$_2$ (along with circulating epinephrine) is a physiologically important endogenous bronchodilator that is particularly important to maintain airway patency (dilation) for most asthmatics. Inhibit this synthesis, with aspirin or another nonselective cyclooxygenase inhibitor/NSAID, and bronchoconstriction or bronchospasm may ensue in that population of asthmatics who often are exquisitely sensitive to these drugs. This aspirin hypersensitivity phenomenon is relatively uncommon in children with asthma, but more prevalent in adults. Estimates that it affects between 10% and 25% of adult asthmatics with so-called "triad asthma": asthma plus nasal polyps and chronic urticaria.

Virtually all other NSAIDs that nonselectively inhibit cyclooxygenases may cross-react, although the incidence of severe pulmonary reactions seems the highest with aspirin itself. Selective COX-2 inhibitors (e.g., celecoxib) pose less of a problem because they are less likely to inhibit bronchodilator prostaglandins, which are formed by the COX-1 pathway, but they are not absolutely free from the potential problem. If one needs a drug to manage fever or mild pain in an asthmatic, acetaminophen is preferred: it does not cross-react; owing to negligible effects on prostaglandin synthesis via cyclooxygenase-dependent pathways, it is not classified as an NSAID.

295. The answer is b. (*Craig, p 327; Brunton, pp 122, 578–579; Katzung, p 512.*) Dextromethorphan is a centrally acting antitussive drug that is about as efficacious a cough-suppressant as codeine. However, unlike codeine (c) and hydrocodone (d; another useful antitussive in some cases), dextromethorphan is not an opioid and lacks analgesic effects or the potential for ventilatory suppression or abuse. Diphenhydramine (c) and promethazine (e) also have antitussive action. However, they, too, can cause generalized CNS and ventilatory depression. They also exert significant antimuscarinic effects. Although that may be good in terms of inhibiting ACh-mediated bronchoconstriction, it may also cause thickening of airway mucus, favoring mechanical plugging of the airways with viscous mucus deposits that cannot be removed normally by mucociliary transport or coughing. Note warnings for all pediatric patients, specifically because of the risk of serious (and sometimes fatal) respiratory depression. This warning was not specifically targeted at pediatric patients with asthma. Nonetheless, asthma patients (and younger ones especially) are particularly vulnerable to drugs that suppress ventilatory drive, and so the warning should elicit extra vigilance.

296. The answer is c. (*Brunton, pp 361–362, 407; Craig, pp 295–296, 355–360; Katzung, pp 319–322.*) The term asthma derives from a Greek word that means, literally, "to pant." In severe asthma attacks such as the one we describe here the hyperpnea precedes the likely development of ventilatory depression and, ultimately, ventilatory arrest. It is a sometimes successful and sometimes futile physiologic response elicited to increase ventilatory oxygen uptake and eliminate excess CO_2, although it may be insufficient to raise arterial O_2 saturation adequately and more than sufficient to induce metabolic alkalosis from excess CO_2 loss. Nonetheless, it is a "protective" response, and breathing too quickly, even inefficiently, is better than not breathing at all. This leads to the admonition: Never give a drug that can depress ventilation or the normal ventilatory drive to an asthma patient unless he or she has a protected airway and ventilation can be controlled and supported mechanically. IV midazolam (or the IV administration of virtually any other benzodiazepine, opioid, or barbiturate) will allay anxiety, but will also tend to suppress ventilatory drive and hasten the onset of ventilatory arrest. In the scenario described here, diazepam is the wrong drug to give.

Albuterol (a) or a similar β_2 agonist bronchodilator, whether given by inhalation or parenterally, would not be expected to worsen the boy's ventilatory status. They should not be the only drugs relied on, but they would be appropriate adjunctive treatments, as would be all the rest for the stated purposes. As an important aside, you may recall that atropine (b) and other drugs with antimuscarinic activity have bronchodilator activity, but also tend to make airway mucus secretions more viscous, leading to airway mucus plugging. In the context of this scenario, with the administration of other drugs that we listed, and the availability of airway suctioning devices as needed, the mucus-thickening effects of an antimuscarinic should not be a problem with which we cannot easily deal by way of airway suctioning and the administration of mucus-thinning (mucolytic) drugs. Glucocorticoids (d) and nebulized saline would be valuable, if not essential, adjuncts to this boy's therapy.

297. The answer is c. (*Brunton, pp 721–722, 1598–1599, 1603–1604; Craig, pp 464–465; Katzung, pp 328–329, 332.*) It usually takes a couple of weeks of inhaled corticosteroid use "as directed" to suppress airway inflammation, and the resulting bronchoconstriction, well enough that the patient can sense clinical improvement (fewer or milder asthma symptoms). Unless the patient is forewarned about this slow onset, and urged to remain compliant, they are likely to believe the drug is ineffective and therefore not worth taking. Clearly, inhaled corticosteroids do not cause the obvious "rush"—the prompt, dramatic, and unmistakable symptom relief that typically occurs with adrenergic bronchodilators. Nonetheless, given adequate time, the inhaled steroids usually prove to be the key to effective long-term control of asthma. Inhaled corticosteroids act locally; little enters the systemic circulation; such side effects as fluid retention, weight gain (e), and hyperglycemia, that are typical with systemic steroids (e.g., prednisone), rarely occur or become problematic. Inhaled steroids do not cause cardiac stimulation (a), diarrhea (b), or drowsiness (d).

298. The answer is e. (*Brunton, pp 728–730; Craig, p 463; Katzung, pp 325–327.*) Theophylline, a methylxanthine, is a caffeine–like drug that is becoming outmoded as therapy for asthma in most adolescents and adults. It should probably not be prescribed by any physician other than a pulmonologist who is familiar with the limitations and problems with this class of drugs. A low margin of safety, extreme dependence on adequate liver function (for metabolism), susceptibility to numerous clinically significant drug interactions, and a lack of airway anti inflammatory activity, are among the reasons why without proper dosage adjustments and monitoring it is all too easy, and common, for blood levels to fall into subtherapeutic ranges or, as we see here, into toxic ranges. The earliest signs and symptoms of excess involve CNS stimulation (jitteriness, tremors, difficulty sleeping, anxiety). As blood levels rise the CNS is increasingly stimulated. Seizures may occur, and when they do the inability to breathe during the seizures is the main cause of death. Thus, answer b is incorrect. Theophylline tends to cause tachycardia, increases of cardiac contractility and, potentially, tachyarrhythmias. Bradycardia (a) is not at all likely. Theophylline is not hepatotoxic (c); it does not cause paradoxical bronchospasm (d), even when serum levels are very high or truly toxic.

299. The answer is a. (*Craig, pp 87, 93, 115–116, 124–125, 130; Brunton, pp 187–188, 193–194, 208–209; Katzung, p 297.*) By now you should be able to recall the classifications and actions of the drugs listed in this question. Acetylcholinesterase inhibitors and such muscarinic agonists as pilocarpine are sometimes used as topical miotics for managing glaucoma (mainly angle-closure/narrow angle forms of the disease). Certain topical β blockers are used for open-angle glaucoma, probably working by inhibiting aqueous humor production. However, all these drugs (and others in these classes, used systemically for a host of other common medical conditions) are contraindicated for asthma patients—even if or when they are used topically on the eye(s). An important element in the pathophysiology of asthma is airway smooth-muscle hyperresponsiveness to various bronchoconstrictor stimuli, ACh clearly among them.

You may recall that the choline ester, methacholine, is used to help diagnose asthma when the diagnosis is otherwise questionable. The basis of this "methacholine challenge" centers on the concept that airway smooth muscles of people with asthma are much more sensitive (hyperreactive) to choline esters (and several other drugs) than those of people who do not have asthma. Very low doses of methacholine are given, by inhalation, while pulmonary function tests are recorded. Asthmatics experience significant (sometimes dangerous) bronchoconstrictor responses to methacholine doses that are far lower than those that would provoke even slight changes in nonasthmatics.

Recall too that ACh esterase inhibitors cause what amounts to a "build up" of ACh at the neuroeffector junction. These drugs, whether used for glaucoma or such other conditions as myasthenia gravis, can have lethal effects for some asthma patients. (Note, too, that ACh esterase inhibitors are found in some insecticides, so there is a risk to the asthma patient in agricultural or gardening/lawn care activities.) Muscarinic agonists, whether those used for glaucoma or for stimulating the gut or urinary tract (e.g., bethanechol for functional urinary retention) may prove lethal too. Finally, asthmatics tend to be extremely dependent on the bronchodilator actions of circulating epinephrine. Block the β_2 receptors that mediate that effect and the outcome can be disastrous. Even the so-called "cardioselective" β blockers (atenolol, metoprolol) can cause serious problems for asthmatics. That is because their ability to block β_1 receptors is relative and dose-dependent, not absolute: they may pose no pulmonary problems for persons without asthma, but may be deadly in those who do.

300. The answer is b. (*Brunton, p 722; Craig, p 467; Katzung, pp 127, 325, 332.*) When pulmonary function deteriorates so much that respiratory acidosis ensues (because sufficient amounts of CO_2 aren't being eliminated by ventilation) and severe hypoxia develops (because of inadequate oxygen transfer), acute tolerance (in essence, desensitization) develops to the bronchodilator effects of drugs with β_2- agonist activity—all of them. If this point is forgotten, repeated administration of a β_2 agonist will lead to increasing degrees of cardiac stimulation (rate, contractility, automaticity, conduction) because under these conditions they lose their selectivity for β_2 receptors and also begin activating β_1 receptors very effectively. (They become isoproterenol-like in their profiles.)

Even epinephrine won't work as an efficacious bronchodilator under these conditions, and repeated injections of it will do little more than cause further cardiac stimulation plus vasoconstriction via α activation. Through mechanisms that are not quite clear, administering suitable doses of a parenteral steroid under these conditions of acidosis and hypoxia "restores" a substantial degree of airway responsiveness to β agonists. Giving a steroid (plus oxygen, which helps correct the underlying blood gas and pH changes) is essential.

Giving diphenhydramine, even though it blocks the bronchoconstrictor effects of both ACh and histamine, will not do much good for the acute and life-threatening signs and symptoms. Giving cromolyn will prove largely worthless and certainly not life-saving.

Local Control Substances: Autacoids and Drugs for Inflammatory Processes

Histamine receptor antagonists
Serotonin agonists
Serotonin antagonists
Hyperuricemia, gout
Ergot alkaloids

Prostaglandins and related
  eicosanoids
NSAIDS (and other eicosanoid
  synthesis inhibitors)

Questions

DIRECTIONS: Each item contains a question or incomplete statement that is followed by several responses. Select the **one best** response to each question.

301. Arachidonic acid is metabolized by two main pathways: cyclooxygenase and lipoxygenase. Which of the following is a main end-product of the lipoxygenase pathway?

a.   Leukotrienes
b.   Platelet-activating factor (PAF)
c.   Prostacyclin (PGI_2)
d.   Prostaglandins
e.   Thromboxanes
f.   Uric acid

302. A patient has mild cutaneous and systemic manifestations of an allergic response. Before you prescribe a short course of diphenhydramine for symptom relief, you should realize that this drug has one mechanism of action resembling, causes many side effects similar to, and shares many contraindications, that apply to an "autonomic" drug with which you should be very familiar. Which of the following is that drug?

a. Atropine
b. Bethanechol
c. Norepinephrine
d. Phentolamine
e. Physostigmine
f. Propranolol

303. A patient with an allergic disorder experiences significant bronchoconstriction and urticaria. Histamine, released from mast cells, is incriminated as an important contributor to these responses. Which of the following drugs may pose extra risks for this patient—not because it has any bronchoconstrictor effects in its own right, but because it quite effectively releases histamine from mast cells?

a. Atropine
b. Isoproterenol
c. Neostigmine
d. Pancuronium
e. Propranolol
f. d-Tubocurarine

304. A patient presents with a history of frequent and severe migraine headaches. When we give one of the more commonly used drugs for abortive therapy, sumatriptan, upon which of the following "local control substances" is it mainly acting?

a. Histamine
b. $PGF_{2\alpha}$
c. Prostacyclin
d. Serotonin
e. Thromboxane A_2

305. A male patient with severe arthritis will be placed on long-term therapy with indomethacin. We recognize the risk of NSAID-induced gastrointestinal ulceration and want to prescribe another drug for ulcer prophylaxis. Which of the following drugs should we choose?

a. Celecoxib
b. Cimetidine
c. Diclofenac
d. Diphenhydramine
e. Misoprostol

306. Aspirin causes significant bronchoconstriction and bronchospasm in a patient who was subsequently identified as being "aspirin-sensitive." Which of the following mechanisms summarizes best why aspirin provoked the respiratory problems in this patient?

a. Drug-mediated hypersensitivity of H_1 receptors on airway smooth muscles
b. Drug-mediated hypersensitivity of muscarinic receptors on airway smooth muscles
c. Enhanced formation of antibodies directed against the salicylate on airway mast cells
d. Inhibited synthesis of endogenous prostaglandins that have bronchodilator activity
e. Reduced (blocked) epinephrine binding to β_2-adrenergic receptors on airway smooth-muscle cells

307. A child takes what comes close to being a lethal dose of acetaminophen. Which of the following is the most likely pathology involved in this drug overdose?

a. Acute nephropathy
b. A-V conduction disturbances, heart block
c. Liver failure
d. Status asthmaticus
e. Status epilepticus

308. A patient with asymptomatic hyperuricemia is started on probenecid. In a couple of days he develops acute gout. Which of the following is the best explanation of how probenecid triggered this acute gouty arthritic episode?

a. Accelerated synthesis of uric acid by the probenecid
b. Coprecipitation of probenecid and urate in the joints
c. Idiosyncratic response
d. Probenecid-induced systemic acidosis, favoring uric acid crystallization
e. Reduced renal excretion of uric acid

309. A 29-year-old woman has recently developed migraine headaches. For various reasons you cannot prescribe a triptan for abortive therapy, so you prescribe ergotamine. Which of the following is the main mechanism of action of this drug in terms of the migraine?

a. Activates serotonin receptors
b. Inhibits thromboxane synthesis/improves cerebral blood flow
c. Propranolol-like blockade of β-adrenergic receptors
d. Reduces cerebral metabolic rate (reduced oxygen demand)
e. Strong antimuscarinic activity

310. Such drugs as methotrexate, hydroxychloroquine, or penicillamine are often turned to for managing rheumatoid arthritis that is not controlled adequately with "traditional" NSAIDs (e.g., aspirin, ibuprofen, or indomethacin). Which of the following statements best summarizes how those drugs differ from a typical NSAID?

a. Activate the immune system to neutralize inflammatory mediators
b. Are primary therapies for gouty arthritis
c. Are remarkably free from serious toxicities
d. Provide much quicker relief of arthritis signs, symptoms
e. Slow, stop, possibly reverse joint pathology in rheumatoid arthritis

311. For quite a while the "coxibs" (selective COX-2 inhibitors) were pre-scribed in preference to nonselective cyclooxygenase inhibitors for manag-ing such conditions as rheumatoid arthritis. Which of the following statements best describes an action or property of these COX-2 inhibitors?

a. Are associated with a lower risk of gastric or duodenal ulceration
b. Cure arthritis, rather than just give symptom relief
c. Effectively inhibit uric acid synthesis
d. Have a lower risk of adverse or fatal cardiac events
e. Have significantly faster onsets of action

312. We have a patient with drug-induced hyperuricemia. Our pharma-cologic approach for managing this will be to inhibit uric acid synthesis. Which of the following enzymes do we want to target with our drug?

a. 5'-Lipoxygenase
b. Cyclooxygenase 1
c. Cyclooxygenase 2
d. Phospholipase A_2
e. Xanthine oxidase

313. Our clinical goal (as noted in Question 312) is to inhibit uric acid synthesis. Which of the following drugs will do that?

a. Allopurinol
b. Aspirin
c. Celecoxib
d. Corticosteroids (glucocorticoids)
e. Probenecid
f. Zileuton

314. We administer a drug that interrupts/inhibits eicosanoid formation and causes significant anti inflammatory effects, by nonselectively inhibiting both cyclooxygenase-1 and -2 (COX-1 and -2). Which of the following drugs did we give?

a. Acetaminophen
b. Allopurinol
c. Celecoxib
d. Indomethacin
e. Misoprostol
f. Monteleukast

315. Glucocorticoids are widely used for a host of inflammatory reactions and the diseases they cause. In terms of inflammatory responses and underlying metabolic reactions, which of the following enzymes or processes is the main target of these drugs when they are given at pharmacologic (supraphysiologic) doses?

a. Cyclooxygenases (COX-1 and -2)
b. Histidine decarboxylase
c. 5'-lipoxygenase
d. Phospholipase A_2 (PLA$_2$)
e. Xanthine oxidase

316. Bradykinin plays important roles in local responses to tissue damage and a variety of inflammatory processes. It also has vasodilator activity. Which of the following statements is correct about this endogenous peptide?

a. Captopril inhibits its metabolic inactivation
b. Drugs that are metabolized to, or generate, nitric oxide, counteract bradykinin's vascular effects
c. Increased blood pressure is the predominant cardiovascular response
d. Newer histamine H_1 blockers (e.g., fexofenadine; "second-generation" antihistamine) also competitively block bradykinin receptors
e. The main renal responses to endogenous bradykinin are arteriolar constriction and reduced GFR

317. A newborn has blood gas and hemodynamic problems because of a patent (open) ductus arteriosus. Which of the following drugs would be administered in an attempt to close the ductus?

a. Cimetidine
b. Diphenhydramine
c. Indomethacin
d. Misoprostol
e. Prostaglandin E_1 (PGE_1; alprostadil)

318. A 29-year-old woman develops frequent, debilitating migraine headaches. Sumatriptan is prescribed for abortive therapy. Not long after taking the drug she is rushed to the hospital. Her vital signs are unstable, and she has muscle rigidity, myoclonus, generalized CNS irritability and altered consciousness, and shivering. You learn that for several months she had been taking another drug with which the triptan interacted. Which of the following was the most likely drug?

a. Acetaminophen
b. Codeine
c. Diazepam
d. Fluoxetine
e. Phenytoin

319. A patient suffers badly from a variety of upper respiratory responses during "hay fever" (seasonal allergy) seasons, and his asthma is provoked. We prescribe orally inhaled nedocromil for prophylaxis. Which of the following is the main mechanism by which nedocromil causes its desired effects?

a. Competitively blocks histamine H_1 receptors, thereby blocking bronchoconstriction
b. Decongests mucous membranes via a local vasoconstrictor action
c. Directly binds antigens, preventing them from interacting with mast cell antibodies
d. Inhibits mediator release from immunologically sensitized mast cells
e. Inhibits synthesis of histamine and leukotrienes

320. A patient (assume he is taking no other drugs) has been taking doses of aspirin that are too high for several weeks. Low-grade aspirin toxicity (salicylism) develops. Which of the following signs or symptoms would be most indicative of the salicylism and the high salicylate levels that caused it?

a. Constipation
b. Cough
c. Hypertension
d. Myopia
e. Tinnitus

321. Aspirin generally should be avoided as an anti-inflammatory, analgesic, or antipyretic drug by patients with hyperuricemia or gout. That is because it counteracts the effects of one important drug the hyperuricemic patient may be taking. Which of the following drugs has its desired effects reduced or eliminated by this prototypical NSAID?

a. Acetaminophen
b. Allopurinol
c. Colchicine
d. Indomethacin
e. Naproxen
f. Probenecid

322. Misoprostol, an analog of PGE_1, is sometimes used adjunctively to stimulate gastric mucus production and help reduce the incidence of gastric ulcers associated with long-term or high-dose NSAID therapy for arthritis. Which of the following is the other main use for this lipid-derived autacoid?

a. Closure of a patent ductus arteriosus in newborns
b. Contraception in women who should not receive estrogens or progestins
c. Induction of abortion in conjunction with mifepristone ("RU486")
d. Prophylaxis of asthma *in lieu* of a corticosteroid
e. Suppression of uterine contractility in women with premature labor

323. Bradykinin is a nonapeptide that acts on at least two distinct receptors, named B_1 and B_2. Among bradykinin's main physiologic or pathophysiologic effects are mediation of sensory/peripheral pain, bronchoconstriction, inflammation, and cardiovascular/hemodynamic function via a vasodilator effect on the peripheral vasculature. Which of the following drugs inhibits metabolic inactivation of bradykinin?

a. Acetaminophen
b. Captopril
c. Cimetidine
d. Ketoconazole
e. Phenelzine

324. An intradermal injection of histamine has important effects on vascular smooth muscle tone. Which of the following pathways mediates this response to H_1 histamine receptor activation?

a. Activation of cellular Na^+ influx
b. Activation of tyrosine kinases
c. Elevation of intracellular cyclic AMP (cAMP) levels
d. Increased formation of inositol triphosphates (IP_3)
e. Inhibition of adenylate cyclase activity

325. A patient who was transported by ambulance to the emergency department took a potentially lethal overdose of aspirin. Which of the following drugs would be a helpful adjunct to manage this severe aspirin poisoning?

a. Acetaminophen
b. Amphetamines (e.g., dextroamphetamine)
c. N-acetylcysteine
d. Phenobarbital
e. Sodium bicarbonate

326. We look at data that summarize the actions of two prototypic histamine receptor blockers—diphenhydramine as the exemplar of the older antihistamines (competitive histamine receptor antagonists) and fexofenadine as a representative agent of the "second generation" antihistamines. Which of the following statements best describes, compares, or contrasts these drugs or the pharmacologic groups to which they belong?

a. Diphenhydramine and other drugs in its class (ethanolamines) tend to cause drowsiness more often than fexofenadine and related second generation antihistamines
b. Diphenhydramine is a preferred antihistaminic for patients with prostate hypertrophy or angle-closure glaucoma, whereas fexofenadine and related drugs are contraindicated
c. Diphenhydramine overdoses tend to cause bradycardia, whereas fexofenadine overdoses tend to cause significant increases of heart rate
d. Fexofenadine and related second generation histamine antagonists have intrinsic bronchodilator activity, which makes them suitable as primary/sole therapy for people with asthma
e. Fexofenadine, and drugs in its class, have better efficacy in terms of suppressing histamine-mediated gastric acid secretion

327. A patient has been taking one of the drugs listed below for about 4 months and is experiencing the desired therapeutic effects from it. The MD now prescribes indomethacin to treat a particularly severe flare-up of rheumatoid arthritis. Within a matter of days the therapeutic effects of the first drug wane dramatically, its actions antagonized by the indomethacin. Which of the following was the most likely drug affected by the indomethacin?

a. Allopurinol, given for prophylaxis of hyperuricemia
b. Captopril, given for essential hypertension
c. Fexofenadine, given for managing seasonal allergy responses
d. Sumatriptan, given for abortive therapy of migraine headaches
e. Warfarin, given for prophylaxis of venous thrombosis

328. A patient takes an acute, massive overdose of aspirin that, without proper intervention, will probably be fatal. Which of the following would you expect to occur in the advanced (late) stages of aspirin (salicylate) poisoning?

a. Hypothermia
b. Metabolic alkalosis
c. Respiratory alkalosis
d. Respiratory plus metabolic acidosis
e. Ventilatory stimulation

329. A patient presents in the emergency department with an overdose of a drug. The MD knows what the drug is and so orders appropriate "symptomatic and supportive care," plus multiple doses of N-acetylcysteine. Assuming the MD's treatment plan is correct, which of the following drugs was the most likely cause of the overdose?

a. Acetaminophen
b. Aspirin
c. Colchicine
d. Diphenhydramine
e. Loratadine
f. Methotrexate

330. A patient has acute gout. The physician initially thinks about prescribing just one or two oral doses of colchicine, 12 h apart, but then decides otherwise. The main reason for avoiding colchicine, even with a very short oral course, is the development of which of the following?

a. Bone marrow suppression
b. Bronchospasm
c. GI distress that is almost as bad as the acute gout discomfort
d. Hepatotoxicity
e. One or two oral doses seldom relieve gout pain
f. Refractoriness/tolerance with just a dose or two

331. A patient with hyperuricemia is placed on an "antigout" drug. Before starting the drug you measure the total uric acid (amount, not concentration) in a 24-h urine sample and then do the same several weeks after continued drug therapy at therapeutic doses. The posttreatment sample shows a significant reduction in urate content. There were no new pathologies developing during therapy, and the patient's daily purine intake did not change at all. Which of the following drugs was given?

a. Acetaminophen
b. Allopurinol
c. Colchicine
d. Indomethacin
e. Probenecid

332. A patient with annoying hay fever (seasonal allergy) symptoms goes to the store, intent on purchasing an oral medication to make them more comfortable. They see the prices for loratadine and related second generation antihistamines and are shocked about how high they are. Nearby on the shelf they see store-brand allergy relief pills that are much cheaper. The active ingredient is diphenhydramine. If they were to take full therapeutic doses of the diphenhydramine, based on label directions, which of the following effects or side effects are they most likely to experience as an additional price to be paid for their allergy relief?

a. Bradycardia
b. Diarrhea
c. Drowsiness, somnolence
d. "Heartburn" from increased gastric acid secretion
e. Urinary frequency

333. A patient develops acute gout. Which of the following is an accurate description of how uric acid causes the arthritic response?

a. Activates microtubular formation in leukocytes
b. Directly activates leukotriene B_4 receptors
c. Has intrinsic tumor necrosis factor (TNF) activity
d. Mechanically damages articulating surfaces of the joints
e. Uncouples oxidative phosphorylation leading to tissue damage

334. Your patient has rheumatoid arthritis that has been refractory to diclofenac, ibuprofen, indomethacin, and sulindac. In addition, she has experienced numerous GI bleeds in response to those drugs. We start her on therapy with etanercept. Which of the following is the most likely mechanism by which etanercept suppresses the signs, symptoms, or underlying pathophysiology of rheumatoid arthritis?

a. Inhibits eicosanoid synthesis by inhibiting phospholipase A_2
b. Inhibits leukocyte migration by blocking microtubular formation
c. Neutralizes circulating tumor necrosis factor (α-TNF)
d. Selectively and effectively inhibits COX-2
e. Stimulates collagen and mucopolysaccharide synthesis in the joints

Local Control Substances: Autacoids and Drugs for Inflammatory Processes

Answers

301. The answer is a. (*Brunton, pp 655–657; Craig, p 425; Katzung, pp 298–301, 581.*) The arachidonic acid (AA) "cascade" begins with AA synthesis from membrane phospholipids by phospholipase A_2. Once arachidonic acid is formed, the metabolic pathways diverge into the lipoxygenase pathway that forms cysteinyl leukotrienes (LTs) and the cyclooxygenase pathways that synthesize prostaglandins, including prostacyclin and thromboxane A_2. One important intermediate early on in the LP pathway is LTA_4. From that we get LTB_4, which mainly regulates chemotaxis (cytokine activity) and activates phagocytosis in white blood cells. Also derived from LTB_4 are, sequentially, LTC_4, LTD_4, and LTE_4 (cysteinyl leukotrienes, historically and collectively called SRS-A, for slow-reacting substance of anaphylaxis), which cause mainly bronchoconstriction. Leukotriene synthesis can be inhibited by zileuton (once used clinically), a 5'lipoxygenase inhibitor. The leukotriene receptors can be blocked by montelukast and zafirlukast, which are used prophylactically to suppress airway inflammation and bronchoconstriction in asthma.

302. The answer is a. (*Brunton, pp 637–640, 642, 1004; Craig, p 454; Katzung, pp 266, 319–321.*) Diphenhydramine, an older or "first-generation" antihistamine, is a competitive antagonist of histamine's effects on H_1 receptors and also strongly blocks muscarinic cholinergic receptors. Other older H_1 blockers (but none of the second-generation H_1 blockers, such as fexofenadine) possess this atropine-like effect, often to a lesser degree than diphenhydramine. (If you wished to argue that because diphenhydramine was more like scopolamine, because it causes not only anticholinergic effects but also a considerable degree of sedation, you would be correct.) Thus, common side effects related to antimuscarinic activity include sedation, dry mouth, photophobia, and cycloplegia (paralysis of accommodation). Key contraindications include prostatic hypertrophy, bowel or bladder obstruction or hypomotility, tachycardia, and narrow-angle (angle-closure) glaucoma.

To refresh your memory about the other drugs listed, bethanechol (b) is a muscarinic agonist, norepinephrine (c) is an effective agonist for β_1- and α-adrenergic receptors, phentolamine (d) is a nonselective α blocker, physostigmine (e) is an acetylcholinesterase inhibitor, and propranolol (f) is, of course, the prototypic nonselective β-adrenergic blocker.

303. The answer is f. (*Brunton, pp 226, 632; Craig, p 451; Katzung, pp 260, 438.*) Tubocurarine, arguably the prototypic nondepolarizing skeletal neuromuscular blocker (competitive antagonist of the effects of ACh on skeletal muscle nicotinic receptors), differs from most of the other nondepolarizing neuromuscular blockers (including pancuronium) because it quite effectively triggers histamine release. It is a "direct" effect on mast cells, not one involving activation of antibodies on the mast cells. This effect is not clinically significant for patients who do not have asthma, but for many who do, the bronchoconstriction can be problematic (even though the patient is intubated while they are receiving the blocker). In the absence of (released) histamine, curare and the other neuromuscular blockers would have no effect on airway smooth-muscle activity.

(Note: In addition to tubocurarine, morphine, and several intravascular contrast media used in diagnostic radiology—particularly some of the iodinated compounds—also have a reputation as "histamine-releasers." Some venoms and other animal toxins also cause mast cell degranulation, a component of which is histamine release.)

Atropine causes bronchodilation by blocking muscarinic receptors on airway smooth muscle cells. Isoproterenol, the β_1/β_2 agonist, is a bronchodilator. Propranolol triggers airway smooth-muscle contraction in asthmatics, but that is due to blockade of epinephrine's agonist (bronchodilator) actions on β_2 receptors. Histamine is not involved in the responses to any of these drugs.

304. The answer is d. (*Brunton, pp 300t, 305–308, 334; Craig, pp 283–284; Katzung, pp 268–272.*) Acute migraine therapy often involves giving a drug that mimics the effects of endogenous serotonin, thereby reversing the cerebrovasodilation that contributes significantly to migraine signs and symptoms. A good example is sumatriptan (member of a small group of drugs called triptans). These are 5-HT$_{1B/2D}$ receptor agonists. Histamine and, to a lesser extent, prostacyclin [PGI$_2$] are vasodilators, too, but they don't seem to have appreciable roles in migraine, nor are they targets of antimigraine drug activity. Activation of β$_2$-adrenergic receptors in the cerebral vasculature also leads to vasodilation and migraine symptoms. The β-adrenergic blockers (particularly propranolol) are useful for some migraineurs, but only for prophylaxis, not for abortive therapy.

305. The answer is e. (*Brunton, pp 665, 973, 979; Craig, p 481; Katzung, pp 299, 309, 1043.*) Misoprostol is a long-acting synthetic analog of PGE$_1$, and its only use (outside of reproductive medicine) is prophylaxis of NSAID-induced gastric ulcers. Its main effects are suppression of gastric acid secretion and enhanced gastric mucus production (a so-called mucotropic or cytoprotective effect). The need for the drug arises, of course, because such drugs as indomethacin (and most other COX-nonselective inhibitors) inhibit PGE$_1$ synthesis as well as that of other prostaglandins, prostacyclin, and thromboxane A$_2$.

Although cimetidine (b) might help reduce gastric acid secretion (via H$_2$ blockade) and diphenhydramine (c) may too (via antimuscarinic effects), their antisecretory effects are weak and nonspecific in this situation, and they don't increase formation of the stomach's protective mucus nor adequately suppress gastric acid secretion.

Celecoxib (a; and other coxibs) are associated with a lower risk or incidence of peptic ulcers than more traditional NSAIDs, mainly because the former are relatively selective COX-2 inhibitors: it is the COX-1 pathway that, when inhibited, mainly allows gastric HCl secretion to rise and mucus production to fall. However, we asked about which drug would be an add-on to indomethacin therapy, and adding a COX-2 inhibitor would be irrational. Diclofenac (c) is an NSAID that, when used long-term (e.g., as an alternative to indomethacin or any of the other reasonable options), may cause ulcers just as indomethacin may. In fact, a fixed-dose combination product containing diclofenac and misoprostol is available.

306. The answer is d. (*Brunton, pp 664, 683, 685, 689–690; Craig, pp 425–426; Katzung, p 581.*) Inhibited synthesis of prostaglandins that are bronchodilators (mainly PGE$_2$) are thought to be responsible for severe or fatal responses to aspirin in some asthmatics. Note that aspirin inhibits the synthesis of $PGF_2\alpha$ and of TXA_2, both of which are bronchoconstrictors. As a result, one would predict reduced bronchoconstriction with aspirin. However, in those patients with aspirin-sensitive asthma (indeed, in many asthmatics overall), the adverse effects arising from inhibited PGE_2 synthesis tend to predominate, and so aspirin and other efficacious NSAIDs are generally contraindicated.

307. The answer is c. *(Brunton, pp 83, 694, 1741; Craig, pp 66, 314; Katzung, pp 595–596.)* The primary cause of death from acetaminophen overdoses is hepatic necrosis. The drug's main toxic metabolite is N-acetyl-benzoqinoneimine. It reacts with sulfhydryl groups that are constituents of key macromolecules and metabolic cofactors (e.g., glutathione) in the liver. If acetaminophen doses are low, glutathione conjugates the metabolite. With toxic doses, however, glutathione is depleted and other –SH groups on hepatocyte proteins are attacked and irreversibly altered. Concomitant with overall hepatic damage we find, eventually, profound hypoglycemia (as the liver's stores of glycogen are depleted) and coagulopathies (as hepatic clotting factor synthesis stops and the patient begins bleeding spontaneously).

Nephropathy (a) is not a primary or important consequence of acetaminophen toxicity. If A-V conduction disturbances, heart block, or other cardiac electrophysiologic anomalies (b) occur, they are secondary to hepatic dysfunction. Status asthmaticus (d) and acute seizures (e) are not likely or direct consequences of acetaminophen poisoning.

308. The answer is e. *(Brunton, pp 710–711; Craig, pp 444–445; Katzung, pp 597–598.)* It has been said that the initial phase of uricosuric therapy is the most worrisome period. Probenecid is a uricosuric drug, but that effect depends on having high (therapeutic) blood levels that are sufficient to inhibit active tubular reabsorption of urate. At subtherapeutic blood levels the main effect is inhibition of tubular secretion of urate, which reduces net urate excretion and raises serum urate levels (sometimes to the point of causing clinical gout). It is only once drug levels are therapeutic that the desired effects to inhibit tubular reabsorption of urate predominate. Thus, and intuitively, once a patient starts probenecid therapy drug levels must pass through that stage in which urate excretion will actually go down.

Some texts suggest using a short course of colchicine or another (nonaspirin) NSAID that is indicated for gout when probenecid therapy is started. That is for prophylaxis of acute gout that might occur. Although this may be acceptable, other rules are perhaps more important: (1) do not administer a uricosuric during a gout attack; (2) if the patient has had a gout attack recently, suppress the inflammation for 2 to 3 months with a suitable anti-inflammatory and consider starting a uricosuric only after that 2- to 3-month symptom-free interval; and (3) do not use uricosurics for patients with "severe hyperuricemia" and/or poor renal function. Doing otherwise is associated with a great risk of potentially severe renal tubular damage as the uricosuric shifts large amounts of uric acid from the blood (with its large volume, that keeps urate relatively "dilute") into a small volume of acidic urine, which concentrates urate and lowers its solubility via pH-dependent mechanisms.

(The patient who skips doses of probenecid also becomes very vulnerable to the "paradoxical" extra risk, because doing this may allow drug levels to fall into that subtherapeutic range in which more urate is retained than eliminated.)

309. The answer is a. *(Brunton, pp 308–310; Craig, pp 718–719; Katzung, pp 273–278.)* Ergotamine has several pharmacologic properties. The one that seems to be responsible for its efficacy in migraines is activation (as a typical agonist) of serotonin receptors (5-HT$_{D1}$) in the cerebral vasculature, thus causing a triptan-like effect (but the drug should not be used with a triptan). The drug works best in prodromal phases (classical signs and symptoms the migraineur should learn to recognize before a full-blown migraine attack develops). It's less effective once the full onslaught of migraine has developed. It lacks intrinsic sedative or analgesic activity.

In addition to the effects just mentioned, toxic doses of ergotamine cause peripheral vasoconstriction intense enough to cause hypertension and tissue ischemia (including gangrene of such structures as the fingers and toes). The syndrome of poisoning is called ergotism.

The ergot alkaloids, as a group, also cause intense, prolonged uterine-contracting effects. This contraindicates their use during pregnancy, but explains the use of the related drugs ergonovine and methylergonovine postpartum to control uterine bleeding (bleeding is reduced by the strong uterine contractions).

310. The answer is e. *(Brunton, pp 690, 706, 1336; Craig, pp 432–437; Katzung, pp 588–594.)* Methotrexate, gold salts, and penicillamine are members of a diverse group of drugs called DMARDs (disease-modifying antirheumatic drugs) or SAARDs (slow-acting antirheumatic drugs). The former term derives from the ability of these drugs to slow, stop, or in some cases reverse joint damage associated with rheumatoid arthritis (RA). They do more than merely mask or relieve RA symptoms, which is mainly what the traditional NSAIDs do. The second acronym derives from the fact that it may take a month (or a couple more) for meaningful symptom relief to develop; they are not at all quick-acting drugs. Their actions probably are due to suppression of immune responses that often contribute to the etiology of RA.

Their toxicities can be serious, which is one reason why, until not long ago, these agents were considered third-line or even last resort treatments for refractory rheumatoid disease. (Methotrexate is now being used much earlier, and safely, for RA, now that we know better how to use it and monitor for serious toxicities; see the chapter, "Cancer Chemotherapy and Immunosuppressants.") Most of these drugs can cause serious blood dyscrasias; in addition, penicillamine can cause renal and pulmonary toxicity; hydroxychloroquine is associated with vision impairments/retinopathy.

311. The answer is a. (*Brunton, pp 657–658, 671, 681, 684, 702–705; Craig, p 431; Katzung, pp 582–584.*) Celecoxib and related drugs, by virtue of their selective COX-2 inhibition, do not interfere as much with synthesis of PGE_2, which normally suppresses a component of gastric acid secretion and stimulates gastric mucus production. Overall, then, the risks of gastric and duodenal ulcers are reduced. The selectivity also means that the COX-2 inhibitors do not interfere with the production of other eicosanoids, such as TXA_2. That is both good and bad, clinically. On the good side, this means that COX-2 inhibitors don't cause antiplatelet effects and increase the risk of excessive or spontaneous bleeding. On the other hand, this lack of effect renders them unsuitable for causing desired antiplatelet-aggregatory effects, as might be wanted when we administer aspirin. This may explain the finding that some COX-2 inhibitors have been associated with (cause?) a higher risk of sudden cardiac death (d) in vulnerable patients, and why some have been pulled off the market and are subjects of considerable litigation.

COX-2 inhibitors, like the nonselective alternatives, aren't cures for arthritis (b); they alleviate signs and symptoms but seem to have no demonstrable impact on the underlying pathophysiology. They have no effect on uric acid metabolism (c) or excretion. Their onsets of action are, overall, no faster (e) than those of a typical NSAID.

312. The answer is e. (*Brunton, pp 708–709; Craig, pp 445–446; Katzung, p 599.*) Xanthine oxidase catalyzes the last two steps in (human) purine degradation: the conversion of hypoxanthine to xanthine and the conversion of xanthine to uric acid. The enzyme can be inhibited by allopurinol. This pathway is not part of the arachidonic acid-cyclooxygenase-lipoxygenase pathways.

313. The answer is a. (*Brunton, pp 708–709; Craig, pp 445–446; Katzung, pp 598–599.*) Allopurinol (through its active metabolite, oxypurinol, which is a xanthine oxidase substrate) inhibits xanthine oxidase and so blocks synthesis of xanthine and its metabolite, uric acid. Purine degradation stops at the production of hypoxanthine, which is more soluble in body fluids than the two subsequent products of xanthine oxidase activity, xanthine, and uric acid.

Allopurinol has no effect on other inflammatory pathways or arthritides other than those related to hyperuricemia, nor does it directly affect renal function to enhance or inhibit urate excretion.

314. The answer is d. (*Brunton, pp 671, 675t, 695–696; Craig, p 427; Katzung, pp 299, 577–582.*) Indomethacin (and aspirin and many other NSAIDs) inhibits both COX-1 and COX-2. This differs from the "coxibs" (e.g., celecoxib; c), which are relatively selective for inhibiting COX-2.

Acetaminophen (a) has antipyretic and analgesic effects that somehow involve inhibition of prostaglandin metabolism, but it has little or no clinically useful anti-inflammatory activity. Misoprostol (e) is a synthetic analog of PGE_1, and has no synthesis-inhibitory actions. It is mainly used as prophylaxis against NSAID-induced gastric ulceration; and is also used as an abortifacient because of its significant uterine-stimulating activity. Monteleukast blocks leukotriene receptors. It does not inhibit 5'-lipoxygenase (leukotriene synthesis) or any other pathways involved in the biosynthesis of inflammatory mediators. It is occasionally used for oral prophylaxis of asthma (owing to its airway anti-inflammatory activity; and mainly as an alternative to the related lipoxygenase inhibitor, zafirlukast, which interacts significantly with other drugs, warfarin being a noteworthy one. Allopurinol (b) inhibits xanthine oxidase, which is not part of the arachidonic acid metabolic pathways but rather of purine metabolism and the ultimate formation of uric acid. It is used for prophylaxis of hyperuricemia of various etiologies, including that which is associated with leukemias or is drug-induced (e.g., by drugs used to treat leukemias or other disseminated cancers; thiazide and loop diuretics).

315. The answer is d. *(Brunton, pp 721–722, 1407, 1594–1596, 1599–1600; Craig, p 425; Katzung, pp 577, 580, 643–646.)* Anti-inflammatory doses of glucocorticosteroids inhibit phospholipase A_2 activity. In doing so, they inhibit arachidonic acid synthesis and, therefore, synthesis of all subsequent products of the cyclooxygenase and lipoxygenase pathways, both of which originate with arachidonic acid. This action of glucocorticoids is indirect because their initial or direct effect is induced synthesis of annexins (previously called lipocortins), which are the moieties that directly inhibit PLA_2 activity. Glucocorticoids have no intrinsic or direct inhibitory effects on later steps in AA metabolism, that is, no effects on cyclooxygenase or lipoxygenase activity.

Cyclooxygenases (a) are inhibited by NSAIDs such as aspirin (nonselective COX-1 and -2 inhibitors) or the "coxibs" (celecoxib), which relatively selectively inhibit COX-2. We have no clinically useful inhibitors of histamine synthesis which involves histidine decarboxylase activity; b. As noted elsewhere, zileuton inhibits 5'-lipoxygenase (c) and the subsequent formation of leukotrienes. Allopurinol inhibits the synthesis of xanthine and uric acid by inhibiting xanthine oxidase (e).

316. The answer is a. *(Brunton, pp 646, 648–649, 800–801; Craig, pp 212–215; Katzung, pp 177, 285–288.)* Bradykinin is metabolized to biologically inactive peptides by an enzyme that has three names: angiotensin-converting enzyme (ACE)—recall that the prototype ACE inhibitor is captopril), bradykininase, and kininase II.

Bradykinin, whether injected experimentally or derived from endogenous sources (kininogens cleaved by specific proteases called kallikreins), exerts significant vasodilator effects that can lower systolic and diastolic blood pressures. Although this may not be an important pressure-regulating mechanism in normotensive individuals, it probably is in many (most?) patients with essential hypertension.

Recall that ACE inhibitors lower blood pressure in many hypertensive patients. One mechanism involves "preserving" bradykinin by inhibiting its enzymatic inactivation. Bradykinin also causes prerenal arteriolar vasodilation and increases GFR, leading to diuretic effects.

The peptide's vascular effects are mediated by endothelial cell–derived nitric oxide, and they are enhanced by other drugs that cause vasodilation by a nitric oxide–related mechanism.

Bradykinin receptor blockers prevent the peptide's vasodilator effects.

317. The answer is c. *(Brunton, p 695; Craig, p 721; Katzung, p 585.)* The ductus arteriosus in neonate may remain patent largely because of the vasodilator effects of endogenous PGE_1, formed *via* the cyclooxygenase pathway. When the goal is to close a patent ductus after birth we generally use the very efficacious prostaglandin synthesis (COX-1/-2) inhibitor, indomethacin. Conversely, there are times when surgical procedures are required on a congenitally anomalous heart in newborns, and we want to keep the ductus open until surgery. In that case, alprostadil (PGE_1) may be administered. Administration of H_1 or H_2 histamine receptor blockers (diphenhydramine, cimetidine, respectively) will be of no benefit. Misoprostol (d) is a prostaglandin analog. Giving it to a newborn with a patent ductus is likely to keep the lesion open, not close it.

318. The answer is d. *(Brunton, pp 305–308, 334, 450; Katzung, pp 271, 483, 492–494, 991.)* This patient has what is almost certainly the serotonin syndrome. The triptan "adds" serotonin to the circulation, and its neuronal reuptake will be blocked by fluoxetine (or sertraline, others), which is classified as a selective serotonin reuptake inhibitor (SSRI) antidepressant. When sumatriptan (or other triptans used for migraine) is added, rapid accumulation of serotonin and/or the triptan in the brain can occur. The other drugs listed are not likely to interact with this serotoninergic drug.

319. The answer is d. *(Brunton, pp 726–727; Craig, pp 455, 466–467; Katzung, pp 329–330.)* The precise mechanism of action by which nedocromil or the related drug cromolyn works is not known, but the most likely explanation is "stabilization" of immunologically sensitized mast cells. This may involve calcium channel blockade: calcium entry into mast cells is a critical step in their immunologically mediated activation. There is no direct or indirect interaction with antigens (c) or mast cell antibodies, but the drug does suppress the release of preformed mast cell mediators. Nedocromil and cromolyn have no histamine receptor-blocking activity (a), nor vasoconstrictor or other decongestant effects (b). They do not inhibit synthesis of histamine, leukotrienes, or other vasodepressor, bronchoconstrictor, or inflammatory mediators in mast cells or elsewhere.

320. The answer is e. *(Brunton, p 691; Craig, p 429; Katzung, pp 581–582.)* Tinnitus, along with a feeling of dizziness or lightheadedness, GI upset (including nausea and some pain or other discomfort, and diarrhea more so than constipation), and such visual changes as blurred or double vision, all or collectively are part of a low-grade aspirin "toxicity" called salicylism. It is not necessarily worrisome (to the physician, provided he/she prescribed the drug at dosages likely to produce the syndrome), dangerous, or indicative of imminent and severe toxicity. Indeed, some patients experience one or more signs or symptoms of salicylism in response to high (antiarthritic) doses of aspirin.

321. The answer is f. *(Brunton, pp 673–693, 707; Craig, p 445; Katzung, pp 299, 309, 999t, 1043.)* Probenecid and the related drug, sulfinpyrazone are classified as uricosurics: at sufficiently high (therapeutic) doses they enhance the renal elimination of uric acid by inhibiting tubular reabsorption of filtered urate. Aspirin significantly impairs the uricosurics' actions.

Important note: Aspirin (given alone) has blood level–dependent effects on urate elimination by the kidneys. At "low doses" perhaps up to about 1 g/day, it selectively inhibits tubular secretion of urate and so can raise serum urate levels. At doses much higher than that (including doses sometimes prescribed for arthritis other than gout), the predominant effect (and the net, or overall, effect) is uricosuria due to blockade of tubular reabsorption of urate; this effect is greater than the drug's inhibitory effect on tubular secretion of urate. Nonetheless, aspirin is not used as a uricosuric drug because the doses/serum levels needed to cause that are sufficiently high to cause significant side effects (e.g., salicylism; see Question 312) that don't arise with the traditional uricosurics such as probenecid.

322. The answer is c. *(Brunton, pp 665, 973; Craig, pp 481, 719; Kaztung, pp 177, 177f, 178, 285, 285i, 286–287.)* In addition to misoprostol's use as a cytoprotective/mucotropic drug for some patients taking NSAIDs, misoprostol is also used as an adjunct to mifepristone to induce therapeutic abortion. This capitalizes on the prostaglandin analog's strong uterine-stimulating effects (thus, answer e is incorrect). The drug is sometimes used to maintain patency of an open ductus arteriosis, not to close it (a). It is not a contraceptive in the typical sense, such as we would associate with estrogen-progestin oral contraceptives. Given the drug's abortifacient effects, it is contraindicated for women who are pregnant, or wish to become pregnant (b). Misoprostol has bronchodilator activity, but it is relatively weak and the drug is not suitable as a substitute for corticosteroids (d) or other typical asthma medications.

323. The answer is b. (*Brunton, pp 646, 648–649, 800–801; Craig, pp 155–156, 210–215; Katzung, pp 172–174, 299.*) Bradykininase, the enzyme that metabolically inactivates bradykinin, is identical to angiotensin converting enzyme (ACE), and captopril is the prototypic inhibitor of both enzymes even though it is commonly classified as an ACE inhibitor. Inhibition of bradykinin metabolism by ACE inhibitors may contribute to their antihypertensive and cardioprotective effects, and may also explain the admittedly rare occurrence of angioedema in response to those drugs. Acetaminophen (a) has no effects on bradykinin metabolism or its interactions with cellular receptors. Cimetidine (c) is a competitive histamine receptor blocker (H_2 receptors). It is an efficacious cytochrome P450 inhibitor, but it apparently does not affect bradykinin metabolism or cellular responses. Ketoconazole (d) is another efficacious P450 inhibitor, and a participant in many clinically significant drug interactions, but not with or involving bradykinin. Phenelzine (e) is a monoamine oxidase inhibitor. It does not affect bradykinin metabolism.

324. The answer is d. (*Brunton, pp 629–636; Craig, p 452; Katzung, pp 260–261.*) Activation of H_1 receptors appears to be linked to phospholipase C and increased intracellular formation of inositol-1,4,5-triphosphate (IP_3) and 1,2-diacylglycerol. IP_3 binds to an endoplasmic reticulum receptor, triggering release of Ca^{2+} into the cytosol, where it activates Ca-dependent protein kinases. Diacylglycerol activates protein kinase C. Additionally, stimulation of H_1 receptors may activate phospholipase A_2 and trigger the arachidonic acid cascade, leading to prostaglandin production.

The H_2 receptors are the ones associated with adenylate cyclase; activating them increases cytosolic cAMP levels and activates cAMP-dependent protein kinase.

325. The answer is e. (*Brunton, pp 686–689, 691–692; Craig, pp 262–263, 312–314; Katzung, pp 581–582, 991.*) Sodium bicarbonate (IV) can be an important adjunct to managing severe salicylate poisoning for two main reasons: (1) it helps raise blood pH, which as stated earlier is profoundly reduced from metabolic plus respiratory acidosis; (2) it alkalinizes the urine, which (via a pH-dependent mechanism, *a la* Henderson-Hasselbach) converts more aspirin molecules into the ionized form in the tubules, thereby reducing tubular reabsorption of a substance we want to eliminate from the body as quickly as possible.

Acetaminophen (a), even though it is usually an effective antipyretic, is not good for managing fever of severe aspirin poisoning. It would add yet another drug that might complicate the clinical picture, and ordinary (and ordinarily safe) doses aren't likely to do much to lower temperature quickly or sufficiently. (Thus, we use physical means to lower body temperature.) *N*-acetylcysteine (c), the antidote for acetaminophen poisoning, does nothing for salicylate poisoning. Amphetamines (b) might seem rational for managing ventilatory depression that characterizes late stages of severe aspirin poisoning. The more likely outcome of giving an amphetamine is simply to hasten the onset of seizures. Phenobarbital (d), or other CNS depressants, would aggravate an already bad state of CNS/ventilatory depression. (However, if seizures develop they must be managed—for example, with IV lorazepam and phenytoin, even though they cause CNS depression. Without them, the patient may quickly die from status epilepticus.)

326. The answer is a. (*Brunton, pp 639–640; Craig, p 453; Katzung, pp 264–268.*) One of the main advantages of the first generation antihistamines (fexofenadine, loratadine, others) over the older (second generation) H_1 antagonists such as diphenhydramine, is a relative lack of CNS depressant (sedating) effects when administered at usual recommended doses. The implication of this difference is that the newer agents are much less likely to cause daytime drowsiness or other problems that might interfere with daytime activities requiring alertness. Sedation is a particular problem with diphenhydramine, doxylamine, and other members of the ethanolamine class of first generation antihistamines, yet it also provides a clinically useful effect based on this action: they are useful as OTC (diphenhydramine, doxylamine) and prescription (diphenhydramine) sleep-aids.

Diphenhydramine and to a large degree all the other first generation antihistamines, tend to cause appreciable muscarinic receptor-blocking (atropine-like) effects, and so they are unsuitable or potentially dangerous for patients with such atropine-related comorbidities as prostatic hypertrophy, hypomotility disorders of the urinary or GI tracts, tachycardia, or angle-closure glaucoma. So, answer b is not correct. Owing to antimuscarinic effects, diphenhydramine overdoses are more likely to cause tachycardia (by blocking parasympathetic-ACh-muscarinic receptor influences on the SA node) than bradycardia (c). The second generation antihistamines do block histamine-related bronchoconstriction, but in the absence of histamine they have no intrinsic bronchodilator activity. More important is the fact that these drugs play no role as primary therapy for asthma. They may be preferred to older antihistamines (largely because they lack the antimuscarinic-related mucus-thickening effects of such drugs as diphenhydramine), but they should be used only as adjuncts to more appropriate asthma drugs such as inhaled corticosteroids (to suppress airway inflammation) and inhaled β-adrenergic drugs for control or rescue therapy.

None of the H_1 blockers—first generation or second generation agents—have H_2 blocking activity which is necessary to suppress histamine-mediated acid secretion by gastric parietal cells.

327. The answer is b. (*Brunton, pp 123, 695, 851; Craig, pp 249–250; Katzung, pp 177, 177f, 178, 210, 284.*) A major component of the antihypertensive actions of captopril and other ACE inhibitors is prostaglandin-dependent. That element of drug action is antagonized by indomethacin due to its great efficacy to inhibit prostaglandin synthesis. Other drugs with actions that may be inhibited by prostaglandin synthesis inhibitors such as indomethacin include the thiazide and loop diuretics and (allegedly) many if not most of the β blockers. The actions of none of the other drugs listed are antagonized by indomethacin. We should note, however, that giving indomethacin to a patient taking warfarin or any of the antiplatelet drugs (used for prophylaxis of arterial thrombosis) is risky. One of the major toxicities of the NSAIDs is gastric mucosal damage and the risk of GI bleeds. In the presence of anticoagulants or antiplatelet drugs the risk of a serious GI bleed, perhaps progressing to hemorrhage, goes up markedly. However, this is not due to a typical pharmacodynamic or pharmacokinetic interaction between the drugs, and the anticoagulants' effects certainly are not inhibited by the NSAID.

328. The answer is d. (*Brunton, pp 686, 691–692; Craig, p 313; Katzung, pp 581–582, 991.*) Late, severe aspirin poisoning is characterized by a combination of respiratory and metabolic acidosis. In early stages of aspirin poisoning (or even with high "therapeutic" doses of the drug), ventilatory stimulation occurs. That induces a respiratory alkalosis (c; net CO_2 loss, relative HCO_3 retention). The kidneys compensate for this by increasing HCO_3 excretion to help normalize blood pH and causing what has been called "compensated respiratory alkalosis." As serum levels of aspirin rise, however, blood pH falls precipitously. Part of that is due to the accumulation of acidic salicylic acid in the blood, and part is due to inhibited oxidative phosphorylation that shifts metabolism from oxidative to glycolytic (with lactic acid being the key end product). No longer synthesizing ATP effectively, the mitochondria generate metabolic heat, which contributes to fever (not hypothermia; a). Ventilatory failure (not stimulation; e) ensues, leading to respiratory acidosis (from CO_2 retention) along with the metabolic acidosis. Cardiovascular collapse and seizures eventually cause death. Note that hepatotoxicity is not a component of this: that is the main cause of morbidity and mortality with acetaminophen poisoning.

329. The answer is a. (*Brunton, pp 83, 694–695, 1741; Craig, p 314; Katzung, pp 57–58, 59i, 595–596, 988, 989t.*) Acetaminophen's main toxic metabolite is N-acetyl-benzoqinoneimine. It reacts with sulfhydryl groups (particularly with glutathione) in hepatocytes, ultimately leading to hepatic necrosis when acetaminophen levels are sufficiently high. N-acetylcysteine is rich in–SH groups. It therefore reacts with the imine, hopefully sparing endogenous sulfhydryl compounds from further attack and, hopefully, allowing time for the hepatocytes to recover from the biochemical stress. This foul-smelling antidote must be given early after acetaminophen poisoning occurs or is likely (it is usually given orally), and it must be given repeatedly (see specialty texts for more information). It is a preventative against hepatotoxicity, not a reversing agent. As an aside, various nomograms are available to give some reasonable of whether a particular acetaminophen dose (more precisely, blood level) is likely to be hepatotoxic or not. They plot plasma acetaminophen levels as a function of time after drug ingestion (yielding, basically, an elimination rate and an elimination half-life). If the patient's acetaminophen level at a specified time following intake is above the line, hepatotoxicity is probable. Such a finding, however, does not mean that N-acetylcysteine administration will be without benefit and so should not be done. (See the explanation for Question 485 for more information, and a look at this issue from a somewhat different perspective.)

All of the other drugs listed can exert toxic effects (often serious) with overdoses, but N-acetylcysteine is not an appropriate or effective antidote for any of them.

330. The answer is c. (*Brunton, pp 707–708; Craig, pp 443–444; Katzung, pp 596–597.*) The main reason why many physicians are shunning oral colchicine for acute gout is that many patients develop horrible GI discomfort, vomiting, diarrhea, and the like. For some, the "cure" is almost as bad as the disorder for which the drug is given. This GI distress can be alleviated somewhat by giving colchicine IV, but more serious systemic responses can develop if the IV dose is too great or too many IV doses are given in a short period of time. Indomethacin seems to have become one of the preferred alternatives for anti-inflammatory therapy of acute gout or prophylaxis of recurrences. (And clearly indomethacin is not without side effects or toxicities; the risks and discomforts are simply more acceptable, for some patients, with it.)

But when colchicine does work in acute gout, relief may be dramatic and occur literally "overnight" with just a dose or two. The likely mechanism of action involves impaired microtubular assembly or function in leukocytes, which limits their migration to the area of crystal deposition and so limits their ability to amplify the inflammatory reaction.

Bone marrow suppression can occur, but that is mainly with long-term, high-dose oral or parenteral colchicine administration (the latter of which must be avoided). The same applies to frank gastric damage (with the possibility of gastric bleeding or hemorrhage) and to blood dyscrasias (bone marrow toxicity).

331. The answer is b. (*Brunton, pp 708–709; Craig, pp 445–446; Katzung, pp 598–599.*) You may think that reductions in urate content in a 24-h urine sample would be bad for the hyperuricemic patient, but that is because you probably automatically (and incorrectly) equate less urine urate with increased serum urate. Not necessarily so. Allopurinol inhibits uric acid synthesis by inhibiting xanthine oxidase: less uric acid made, less to be excreted in the urine, and less to be detected there. This is one manifestation of allopurinol "at work." Acetaminophen (a) has no effects on uric acid synthesis, excretion, or solubility. Colchicine (c) is sometimes used for prophylaxis or treatment of gout, but its actions derive from its anti-inflammatory action and, probably, suppression of neutrophil chemotaxis by interfering with microtubular function. It has no effects on urate synthesis or elimination. The same applies to indomethacin (d): anti-inflammatory actions, but no effects per se on uric acid. Probenecid (e) is a uricosuric drug that acts by inhibiting tubular reabsorption of urate when serum levels of the drug are therapeutic. As a result, the more likely outcome of this drug is an increase of urate concentrations in a urine sample. Probenecid does not affect uric acid synthesis.

332. The answer is c. (*Brunton, pp 422, 637–640, 642; Craig, pp 454–455; Katzung, pp 264–266, 1053.*) Diphenhydramine, a member of the ethanolamine class of H_1 antagonists and arguably the prototype of all the older ("first generation" antihistamines), possesses two main properties in addition to effective competitive blockade of H_1 receptors: sedation (c), in part due to the drug's lipophilicity; and muscarinic (cholinergic) receptor blockade that is also competitive. Both effects occur commonly, and can be quite intense. The CNS depressant effects of diphenhydramine are such that this drug is the main (if not only) active ingredient in OTC sleep aids, helping one drift off to sleep even in the absence of allergy signs and symptoms and probably in a way that is unrelated to the drug's peripheral H_1-blocking activity.

The antimuscarinic (atropine-like effects) would be manifest by such side effects as tachycardia (not bradycardia; a); constipation (not diarrhea; b); a suppression of ACh-induced gastric acid secretion (not the opposite; d); and a tendency for urinary retention (not frequency; e). The strong antimuscarinic effects of diphenhydramine earn it the same precautions and contraindications we normally apply to atropine itself, including prostatic hypertrophy and angle-closure glaucoma. Other side effects include xerostomia, blurred vision, paralysis of accommodation, and inhibition of sweating. Diphenhydramine toxicity manifests in ways that are markedly similar to what occurs with atropine poisoning, and is managed in the same way, including the use of physostigmine (ACh esterase inhibitor with actions in both the peripheral and central nervous systems) for severe or life-threatening toxicity.

As an important aside, loratadine, desloratadine, fexofenadine, and related newer (second generation) H_1 blockers (piperidine class) are associated with much less CNS depression (they are advertised as "nonsedating"—usually with a disclaimer, in fine print, "when taken as directed."). Unlike diphenhydramine and most of the older H_1 blockers, the newer agents cause no antimuscarinic effects and have no atropine-related precautions or contraindications.

333. The answer is d. (*Brunton, pp 706–707; Craig, pp 441–442; Katzung, pp 596, 598–599.*) The clinical problems that arise with uric acid relate to its poor solubility in body fluids—solubility that gets less as local pH falls. When a part of the body (e.g., a joint in the great toe, which is a common site of a gout attack) is damaged or otherwise insulted, uric acid crystals concentrate and precipitate in the area. These crystals cause mechanical damage to the joint surfaces and also evoke a typical inflammatory response. Leukocytes are attracted to the area, and in an attempt to phagocytize the crystals they release acidic metabolites that lower local pH, favoring precipitation of even more uric acid and amplifying the entire unwanted series of pathologic reactions.

334. The answer is c. (*Brunton, pp 1017, 1419; Craig, pp 435, 438; Katzung, pp 593, 948.*) Etanercept (and the related drug infliximab) binds to and neutralize TNF-α, which is one of the primary pathophysiologic mediators in rheumatoid arthritis and Crohn's disease. It functions, then, as an antibody. Etanercept has no effect on eicosanoid synthesis (a, d) or leukocyte migration (b). It does not stimulate collagen, mucopolysaccharide, or synovial fluid synthesis.

The Gastrointestinal System and Nutrition

Acid secretion inhibitors
   (H₂ blockers, proton pump
   inhibitors, others)
Antacids
Antidiarrheals
Emetics, antiemetics
Gallstone-dissolving drugs

Inflammatory bowel disease drugs
Laxatives, cathartics
Mucosal protective drugs
Pancreatic enzyme replacement
Prokinetic agents
Vitamins

Questions

DIRECTIONS: Each item contains a question or incomplete statement that is followed by several responses. Select the **one best** response to each question.

335. A patient has severe gastroesophageal reflux disease (GERD). In addition to providing some immediate symptom relief, for which we will prescribe usually effective doses of an OTC combination antacid product, we want to suppress gastric acid as fully as possible. Which of the following drug is most likely to meet that criterion?

a. Atropine
b. Calcium carbonate
c. Cimetidine
d. Esomeprazole
e. Misoprostol
f. Propantheline

336. A patient with multiple medical problems is taking several drugs, including theophylline, warfarin, quinidine, and phenytoin. Despite the likelihood of interactions, dosages of each are adjusted carefully so their serum concentrations and effects are acceptable. However, the patient suffers some GI distress and starts taking a drug provided by one of his "well-intentioned" friends. He presents with excessive or toxic effects from *all* his other medications, and blood tests reveal that their serum concentrations are high. Which was the drug the patient most likely self-prescribed and took?

a. Cimetidine
b. Esomeprazole
c. Famotidine
d. Nizatidine
e. Ranitidine

337. We have two patients. One requires suppression of emesis caused by an anticancer drug that causes a high incidence and severity of vomiting (a highly emetogenic drug). Another patient has severe diabetic gastroparesis and gastroesophageal reflux, which requires relief. Which drug would be most suitable for both indications (assuming no specific contraindications)?

a. Diphenoxylate
b. Dronabinol
c. Loperamide
d. Metoclopramide
e. Ondansetron

338. A patient with multiple GI complaints is receiving chenodeoxycholic acid (chenodiol) as part of his drug regimen. Which of the following is the most likely purpose for which this drug is being given?

a. Dissolving cholesterol stones in the bile ducts
b. Enhancing intestinal digestion and absorption of dietary fats
c. Helping to reverse malabsorption of fat-soluble vitamins from the diet
d. Stimulating gastric acid secretion in achlorhydria
e. Suppressing steatorrhea and its consequences

339. A patient who has been a high-dose alcohol abuser for many years presents with hepatic portal-systemic encephalopathy. Which of the following drugs, given in relatively high doses, would be most suitable for the relief of signs and symptoms of this condition, and the likely underlying biochemical anomalies?

a. Diphenoxylate
b. Esomeprazole
c. Lactulose
d. Loperamide
e. Ondansetron

340. Fat-soluble vitamins, compared with their water-soluble counterparts, generally have a greater potential toxicity to the user when taken in excess. Which of the following most accurately states the main reason for this finding?

a. Administered in larger doses
b. Avidly stored by the body
c. Capable of dissolving membrane phospholipids
d. Involved in more essential metabolic pathways
e. Metabolized much more slowly

341. A patient presents with malaise and skin and mucous membranes appear pale. Among the key findings from blood work are hypochromic, microcytic red cells, and reduced red cell count; reduced hematocrit; reduced reticulocyte count; and reduced total hemoglobin content. Assuming the most likely diagnosis is correct, which of the following drugs would be most proper to administer?

a. Cyanocobalamin (B_{12})
b. Folic acid
c. Iron
d. Vitamin C
e. Vitamin D

342. We have a patient who will start taking one of the drugs listed. As we hand them the prescription we advise them not to take supplemental vitamin B_6 (pyridoxine), whether alone or as part of a multivitamin supplement, because the vitamin is likely to counteract a desired effect of the prescribed drug. To which of the following drugs does this advice apply?

a. Captopril for heart failure or hypertension
b. Haloperidol for Tourette's syndrome
c. Levodopa/carbidopa for Parkinson's disease
d. Niacin for hypertriglyceridemia
e. Phenytoin for epilepsy

343. You have a patient who has been consuming extraordinarily large amounts of alcohol for several years. He goes into acute withdrawal and manifests nystagmus and bizarre ocular movements and confusion (Wernicke's encephalopathy). Although this patient's alcohol consumption pattern has been accompanied by poor nutrient intake overall, you need to manage the encephalopathy. Which of the following drugs is most appropriate for this use?

a. α-Tocopherol (vitamin E)
b. Cyanocobalamin (vitamin B_{12})
c. Folic acid
d. Phytonadione (vitamin K)
e. Thiamine (vitamin B_1)

344. A patient with tuberculosis is being treated with isoniazid. She develops paresthesias, muscle aches, and unsteadiness. Which of the following vitamins needs to be given in supplemental doses in order to reverse these symptoms—or used from the outset to prevent them in high-risk patients?

a. Vitamin A
b. Vitamin B_1 (thiamine)
c. Vitamin B_6 (pyridoxine)
d. Vitamin C
e. Vitamin K

345. An opioid abuser, seeking something to self-administer for subjective responses, gets a large amount of diphenoxylate and consumes it all at once. He is not likely to do this again because he has consumed a combination product that contains not only the opioid but also another drug that causes a host of unpleasant systemic responses. Which of the following is, most likely, that other drug found in combination with the diphenoxylate?

a. Apomorphine
b. Atropine
c. Ipecac
d. Magnesium sulfate
e. Naltrexone

346. During a regular checkup, your patient states "You know, doc, sometimes after eating I get heartburn . . . you know, acid-indigestion." Since the symptoms seem to be mild and infrequent, you suggest an empiric trial of an OTC antacid for prompt symptom relief. You recommend several brands for the patient to try. All the products you list are combination products that contain a magnesium salt and an aluminum salt. Which of the following is the most likely reason why the vast majority of these products contain these two particular drugs or salts?

a. Al salts counteract the gastric mucosal-irritating effects of Mg salts
b. Al salts require activation by an Mg-dependent enzyme in order to inhibit the parietal cell proton pumps
c. Mg salts cause a diuresis that helps reduce systemic accumulation of the Al salt by increasing renal Al excretion
d. Mg salts potentiate the ability of Al salts to inhibit gastric acid secretion
e. Mg salts tend to cause a laxative effect (increased motility) that counteracts the tendency of an Al salt to cause constipation

347. A patient presents with severe abdominal pain and a "burning" sensation in the upper abdomen. Endoscopy reveals several benign ulcers in the antral mucosa of the stomach. Which of the following drugs is most likely to provide the fastest—albeit probably the briefest—relief of the discomfort with just a single dose?

a. Antacids
b. Belladonna alkaloids
c. Cimetidine or another H_2 blocker
d. Misoprostol
e. Propantheline

348. On your first day on a general medicine clerkship you encounter a patient who is taking a proton pump inhibitor, bismuth, metronidazole, and tetracycline. Which of the following is the most likely purpose for administering this drug combination?

a. Antibiotic-associated pseudomembranous colitis
b. Irritable bowel syndrome (IBS)
c. Refractory or recurrent, and severe, gastric or duodenal ulcers secondary to *H. pylori*
d. "Traveler's diarrhea," severe, *Escherichia coli*–induced, from drinking contaminated water
e. Ulcers that occur in response to long-term, high-dose NSAID therapy for arthritis

349. We have just confirmed that our patient is pregnant, and give her a strong warning to avoid taking supplements of a vitamin, especially in high doses, because the substance is highly teratogenic. We also avoid administering any drugs that are derivatives of this nutrient during pregnancy, for the same reason. To which of the following vitamins does this precaution apply?

a. A
b. B_{12}
c. C
d. E
e. Folic acid

350. A patient has multiple gastric ulcers but has done nothing about them. Shortly after consuming a large meal and large amounts of alcohol, he experiences significant GI distress. He takes an over-the-counter heartburn remedy. Within a minute or two he develops what he will later describe as a "bad bloated feeling." Several of the ulcers have begun to bleed and he experiences searing pain.

The patient becomes profoundly hypotensive from upper GI blood loss and is transported to the hospital. Endoscopy confirms multiple bleeds; the endoscopist remarks that it appears as if the lesions had been literally stretched apart, causing additional tissue damage that led to the hemorrhage. Which of the following drugs or products did the patient most likely take?

a. An aluminum salt
b. An aluminum-magnesium combination antacid product
c. Magnesium hydroxide
d. Ranitidine
e. Sodium bicarbonate

351. A patient to be seen in the general medicine clinic is being treated with a number of prescription drugs, one of which is misoprostol. Which of the following is the most likely purpose for which this drug is being administered?

a. Routine management of gastroesophageal reflux disease (GERD)
b. Prophylaxis of GI ulcers during long-term therapy with some nonsteroidal anti-inflammatory drugs
c. Eradicating *Heliobacter pylori* in patients with acute and recurrent gastric ulcers
d. Prevention of acute stress ulcers (e.g., in the postoperative setting)
e. Managing ulcers that tend to develop during pregnancy

352. A patient has steatorrhea due to pancreatic insufficiency secondary to cystic fibrosis. Which of the following drugs usually is considered the most reasonable and usually effective drug for managing the steatorrhea?

a. Atorvastatin (statin-type cholesterol-lowering drug)
b. Cimetidine (or an alternative, e.g., famotidine)
c. Bile salts
d. Metoclopramide
e. Pancrelipase

353. A 26-year-old woman realizes she is losing her hearing. She consults a web-based "support group" for the hard of hearing and reads anecdotes claiming that nicotinic acid (niacin), a water-soluble B-complex vitamin, can improve cochlear blood flow and ward-off further hearing loss. She isn't intrigued about getting hearing aids that were recommended by her ENT doctor so she goes to the health food store and purchases the nutrient in response to what she's read on the web. Believing that if the recommended dose of niacin is good, and doubling the dose would be better, she starts taking excessive doses. Which of the following side effects is this young woman most likely to experience shortly after starting to consume this vitamin complex?

a. Bradycardia
b. Facial flushing and pruritus
c. Hypercholesterolemia, hypertriglyceridemia
d. Hypoglycemia
e. Photophobia due to intense mydriasis

354. Several brand-name and store-brand "pink medications," administered orally and available without prescription, are widely used to help alleviate occasional and short-lived nausea and vomiting, nonspecific GI distress, and diarrhea. They are also recommended for prophylaxis of "traveler's diarrhea," which typically is caused by ingestion of foods or beverages contaminated with *E. coli*. These products contain bismuth subsalicylate, and because of the presence of an aspirin-like compound (a salicylate) they should not be taken by or administered to certain patients. Which of the following patient-related factors or comorbidities contraindicates the use of this drug or product?

a. Essential hypertension
b. Flu, chickenpox, or other viral illness in a child or adolescent
c. Hot flashes and other signs/symptoms of menopause
d. Prostatic hypertrophy or glaucoma in elderly men
e. Rheumatoid or osteoarthritis
f. Severe seasonal allergy signs and symptoms

355. A patient being cared for by the gastroenterology service is being treated with sulfasalazine. Which of the following is the most likely purpose for which it is being given?

a. Antibiotic-associated pseudomembranous colitis
b. *E. coli*–induced diarrhea
c. Gastric *H. pylori* infections
d. Inflammatory bowel disease
e. NSAID-induced gastric ulcer prophylaxis

356. A patient with renal failure is undergoing periodic hemodialysis while awaiting a transplant. Between dialysis sessions we want to reduce the body's phosphate load by reducing dietary phosphate absorption and removing some phosphate already in the blood. Which of the following drugs would be most suitable for this purpose?

a. Aluminum hydroxide
b. Bismuth subsalicylate
c. Magnesium hydroxide/oxide
d. Sodium bicarbonate
e. Sucralfate

357. For years students have read about and been tested on the use of pirenzipine as a promising drug for inhibiting acid secretion in patients with peptic ulcer disease or pathologic acid-hypersecretory disorders such as Zollinger-Ellison syndrome. The drug probably inhibits acid secretion by blocking autonomic ganglionic (postsynaptic or postganglionic) muscarinic M_1 receptors, which in turn reduces parietal cell proton secretion normally triggered by parasympathetic nervous system activation.

Given the brief but accurate description of pirenzipine's site and mechanism of action, which of the following statements best summarizes why this drug is unlikely to be approved in the United States for management of GI disorders related to gastric acid hypersecretion?

a. Causes significant rises of blood pressure in most patients
b. Causes significant skeletal muscle weakness by blocking myocyte activation
c. Induces profuse diarrhea and micturition, leading to fluid and electrolyte loss
d. Likely to cause severe reflex tachycardia
e. Low efficacy because it inhibits only one mediator involved in gastric acid secretion

358. A woman has severe, irritable bowel syndrome characterized by frequent, profuse, and symptomatic diarrhea. She has not responded to first-line therapies and is started on alosetron. Which of the following is the most worrisome adverse effect associated with this drug?

a. Cardiac arrhythmias (serious, e.g., ventricular fibrillation)
b. Constipation, bowel impaction, ischemic colitis
c. Parkinsonian extrapyramidal reactions
d. Pulmonary fibrosis
e. Renal failure

359. A patient undergoing cancer chemotherapy gets ondansetron for prophylaxis of drug-induced nausea and vomiting. Which of the following best describes this drug's main mechanism of action in this setting?

a. Activates μ-type opioid receptors in the chemoreceptor trigger zone
b. Blocks central serotonin (5-HT_3) receptors
c. Blocks dopamine receptors
d. Blocks histamine H_1 receptors in the brainstem and inner ear
e. Suppresses gastric motility and acid secretion via muscarinic blockade

The Gastrointestinal System and Nutrition

Answers

335. The answer is d. (*Brunton, pp 967–971; Craig, pp 477–480; Katzung, pp 1035–1038.*) Esomeprazole and related drugs (lansoprazole, omeprazole, rabeprazole, pantoprazole) inhibit the parietal cell H^+,K^+ATPase—the "proton pump"—that is the "final common pathway" for acid secretion triggered by all the major stimuli of gastric acid secretion. As a result, they are the most efficacious, causing near complete anti-acid-secretory activity.

Recall that the main agonists that provoke acid secretion include gastrin; histamine (arises from enterochromaffin-like [ECL] cells), which activates H_2 receptors that can be blocked by cimetidine (and famotidine, ranitidine and nizatidine); and ACh, which activates muscarinic receptors on both ECL cells and parietal cells and which can be blocked by atropine, propantheline, pirenzipine, and several other drugs with antimuscarinic activity. However, blocking only the histaminergic or cholinergic influences (or even both) only partially inhibits acid secretion.

Misoprostol is unique in several ways. One way is that this prostaglandin analog mimics the effects of endogenous prostaglandins (mainly PGE_2) on parietal cell PG receptors. Unlike the agonists noted above, one result of activating parietal cell PG receptors is inhibition of acid secretion. Overall, the anti-acid-secretory effects are relatively weak. (It inhibits a G protein/adenylate cyclase–mediated pathway that is activated when histamine causes acid secretion.)

Ultimately, however, regardless of whether gastrin, ACh, or histamine is present, parietal cell acid secretion ultimately "funnels through" the proton pump. Block the receptors for any of the mediators noted above and you will suppress acid secretion caused only by that mediator—but that is only a fraction of total acid secretion. Block the proton pump and acid secretion will be inhibited nearly fully, no matter which one or more agonists are present.

Calcium carbonate, as well as aluminum and magnesium salts and sodium bicarbonate, are antacids. They have no inhibitory effects on acid secretion. Instead, they neutralize a component of acid that has already been secreted (and aluminum salts also adsorb pepsins).

336. The answer is a. (*Brunton, pp 971–973; Craig, p 479; Katzung, pp 1086–1087, 1128–1129, 1119.*) Cimetidine differs significantly from the other H_2 blockers, famotidine, nizatidine, and ranitidine, in that it is a very effective inhibitor of the hepatic mixed function oxidase (P450) drug-metabolizing enzyme systems. The alternatives have no significant P450-inhibiting activity, nor do they cause side effects as frequent or as problematic as those caused by cimetidine, especially at high doses. The outcome of P450 inhibition, of course, is reduced hepatic clearance of the interactants, leading to excessive serum concentrations and effects if their dosages are not reduced properly. The examples cited in the question—phenytoin, warfarin, quinidine, and theophylline—are among the most important interactants with cimetidine. They, and other interactants such as lidocaine, have rather low margins of safety, so even slight increases in serum levels (reductions of metabolic clearance) may be enough to cause toxicity. Given the fact that the alternative H_2 blockers don't inhibit the P450 system, there's no rational reason or excuse for prescribing cimetidine to patients on multiple drug therapy (and in this case, the patient should have been warned about self-medicating with it).

Esomeprazole and the related proton pump inhibitors participate in no clinically significant interactions with the drugs noted here, or others.

337. The answer is d. (*Brunton, pp 343, 467, 985–986; Craig, pp 472, 477; Katzung, pp 1044–1046.*) Metoclopramide has clinically useful antiemetic and prokinetic actions and would be suitable for either of the patients described in the question. The antiemetic effect arises from blockade of dopamine (and, probably, serotonin) receptors in the brain's chemoreceptor trigger zone (CTZ). The drug is indicated for not only chemotherapy-induced nausea and vomiting, but also that which may occur with radiation therapy, postoperatively, or in response to opioid analgesics or emetogenic toxins.

The enhanced gastric and upper intestinal motility probably reflects an enhancement of the expected effects of ACh on muscarinic receptors found on longitudinal smooth muscle in the GI tract. Metoclopramide raises the lower esophageal sphincter tone and relaxes the pyloric sphincter, which hastens gastric emptying. This helps explain its beneficial effects in both gastroparesis and GERD.

Diphenoxylate is an oral opioid indicated only for managing diarrhea. Typical antidiarrheal doses inhibit bowel motility well but cause no central opioid-like effects (ventilatory depression, analgesia, euphoria, etc.). Loperamide, a meperidine analog, also lacks opioid- or meperidine-like systemic or central effects at usual doses. It probably works not only by suppressing bowel motility, but also fluid secretion into the intestines. Dronabinol is a cannabinoid, and the principal psychoactive chemical in marijuana. It is used to suppress chemotherapy-induced nausea and vomiting. The drug has no role in managing gastroparesis or GERD. Ondansetron, also used exclusively to manage emetogenic drug-induced symptoms, is a serotonin receptor (5-HT$_3$) blocker that acts mainly in the CTZ and on vagal efferents to parts of the upper GI tract.

338. The answer is a. (*Brunton, p 1007; Katzung, p 1058.*) Chenodeoxycholic acid (chenodiol), one of several naturally occurring bile acids, is effective in some patients with cholesterol gallstones. Its main initial action is reduced hepatic cholesterol synthesis. That, in turn, lowers the cholesterol content in the bile, which favors the spontaneous dissolution of cholesterol stones that have formed already and reduces the incidence of new stone formation. Related drugs are ursodiol (ursodeoxycholic acid) and monooctanoin; the former is given orally, the latter by direct infusion into the common bile duct.

339. The answer is c. (*Brunton, pp 992–993; Craig, p 475; Katzung, pp 1046–1047.*) Lactulose is a synthetic, nonabsorbable disaccharide (galactosefructose). In moderate doses, it acts as an osmotic laxative. In higher doses, it binds intestinal ammonia and other toxins that accumulate in the intestine in severe liver dysfunction. These toxins, and perhaps more so the ammonia, contribute to the signs and symptoms of encephalopathy. None of the other drugs listed provide this benefit.

340. The answer is b. (*Brunton, pp 1661, 1666; Craig, pp 778–789.*) Fat-soluble vitamins, especially A and D, can be stored in massive amounts and, hence, have a potential for serious toxicities. (On the bright side, this abundant storage means that relatively brief periods of inadequate intake are not likely to cause clinical signs and symptoms of deficiency.) Water-soluble vitamins are easily excreted by the kidneys and accumulation to toxic levels is much less common. Conversely, inadequate dietary intake will lead to manifestations of deficiency relatively faster.

341. The answer is c. *(Brunton, pp 1442–1450; Craig, pp 782–783; Katzung, pp 531–532.)* The description contains many of the characteristics of "iron-deficiency anemia." Oral iron salts (e.g., ferrous sulfate, gluconate, or fumarate) are usually the first choice for management (after ruling out such causes as blood loss). Diarrhea (or constipation), nausea, and heartburn are common complaints with oral iron salts, but using these drugs is often preferable to (and safer than) using parenteral iron products such as iron-dextran (risk of anaphylaxis) or other iron complexes, which typically involve erythropoietin administration adjunctively.

Megaloblastic anemia (in contrast with the microcytic anemia we described here) would be treated differently. If it is caused by vitamin B_{12} deficiency (vitamin malabsorption due to deficiency of intrinsic factor), we would treat with cyanocobalamin. The other cause, folate deficiency (inadequate dietary intake) is managed with oral folic acid. Deficiencies of vitamin C or D don't typically cause anemias.

342. The answer is c. *(Brunton, pp 530, 533–534; Craig, p 782; Katzung, pp 448–449.)* Recall that DOPA decarboxylase, an enzyme whose activity is dependent on pyridoxine, is responsible for metabolizing orally administered levodopa to dopamine in the gut; and that only unmetabolized levodopa crosses the blood-brain barrier to be efficacious in relieving parkinsonian signs and symptoms. Recall, too, that levodopa is often administered with carbidopa, a drug that inhibits the peripheral decarboxylase, sparing levodopa for entry into the brain and whose actions are antagonized by pyridoxine. Administering supplemental B_6 will reduce the bioavailability of levodopa, thereby counteracting its antiparkinson effectiveness. None of the other drugs listed, whether used for the stated purpose or others, has its effects antagonized by pyridoxine.

343. The answer is e. *(Brunton, pp 594, 598; Craig, pp 415–416, 780; Katzung, pp 368–372.)* Thiamine, administered parenterally with glucose, is the specific intervention for Wernicke's encephalopathy. It dramatically ameliorates the signs and symptoms. Thiamine deficiency is also responsible for Korsakoff's psychosis, another accompaniment of severe, long-term alcohol consumption, especially without adequately nutritional diets. Unfortunately, the signs and symptoms of Korsakoff's (short-term memory problems, a tendency to fabricate, polyneuropathies) are not reversible.

344. The answer is c. *(Brunton, pp 1102, 1206–1207; Craig, pp 558–559, 780, 782; Katzung, p 784.)* Pyridoxine deficiencies arise often during isoniazid therapy because the antimycobacterial drug interferes with metabolic activation of the vitamin. The treatment or prophylaxis for at risk patients is to administer relatively large doses of B_6 (pyridoxine).

345. The answer is b. *(Brunton, pp 194–195, 570; Craig, p 473; Katzung, pp 511, 1047.)* Diphenoxylate is an opioid that has predominant antidiarrheal activity, and that is its sole use. It inhibits peristalsis and, hence, increases the passage time of the intestinal bolus. Typical antidiarrheal doses do not cause ventilatory depression, analgesia, or the euphoria for which opioids are mainly abused. However, should one attempt to take high doses to become euphoric, unpleasant effects will appear. That is because the product contains a small amount of atropine—usually not enough to cause side effects when the proper dose of the product is consumed, but clearly able to cause all the typical antimuscarinic side effects of which you should be aware (see the chapter, "Autonomic Nervous System") when excessive doses are taken. This pharmaceutical manufacturing "trick" discourages diphenoxylate abuse.

Apomorphine and ipecac are dopaminergic emetics (for parenteral and oral administration, respectively) that are used in some poisonings where inducing emesis is desired. Magnesium sulfate (clearly a foul-tasting salt) is used as a laxative or cathartic. Naltrexone, of course, is an opioid antagonist (μ and κ receptors, naloxone-like, but given orally.)

346. The answer is e. *(Brunton, pp 974–975; Craig, p 479; Katzung, p 1046.)* Magnesium salts used alone tend to cause a laxative effect. (Indeed, at dosages higher than those used for acid neutralization, magnesium salts are used for their laxative or cathartic effects.) Aluminum (and calcium) antacids, given alone, tend to cause constipation. Combining a magnesium salt with an aluminum (and/or calcium antacid) is an often successful approach to minimizing antacid-induced changes of net gut motility.

Magnesium salts do not potentiate the antisecretory actions of Al or any other antacid. Indeed, none of the antacids inhibit gastric acid secretion (i.e., they don't have an antisecretory effect to begin with). They merely neutralize acid that has already been secreted (Mg, Ca, sodium bicarbonate) or adsorb acid and pepsins (most of the aluminum compounds).

Although high concentrations of Mg salts may cause gastric irritation, the amounts and concentrations found in antacid products are not sufficient to do that. Regardless, Al salts don't protect against any such potential effect.

Magnesium salts do contribute to a diuresis, but it is not a significant effect. Regardless, Al salts are "nonsystemic" antacids: they are not absorbed to any appreciable degree, and therefore they don't depend on renal processes for their elimination.

Al salts are effective in the form in which they are administered and don't require any enzymatic (or other type of) "activation" to exert their effects (which involves adsorption of acid, pepsins, etc.).

347. The answer is a. (*Brunton, pp 974–975; Craig, p 478; Katzung, pp 1034–1035.*) The typical symptoms of acid-peptic disease are caused by acid. (You might want to remember the "no acid, no pain" concept, but also recognize that the phrase "no pain, no ulcer" is clearly incorrect because ulcers may be present in the absence of symptoms.)

Although antacids seem to have no ability to accelerate ulcer healing, they act almost instantaneously to neutralize acid (provided adequate dosages are given), thereby relieving pain and other discomforts that are due to the acid in a matter of a minute or so.

All the other drugs can, to varying degrees, suppress gastric acid secretion and ultimately get the patient near or to a "no acid, no pain" state. However, it takes some time (variable, but clearly longer than it takes for an antacid to work) for those medications to be absorbed and reach blood levels sufficient to suppress acid production and then reduce symptoms.

Note: You should be familiar with propantheline (e), but in case you're not: it's an old and someone outmoded antimuscarinic drug, used mainly for managing some gut hypermotility conditions. Nonetheless, it shares virtually all the potential systemic side effects, adverse reactions, contraindications, and precautions, that apply to atropine, which is the prototype antimuscarinic drug and one that is derived from belladonna *spp.*

348. The answer is c. (*Brunton, pp 967, 976–980, 1104; Craig, pp 473, 483; Katzung, pp 1035–1038.*) Several professional organizations, including the American College of Gastroenterology, have guidelines for managing severe, refractory, or recurrent duodenal and/or gastric ulcers, in which *H. pylori* clearly plays an important pathophysiologic role. Although several regimens have been suggested, all of them include an anti-acid-secretory drug (usually a proton pump inhibitor, sometimes an H_2 blocker), two or three antibiotics (e.g., amoxicillin, clarithromycin, or tetracycline, usually with metronidazole), and bismuth. In many cases, this so-called eradicative therapy can cause a clinical cure and prevent recurrences after about 8 weeks of treatment. (The treatment is expensive, but pales in comparison with the cost of treating recurrent episodes or potentially serious complications such as GI bleeding or hemorrhage, either pharmacologically or surgically.)

349. The answer is a. (*Brunton, pp 1685–1687; Craig, pp 487–488, 778; Katzung, pp 919, 1023–1024.*) Pregnant women should not take more than a 25% increase in the normal (recommended) daily dietary intake of vitamin A, because it is definitely teratogenic, especially in the first trimester of pregnancy. Note that the vitamin A-like drugs tretinoin and isotretinoin, which are mainly used for treating refractory or severe acne vulgaris, or to relieve wrinkled facial skin, are contraindicated too.

350. The answer is e. (*Brunton, pp 974–975; Craig, p 478; Katzung, pp 1034–1036.*) You've all done the experiment: mix vinegar and baking soda (sodium bicarbonate) and one product is CO_2. This gas is formed when sodium bicarbonate—still used as a lay remedy for heartburn and other acid-related GI disturbances—reacts with HCl.

Normally intragastric pressure is kept in check when the gastroesophageal sphincter opens. However, when pressure can't be relieved quickly enough, or adequately, the stomach will distend. In the presence of ulcers the lesions can be stretched mechanically, favoring further damage that can lead to acute bleeding. Even in the absence of ulcers, any weakness of the gastric wall can lead to gastric rupture. (This ostensibly bizarre outcome, leading to bleeding or rupture, has been documented.)

None of the other antacids listed, whether alone or in combination, lead to production of CO_2 or any other gas that might lead to the outcome described in the scenario.

351. The answer is b. (*Brunton, pp 665, 685, 698, 973; Craig, p 481; Katzung, p 1043.*) Misoprostol is sometimes used as an adjunct to prevent ulcers in the GI tract caused by NSAIDs used for managing such chronic inflammatory disorders as rheumatoid arthritis. (The NSAIDs to which we are specifically referring includes the nonselective COX-1 and -2 inhibitors—that is, all but the "coxibs" [celecoxib, others]) that are selective COX-2 inhibitors.) Misoprostol is not at all used for "routine" management of acid-peptic disorders such as gastric or duodenal ulcers or gastroesophageal reflux disease (GERD).

The NSAIDs can cause mucosal damage by inhibiting prostaglandin synthesis, one consequence of which is reduced formation of mucus that protects the mucosal cells. Misoprostol, a prostaglandin-like agonist, stimulates mucus formation (mucotropic effect), has some weak acid-antisecretory activity, stimulates HCO_3 secretion, and may protect mucosal cells in other ways (cytoprotective effect).

Just as it is important to know this use, it's equally important to know that pregnancy contraindicates using misoprostol for its GI actions. The drug's prostaglandin-like properties can trigger uterine contractions (oxytocic effect) that may lead to premature labor or abortion.

Note that misoprostol is sometimes used in conjunction with either mifepristone (RU 486) or methotrexate as alternatives to surgical termination of early pregnancy. The prostaglandins related to misoprostol, carboprost tromethamine and dinoprostone, are sometimes used instead of the misoprostol for pharmacologic induction of abortion (mainly in the second trimester).

352. The answer is e. (*Brunton, pp 1005–1006; Katzung, p 1058.*) Pancrelipase is an alcoholic extract of hog pancreas that contains lipase, trypsin, and amylase. (The related drug, pancreatin, is similar.) The goal here is not so much to control the diarrhea, but do so by attacking the cause, which is endogenous pancreatic enzyme deficiency (lipases, amylase, chymotrypsin, and trypsin) that leads to impaired fat digestion and absorption. None of the other drugs mentioned have actions that would be as effective or specific as pancrelipase. "Traditional" antidiarrheals, for example, would only treat the symptoms, not the underlying cause.

Note: You may find pancrelipase administered with antacids, or an acid secretion inhibitor (H_2 blocker or proton pump inhibitor). The purpose of combined therapy is not related to preventing adverse effects of acid on the gastric mucosa, but rather to raise gastric pH and prevent the pancrelipase from being hydrolyzed and inactivated by acid.

353. The answer is b. (*Brunton, pp 683–684, 946–956; Craig, pp 272–273, 779–780, 782; Katzung, pp 570–571.*) Niacin, or nicotinic acid, is mainly used therapeutically for dyslipidemias. The drug often is quite effective in lowering elevated total and LDL cholesterol, raising HDL cholesterol, and lowering elevated triglycerides. (Thus, answer c is incorrect.) One of the main limitations to using this "nutrient," however, is the prevalence of severe facial flushing and pruritus, and GI distress that the patient will often describe as heartburn or acid-indigestion. Although these side effects are potentially severe and disturbing, and a major cause of noncompliance, they are dose-dependent, and tolerance develops to them after a couple of weeks of continued therapy. They occur no matter the reason for which the drug is taken, whether for documented favorable effects on lipid profiles, or based on many anecdotal and largely unsubstantiated or untested reports that they improve cochlear blood flow and slow or otherwise reduce the risk of hearing loss.

These niacin-induced side effects can be minimized by keeping dosages relatively low; by using sustained-release (slow-release) formulations; and by pretreatment with aspirin (which suggests that prostaglandins play some role in the unwanted responses). Whether prostaglandin-mediated or not, vasodilation appears to be involved, and that is more likely to trigger reflex tachycardia than bradycardia (a). Therapeutic doses of niacin, regardless of the purpose for which it is given, tends to cause hyperglycemia, not hypo-glycemia (d). The rises of blood glucose levels may be dramatic, and may involve the phenomenon of insulin resistance in parenchymal cells such as adipocytes and skeletal muscle. Nonetheless, the drug should not be admin-istered to patients with diabetes mellitus unless dosages of other antidiabetic drugs are adjusted to account for the problem. Photophobia (e) usually arises in response to α-adrenergic agonists or muscarinic receptor blockers. Niacin affects neither of these receptors, and is not associated with photo-phobia for any other reason.

354. The answer is b. (*Brunton, pp 682, 687; Craig, pp 473, 483; Katzung, p 1044.*) Bismuth salts such as the subsalicylate (best known, perhaps, as the brand-name product Pepto-Bismol) exert antibiotic activity against *H. pylori* and probably against *E. coli* also. They are commonly prescribed for the eradicative therapy of *H. pylori*-induced refractory gastric ulcers, along with an antibiotic and metronidazole. The salicylate in this formula-tion contraindicates its use in children with influenza or any other viral ill-ness, owing to the risk of Reye's syndrome. It is somewhat controversial what the term "children" means in this Reye's-related context. The risk clearly applies to children in their adolescent (and earlier) years of age, but it may also extend to people younger than about 21 years of age. This is important to know, since children experiencing such viral illnesses as influenza, chickenpox, or even a common cold, may report that their "tummy hurts" and they may experience diarrhea for a variety of reasons. The "pink meds" described in the question are quite well known to many parents. Since they are available OTC (that automatically conveys the notion that they are "safe") and effective, it's not unlikely that the unknowing caregiver might give the child precisely the wrong drug. Warnings against the use of these bismuth-containing medications are printed on the labels of these products, but as you probably know by now many people don't (or can't) read product labels.

The salicylate component also poses risks in other situations for which a salicylate should be avoided. Aspirin-sensitive asthma is a prime example.

Bismuth salts (or the salicylate moiety specifically) lack significant effects on blood pressure or the effects of antihypertensive drugs (a). There are no well-documented beneficial or adverse effects on signs and symptoms typically associated with menopause (c). Likewise, there are no known desired or unwanted effects on prostate, urinary tract, or ocular function or disease (d), whether in older men or not; no effects on arthritic disease (the salicylate in bismuth subsalicylate is apparently sufficient to warrant the Reye's syndrome warning, but not sufficient to favorably influence inflammatory diseases such as arthritis); nor affect signs and symptoms of seasonal (or other) allergic responses (f).

The drug has no H_2-blocking or muscarinic receptor–blocking activity. In the absence of any contraindications, bismuth subsalicylate may be useful for managing some cases of diarrhea, such as "traveler's diarrhea" that often is caused by *E. coli*.

355. The answer is d. (*Brunton, pp 691, 1009, 1012–1014; Craig, pp 480–481; Katzung, pp 1053–1055.*) Sulfasalazine, which is a combination of sulfapyridine and 5-aminosalicylic acid (5-ASA) linked covalently (azo bond), is quite effective for managing inflammatory bowel disease (e.g., ulcerative colitis and Crohn's disease). Some of the sulfasalazine is absorbed, and a portion of that is excreted unchanged back into the colon. Colonic bacteria split the azo linkage, releasing the two drugs. The 5-ASA is responsible for local anti-inflammatory activity (suppression of inflammatory mediators, but how, which, is not well understood) and symptom relief. The other metabolite, sulfapyridine, is primarily responsible for side effects associated with this "two drugs in one" combination: nausea, vomiting, and headaches (dose-dependent); sulfonamide allergic reactions in "sulfa-sensitive" patients; and rare but potentially fatal blood reactions including immune-mediated hemolysis and aplastic anemia.

A related drug, mesalamine, contains only the active 5-ASA. Lacking any sulfapyridine, the side effects and adverse responses are very low compared with sulfasalazine. An even neater strategy is used by olsalazine: the drug comprises of two azo-linked 5-ASA molecules; the bond is cleaved by gut bacteria, releasing two 5-ASA molecules for every molecule of olsalazine administered.

356. The answer is a. (*Brunton, pp 975, 1656; Craig, pp 478–479; Katzung, p 1035.*) Aluminum hydroxide (and all other clinically useful aluminum salts other than the phosphate) has a high affinity for phosphate. In the gut, the aluminum salts bind phosphate and prevent its absorption quite well. They also induce a blood-to-gut gradient that favors elimination of circulating phosphate. (Used inappropriately, it may cause hypophosphatemia: sustained, high-dose use of aluminum-containing antacids is one of the most common causes of hypophosphatemia.) None of the other drugs listed are effective in or used for reducing phosphate absorption or lowering serum levels.

The main limitation to using an aluminum salt by itself is its tendency to cause constipation. This is usually dealt with, when aluminum salts are used as typical "antacids," by coadministering a magnesium salt, which alone tends to cause laxation. (Giving Mg would be inadvisable for patients with renal failure, such as this dialysis patient, who are often unable to excrete Mg at rates sufficient to avoid hypermagnesemia.)

357. The answer is e. (*Brunton, pp 174, 196, 967–968, 975; Craig, pp 477–478; Katzung, pp 114, 1034–1035.*) Acetylcholine, through activation of an H^+,K^+-ATPase on parietal cells in the gastric mucosa, is one of only several agonists that increase gastric acid secretion. Histamine and gastrin are among the other important agonists, and their receptors and prosecretory effects are not blunted or otherwise affected by antimuscarinic or ganglionic-blocking drugs such as pirenzipine.

Blockade of autonomic ganglionic neurotransmission, whether caused by pirenzipine or less selective agents (e.g., trimethaphan, hexamethonium) is most likely to result in hypotension, not rises of blood pressure (a). That is because the sympathetic nervous system exerts primary and dominant resting control over peripheral vasomotor tone, and so ganglionic blockade typically causes hypotension. The drug has little or no affinity for nicotinic receptors on skeletal muscle, and so skeletal muscle weakness (b) is unlikely.

Diarrhea, urinary incontinence, and related problems are unlikely. The parasympathetic nervous system provides predominant resting influences over gut and bladder musculature (sphincters, longitudinal muscle in the gut, trigone and detrusor in the bladder). Block those influences with a drug such as pirenzipine, and the most likely outcomes are constipation and urinary retention, not what was described in answer c. Reflex tachycardia (d), or any other autonomic reflex for that matter, will be blunted by pirenzipine or any other drug that alters ganglionic transmission, whether by interfering with ACh synthesis, release, or its ability to activate cholinergic receptors on postganglionic nerve cell bodies or on cells of the adrenal/suprarenal medulla.

358. The answer is b. (*Brunton, pp 999–1003; Craig, p 473; Katzung, pp 1049–1050.*) Constipation is the most common and most worrisome adverse response to alosetron. This drug's mechanism of desired action involves selective blockade of serotonin receptors (5-HT$_3$) in the gut; the main outcomes include slowing of colonic transport time, increased sodium and water reabsorption from the colon, and reduced secretion of water and electrolytes into the colon.

Although constipation might be viewed as "trivial" or a minor complaint with most drugs, with alosetron it is the most worrisome one. Constipation may (and has) progressed to fecal impaction, bowel perforation or obstruction, and ischemic colitis. Fatalities have occurred.

The risks are such that the drug was pulled from the market in early 2000 and reapproved 2 years later with a limited indication (prolonged, severe diarrhea, predominant IBS in women); abundant warnings in the package insert; and a comprehensive risk-management/avoidance program that includes a requirement for (among other things) a special "sign-off" by both the prescriber and the patient that they understand and acknowledge and can identify the risks and agree to treatment anyway.

359. The answer is b. (*Brunton, pp 1000–1003; Craig, p 477; Katzung, pp 272, 273i, 1049–1052.*) The antiemetic effects of ondansetron—a drug that is widely and effectively used to manage nausea and emesis associated with chemotherapy or surgery—is mainly due to blockade of 5-HT$_3$ receptors in the brain's chemoreceptor trigger zone (and, probably in the solitary tract nucleus and in the stomach and small intestine).

Activation of μ-opioid receptors in the CTZ (a) is what *causes* the nausea and emesis that is so common with such drugs as morphine and other opioid analgesics.

Blockade of central dopamine receptors (c), particularly D$_2$ receptors in the CTZ, is the main mechanism by which phenothiazines (e.g., chlorpromazine, prochlorperazine) cause their antinausea/antiemetic effects. They are useful and effective for some patients with chemotherapy-induced nausea and vomiting, but better suited for prophylaxis of these symptoms due to other causes or for prophylaxis of motion sickness. Central antimuscarinic and antihistaminic actions may contribute to the overall effects.

Blockade of H$_1$ histamine receptors (d) in the brain (brainstem) and vestibular apparatus of the inner ear accounts for the main mechanism of action of such drugs as cyclizine, diphenhydramine (and its derivative, dimenhydrinate), and hydroxyzine. Antimuscarinic effects of these antihistamines may contribute to the overall effect. They are best suited for motion sickness prophylaxis, less effective as "general antiemetics," and not very or specifically effective for chemotherapy-induced symptoms.

Antimuscarinic agents (e; scopolamine can be considered the prototype in terms of motion sickness or emesis control) do not exert their effects via actions on the GI musculature, although suppression of ACh-mediated GI motility and tone certainly occurs. Their effects are primarily central; their clinical utility is mainly limited to prophylaxis or treatment (lower efficacy) of motion sickness.

The Endocrine System, Uterine Stimulants and Relaxants

Anabolic steroids, testosterone, related drugs

Calcium-regulating drugs, including parathyroid hormone and vitamin D

Corticosteroids

Diabetes mellitus and hypoglycemia

Diagnosis, management, of adrenal dysfunction

Erectile dysfunction

Estrogens, progestins, contraceptives, fertility agents

Thyroid disorders

Uterine stimulants and relaxants (oxytocics, tocolytics)

Questions

DIRECTIONS: Each item contains a question or incomplete statement that is followed by several responses. Select the **one best** response to each question.

360. A patient with a previously undiagnosed thyroid cancer presents with thyrotoxicosis (thyroid storm). One drug that is administered as part of early management, and may be lifesaving, is propranolol. Which of the following best summarizes why we give this drug, or what we want it to do?

a. Block parenchymal cell receptors for thyroid hormones
b. Block thyroid hormone release by a direct effect on the gland
c. Inhibit thyroid hormone synthesis
d. Lessen dangerous cardiovascular signs and symptoms of thyroid hormone excess
e. Lower TSH levels

361. A 44-year-old traveling salesman was recently diagnosed with Type 2 diabetes mellitus. The physician prescribed an exercise and diet plan, but this gentleman wouldn't be compliant. He habitually has a morning cup of coffee, gets in his car in the morning, and drives until he gets to his next appointment late afternoon. He says he rarely stops and eats in between.

The next approach is to use a single oral antidiabetic drug, but you are concerned about the drug causing or worsening hypoglycemia in this "meal-skipper." Which of the following drugs poses the greatest relative risk of causing or exacerbating hypoglycemia?

a. Acarbose
b. Glyburide
c. Metformin
d. Pioglitazone
e. Repaglinide

362. A woman deemed at high risk of postmenopausal osteoporosis is started on alendronate. Which of the following is this representative bis-phosphonate's main mechanism of action?

a. Activates vitamin D
b. Directly forms hydroxyapatite crystals in the bone
c. Provides supplemental calcium in the diet
d. Provide supplemental phosphate, which indirectly elevates serum Ca^{2+}
e. Reduces the number and activity of osteoclasts in bone

363. Some patients who are taking high doses of a bisphosphonate for Paget's disease of the bone develop an endocrine-metabolic disorder. Which of the following is the most likely disorder?

a. Cushing's disease (cushingoid symptoms)
b. Diabetes insipidus
c. Diabetes mellitus
d. Hyperparathyroidism
e. Hyperthyroidism

364. Metyrapone is useful in testing hyper- or hypofunction of certain endocrine conditions or biological processes those glands normally control. When we administer this drug for diagnostic purposes, which of the following structures or functions are we most likely assessing?

a. α cells of pancreatic islets
b. β cells of pancreatic islets
c. Leydig's cells of the testes
d. Pituitary-adrenal axis
e. Thyroid gland's response to TSH

365. A 60-year-old man on long-term therapy with a drug develops hypertension, hyperglycemia, and decreased bone density. Blood tests indicate anemia. Stool samples initially were positive for occult blood and then developed a "coffee-grounds" appearance. Which of the following drugs is most likely responsible for the patient's symptoms?

a. Beclomethasone
b. Hydrochlorothiazide
c. Metformin
d. Pamidronate
e. Prednisone

366. A woman with a cardiac arrhythmia is being treated long-term with amiodarone. This drug can cause biochemical changes and clinical signs and symptoms that resemble those associated with which of the following endocrine diseases/disorders?

a. Addisonian crisis
b. Cushing's syndrome
c. Diabetes insipidus
d. Diabetes mellitus
e. Hypothyroidism
f. Ovarian hyperstimulation syndrome

367. An elderly patient with Type 2 diabetes mellitus is being treated with chlorpropamide, prescribed by his elderly primary care doctor. Which of the following adverse responses or side effects is most typical of those expected with administration of chlorpropamide?

a. Cutaneous flushing, headache, after consuming alcohol
b. Hyponatremia
c. Hypertonic (hyperosmolal) urine compared with normal
d. Reduced serum T_3 and T_4 levels, symptomatic hypothyroidism
e. Weight gain unrelated to effects on glycemic status

368. A 22-year-old woman has been sexually assaulted. She requests a postcoital contraceptive. Which of the following usually is the most appropriate drug, assuming no contraindications?

a. Ergonovine (or methylergonovine)
b. Mifepristone
c. Raloxifene
d. Ritodrine
e. Tamoxifen

369. A patient has hyperthyroidism from a thyroid cancer, and the medical team concludes that oral radioiodine (sodium iodide 131 [^{131}I]) is the preferred treatment. The dosage is calculated correctly, and the drug is administered. Which of the following is also correct about this approach?

a. A β-adrenergic blocker should not be used for symptom control if or when ^{131}I is used
b. Hyperthyroidism symptoms resolve almost completely within 24–48 h after dosing with ^{131}I
c. Many patients treated with ^{131}I develop metastatic nonthyroid cancers in response to the drug
d. Oral antithyroid drugs should be administered up to and including the day of ^{131}I administration
e. There is a high incidence of delayed hypothyroidism after using ^{131}I for eradication of a thyroid tumor, and so thyroid hormone supplements may be needed later on

370. A 50-year-old woman at very high risk of breast cancer is given tamoxifen for prophylaxis. Tamoxifen does which of the following in this situation?

a. Blocks estrogen receptors in breast tissue
b. Blocks estrogen receptors in the endometrium
c. Increases the risk of osteoporosis
d. Raises serum LDL cholesterol and total cholesterol, lowers HDL
e. Reduces the risk of thromboembolic disorders

371. A 50-year-old woman is recently diagnosed with Type 2 diabetes mellitus. Exercise and diet do not provide adequate glycemic control, so drug therapy is needed. The physician contemplates prescribing metformin. Which of the following statements about this drug is correct?

a. Beneficial and unwanted actions are unaffected by liver function status
b. Lactic acidosis occurs frequently, but it is seldom serious
c. Metformin-induced hypoglycemia seldom occurs
d. Useful, as monotherapy, for both Type 1 and Type 2 diabetes
e. Weight gain is a common and unwanted side effect

372. A 76-year-old man complains of progressive difficulty starting his urine stream and having to get up several times during each night to urinate. Rectal examination reveals a generally enlarged, smooth-surfaced prostate. Prostatic serum antigen (PSA) titers are elevated. Urine flow increases, and prostate size decreases, in response to finasteride treatment. Which of the following best summarizes the mechanism by which finasteride caused symptom relief?

a. Blocks α-adrenergic receptors
b. Blocks testosterone receptors
c. Inhibits dihydrotestosterone synthesis
d. Inhibits testosterone synthesis
e. Lowers serum testosterone levels by increasing its renal clearance

373. A recalcitrant patient with Type 2 diabetes mellitus is notoriously noncompliant with medication and diet recommendations. However, he thinks he's smart enough to fool the physician into thinking otherwise: he takes his medication and eliminates nearly all carbohydrate intake for a few days before each clinic visit, knowing he will get a finger stick for a spot check of serum glucose levels. The simplest, most cost-effective, and most informative way for the physician to assess for past noncompliance and long-term glycemic control would be to perform or measure which of the following?

a. Glucose concentration in venous blood sample
b. Glucose tolerance test
c. Hb A_{1C}
d. Serum levels of the antidiabetic drug
e. Urine ketone levels (in a sample donated at the time of clinic visit)
f. Urine glucose levels

374. Many therapeutic insulins are often modifications of "regular" insulin. The modifications include substituting some amino acids in the protein using recombinant DNA technology, conjugating insulin with NPH (neutral protamine Hagedorn), or combining it with zinc. For all these insulins, which of the following is the one common result of such changes?

a. Elimination of allergic responses
b. Enabling administration by either subcutaneous or intravenous routes
c. Modification of onsets, durations of action
d. Prevention of cellular K^+ uptake as glucose enters cells
e. Reactivation of endogenous (pancreatic) insulin synthesis
f. Selective effects on glucose metabolism, little/no effects on lipids

375. You have prescribed an oral agent to help control a patient's blood glucose levels. He has Type 2 diabetes. In explaining how the drug works, you describe it as a "starch blocker" that inhibits the intestinal uptake of complex carbohydrates in the diet. You advise also that flatus or some cramping or "grumbling sounds" in the belly may develop. Which of the following drugs best fits this description?

a. Acarbose
b. Any thiazolidinedione ("glitazone")
c. Glipizide
d. Metformin
e. Tolbutamide

376. A young sexually active woman with recurrent, moderate asthma is taking prednisone for suppression of airway inflammation and using two inhaled adrenergic bronchodilators: salmeterol for prophylaxis and albuterol for acute intervention (rescue therapy). She begins taking an oral contraceptive (estrogen-progestin combination). Which of the following summarizes the most likely interaction?

a. Contraceptive failure, pregnancy
b. Glucocorticoid withdrawal syndrome (Addisonian crisis)
c. Hypertensive crisis from enhanced adrenergic drug actions
d. Increased corticosteroid (prednisone) side effects
e. Increased risk of cardiac toxicity from the adrenergic agents
f. Recurrence of airway inflammation (corticosteroid effects antagonized)

377. A patient with Type 1 diabetes is being treated with insulin glargine. Which of the following clinically important properties sets insulin glargine apart, or otherwise differentiates it, from other insulin formulations that might be used instead?

a. Blood levels, hypoglycemic effects, following insulin glargine injection are more accurately described as a plateau rather as a definite "spike" or peak
b. Disulfiram-like reactions (acetaldehyde accumulation from inhibited EtOH metabolism) more common, severe, with insulin glargine
c. Insulin glargine has an extremely fast onset, useful for immediate postprandial control of serum glucose elevations
d. Insulin glargine poses little or no risk of hypoglycemia if the patient skips several meals in a row
e. This insulin sensitizes parenchymal cells to insulin (e.g., the administered insulin itself), not just provides or replaces insulin, thereby enhancing glycemic control

378. A patient presents in the emergency department with a massive overdose of a drug. The most worrisome signs and symptoms include excessive cardiac stimulation (severe tachycardia, palpitations, angina, etc.). The ED physician orders IV administration a β-adrenergic blocker, saying (correctly) it is the only drug likely to normalize cardiac function quickly and save the patient's life. Which of the following was the most likely drug the patient overdosed on?

a. A second-generation sulfonylurea (e.g., glipizide, glyburide)
b. Insulin
c. Levothyroxine
d. Prednisone (oral glucocorticoid)
e. Propylthiouracil

379. A 54-year-old man with other well-treated medical disorders has erectile dysfunction. He takes a dose of sildenafil and shortly thereafter develops acute and severe hypotension. Upon arrival at the emergency department his blood pressure is very low, he is tachycardic, and an EKG shows changes indicative of acute myocardial ischemia. Which other medication was this man most likely taking?

a. Digoxin
b. Glipizide
c. Nitroglycerin
d. Propranolol
e. Testosterone

380. A patient with hypothyroidism following thyroidectomy will require lifelong hormone replacement therapy. Which of the following agents generally would be most suitable?

a. Levothyroxine (T_4)
b. Liothyronine
c. Liotrix
d. Protirelin
e. Thyroid, desiccated

381. A patient develops marked skeletal muscle tetany soon after a recent thyroidectomy. Which of the following drugs is most likely to be chosen to manage this adverse response to surgery?

a. Calcitonin
b. Calcium gluconate
c. Plicamycin (mithramycin)
d. PTH (parathyroid hormone)
e. Vitamin D

382. A 40-year-old man with a symmetrically enlarged thyroid gland associated with elevated levels of T_3 and T_4 is treated with propylthiouracil (PTU). Which of the following best summarizes the principal mechanism of action of PTU?

a. Blocks iodide transport into the thyroid
b. Increases hepatic metabolic inactivation of circulating T_4 and T_3
c. Inhibits proteolysis of thyroglobulin
d. Inhibits thyroidal peroxidase
e. Releases T_3 and T_4 into the blood

383. Your patient, who is taking an oral contraceptive, has heard about and asks about the risk of thromboembolism as a result of taking these drugs. To reduce the risk of this potentially severe adverse hematologic response, but still provide reasonably effective contraception, you would prescribe which of the following?

a. A combination product with a higher estrogen dose
b. A combination product with a higher progestin dose
c. A combination product with a lower estrogen dose
d. A combination product with a lower progestin dose
e. An OC that contains only estrogen

384. A woman goes into premature labor, and the physician administers ritodrine. Which of the following is the main mechanism of action by which this drug slows or suppresses uterine contractions?

a. Blocks prostaglandin synthesis
b. Blocks uterine oxytocin receptors
c. Inhibits oxytocin release from the posterior pituitary
d. Inhibits oxytocin synthesis in the hypothalamus
e. Stimulates α-adrenergic receptors
f. Stimulates β_2-adrenergic receptors

385. A 27-year-old woman is diagnosed with hypercorticism. To determine whether cortisol production is independent of pituitary gland control, you decide to suppress ACTH production by giving a high-potency glucocorticoid. Which of the following glucocorticoids is the best for this indication?

a. Dexamethasone
b. Hydrocortisone
c. Methylprednisolone
d. Prednisone
e. Triamcinolone

386. A patient with Cushing's syndrome is being treated by X-irradiation of the pituitary. It may take several months of treatment for adequate symptomatic and metabolic improvement. Until that time, which of the following might be administered adjunctively to suppress glucocorticoid synthesis?

a. Cimetidine
b. Cortisol (massive doses)
c. Fludrocortisone
d. Ketoconazole
e. Spironolactone

387. A woman who has been taking an oral contraceptive (estrogen plus progestin) for several years is diagnosed with epilepsy and started on phenytoin. Which of the following is the most likely consequence of adding the phenytoin?

a. Agranulocytosis or aplastic anemia, requiring stopping both drugs immediately
b. Breakthrough seizures from increased phenytoin clearance
c. Phenytoin toxicity, significant and of fast onset
d. Profoundly increased risk of craniofacial abnormalities in the fetus
e. Reduced contraceptive efficacy
f. Thromboembolism from the estrogen component of the contraceptive

388. A woman wants a prescription for an oral contraceptive, and your choice is between an estrogen-progestin combination and a "minipill" (progestin only). A main difference is that, compared with the hormone combination products, progestin-only drugs:

a. Are associated with a higher risk of thromboembolism
b. Are directly spermicidal
c. Cause more menstrual irregularities (irregular cycle length, amenorrhea, spotting, etc.)
d. Have better contraceptive efficacy
e. Must be taken on an irregular cycle, rather than daily, so compliance is hindered

389. A woman is taking a combination estrogen-progestin combination oral contraceptive. She experiences a multitude of side effects. Which of the following side effects is most likely due to what can be described as an "estrogen excess," and not likely due to the progestin content of the medication?

a. Fatigue
b. Hypertension
c. Hypomenorrhea
d. Increased appetite
e. Weight gain

390. A patient with an endocrine disorder develops lactic acidosis, and nearly dies, as a result of an uncommon but serious adverse response to therapy with an "endocrine" drug. Which of the following was the most likely cause of this severe problem?

a. Insulin glargine, prescribed for Type 1 diabetes mellitus
b. Levothyroxine, prescribed to maintain euthyroid status following thyroidectomy
c. Metformin, prescribed for Type 2 diabetes mellitus
d. Propylthiouracil, prescribed for hyperthyroidism
e. Spironolactone, prescribed for an adrenal cortical tumor

391. A patient with Type 2 diabetes mellitus begins gaining weight after several months of therapy with an oral antidiabetic agent. A complete workup indicates edema and other signs and symptoms of *heart failure*. Which of the following antidiabetic drug or group was the most likely cause?

a. Acarbose
b. Biguanides
c. Glitazones (thiazolidinediones, such as rosiglitazone)
d. Metformin
e. Sulfonylureas, both first and second generation agents (e.g., tolbutamide, chlorpropamide, glyburide, glipizide)

392. A woman goes into premature labor early enough that there are great concerns about inadequate fetal lung development and the risk of fetal respiratory distress syndrome. Ritodrine therapy is started to slow labor, but parturition seems imminent. Which of the following adjuncts should be administered prepartum, specifically for the purpose of reducing the risks and complications of the newborn's immature respiratory system development?

a. Albuterol (β_2 agonist)
b. Betamethasone
c. Ergonovine (or methylergonovine)
d. Indomethacin
e. Magnesium sulfate

393. We prescribe etidronate for a postmenopausal woman who is at great risk for developing for osteoporosis. Which of the following is the most likely side effect or adverse response to this drug for this patient?

a. Cholelithiasis
b. Esophagitis
c. Fluid/electrolyte loss from profuse diarrhea
d. Hepatic necrosis
e. Renal damage from calcium stone formation
f. Tetany

394. A 75-year-old man had surgery for prostate carcinoma, and local metastases were found intraoperatively. Which of the following is the most appropriate follow-up drug aimed at treating the metastases?

a. Aminoglutethimide
b. Fludrocortisone
c. Leuprolide
d. Mifepristone
e. Spironolactone

395. A 53-year-old woman with Type 2 diabetes mellitus is started on glyburide. Which of the following is a main mechanism by which this drug and others of its class lower blood glucose levels?

a. Decrease insulin resistance by lowering body weight
b. Enhance renal excretion of glucose
c. Increase insulin synthesis
d. Promote glucose uptake by muscle, liver, and adipose tissue via an insulin-independent process
e. Release insulin from the pancreas

396. A 75-year-old woman with diabetes is taking an oral antidiabetic drug. One day she goes without eating for 18 h. Her serum glucose concentration is 48 mg/dL (hypoglycemic) upon arrival at the emergency department, where she is deemed to be in critical condition. Which of the following drugs most likely aggravated this fasting hypoglycemia?

a. Acarbose
b. Glyburide
c. Metformin
d. Pioglitazone
e. Rosiglitazone

397. A man with Type 2 diabetes is receiving a combination of oral drugs to maintain glycemic control. He becomes hypoglycemic and ingests a glucose-containing product marketed to manage such an event. It doesn't work; his blood glucose levels remain low, his symptoms persist. Which of the following antidiabetic drugs was he most likely taking?

a. Acarbose
b. Glyburide
c. Metformin
d. Repaglinide
e. Rosiglitazone

398. A 35-year-old woman has Graves' disease, a small goiter, and symptoms that are deemed "mild-to-moderate." Propylthiouracil is prescribed. Which of the following is the most serious adverse response to this drug, for which close monitoring is required?

a. Agranulocytosis
b. Cholestatic jaundice
c. Gout
d. Renal tubular necrosis
e. Rhabdomyolysis
f. Thyroid cancer

399. A 60-year-old man with Type 2 diabetes mellitus is treated with pioglitazone. Which of the following phrases summarizes best this drug's main mechanism of action?

a. Blocks intestinal carbohydrate absorption
b. Causes glycosuria (increased renal glucose excretion)
c. Increases hepatic gluconeogenesis
d. Increases release of endogenous insulin
e. Increases target tissue sensitivity to insulin

400. A 27-year-old woman with endometriosis is treated with danazol. Which of the following is the most likely drug-induced side effect or adverse response for which you should be monitoring often?

a. Anemia from excessive vaginal bleeding
b. Abnormal liver function tests
c. Psychosis
d. Thrombocytopenia
e. Weight loss

401. A patient with a history of Type 2 diabetes mellitus presents in the emergency department. His complaints include nonspecific gastrointestinal symptoms, including nausea and vomiting. He states he is bloated and has abdominal pain. His appetite has been suppressed for several days. He has malaise and difficulty breathing. His liver is enlarged and tender; liver function tests indicate hepatic damage. Serum bicarbonate is low and lactate levels are high. Kidney function is falling rapidly.

The diagnosis is lactic acidosis, and the suspicion is that it was caused by an antidiabetic drug. Which of the following drugs is this patient most likely to be taking?

a. Acarbose
b. Glipizide
c. Glyburide
d. Metformin
e. Rosiglitazone

402. You are doing summer volunteer work at a health clinic in a very poor region of the world. A 25-year-old man is diagnosed with vitamin D–resistant rickets. Aside from administering high-dose vitamin D and oral phosphate, which of the following might you prescribe as an additional adjunct to "improve bone health" in these rickettsial patients, assuming financial resources were not a limiting factor?

a. Calcitriol
b. Estrogen
c. Hydrochlorothiazide
d. Pamidronate
e. Prednisone

403. A patient is transported to the emergency department shortly after taking a massive overdose of her levothyroxine in an apparent suicide attempt. Which of the following drugs should we administer first for prompt control of the hormone-related effects that are most likely to lead to her death if not correctly managed?

a. Iodine/iodide
b. Liothyronine
c. Propranolol
d. Propylthiouracil
e. Radioiodine (^{131}I)

404. There are two main formulations of oral contraceptives: those that are estrogen-progestin combinations, and those that contain only progestin ("minipill"). Which of the following is the main mechanism by which these drugs exert their desired contraceptive effects?

a. Acidify the cervical mucus, thereby making the mucus spermicidal
b. Displace/detach a fertilized egg from the endometrium
c. Inhibit nidation (implantation of a fertilized ovum)
d. Inhibit ovulation
e. Reduce uterine blood flow such that the fertilized ovum becomes hypoxic and dies

405. A 55-year-old postmenopausal woman develops weakness, polyuria, polydipsia, and significant increases of serum creatinine concentration. A computed tomogram (CT scan) indicates nephrocalcinosis. A drug is considered to be the cause. Which of the following drugs is most likely responsible?

a. Estrogens
b. Etidronate
c. Glipizide
d. Prednisone
e. Vitamin D

406. We have a patient with severe Cushing's disease. Surgery cannot be scheduled for several months, so the MD plans to treat the patient in the interim with a drug that she describes as a "potent inhibitor of corticosteroid synthesis." Which of the following drugs best fits that description?

a. Dexamethasone
b. Hydrocortisone
c. Ketoconazole
d. Prednisone
e. Spironolactone

407. We prescribe bromocriptine for a woman with primary amenorrhea. Normal menstruation returns about a month after starting therapy. Which of the following statements best described the mechanism by which bromocriptine caused its desired effects?

a. Blocked estrogen receptors, enhanced gonadotropin release
b. Increased follicle-stimulating hormone (FSH) synthesis
c. Inhibited prolactin release
d. Stimulated ovarian estrogen and progestin synthesis
e. Stimulated gonadotropin-releasing hormone (GnRH) release

408. A patient has had his parathyroid glands excised during a total thyroidectomy. Which of the following is the main physiologic action or role of parathyroid hormone—one that will require administration of parathormone or other suitable adjuncts?

a. Decreased active absorption of Ca from the small intestine
b. Decreased excretion of phosphate
c. Decreased renal tubular reabsorption of calcium
d. Decreased resorption of phosphate from bone
e. Increased mobilization of calcium from bone

Endocrine System, Uterine Stimulants and Relaxants

Answers

360. The answer is d. (*Brunton, pp 290, 1530; Craig, pp 115, 749–750; Katzung, p 637.*) In thyrotoxicosis, essentially the only effect of administering a β-adrenergic blocker—and it is an important effect, to be sure—is to provide prompt relief of both relatively innocuous manifestations of thyroid hormone excess, such as tremor, and those that are much more dangerous, including significant and potentially life-threatening increases in cardiac rate, contractility, and automaticity. Circulating thyroid hormone levels modulate the responsiveness of β-adrenergic receptors to their agonists (e.g., epinephrine, norepinephrine). When thyroid hormone levels are excessive, so is adrenergic receptor responsiveness. Therefore, we can reduce the adrenergic consequences of the hormone excess using a β blocker. There are no effects on thyroid hormone levels or thyroid gland function or control.

361. The answer is b. (*Brunton, pp 1636–1637; Craig, p 773; Katzung, p 706.*) The most common side effect of the newer sulfonylureas (glyburide, glipizide, glimepiride) is hypoglycemia, and the relative incidence is higher than with any of the other drugs listed.

Normally insulin release peaks in response to a meal. That occurs even when there is a relative insulin deficiency (Type 2 diabetes mellitus). Our hypothetical meal-skipping patient essentially fasts all day. His blood glucose levels will tend to fall as the meal-free interval progresses and during this time physiologic insulin release would be relatively low. However, the newer sulfonylureas—glyburide, glipizide, glimepiride—act by causing insulin release, whether one has eaten or fasted. Thus, the hypoglycemic effect of the drug will enhance the tendency for hypoglycemia that accompanies fasting or that occurs with increased physical activity. This is likely to apply even in the presence of insulin resistance, which is common.

Acarbose (a) is an α-glucosidase inhibitor. The main effect of that drug is a slowed rate of carbohydrate absorption from the gut. This blunts the insulin response to rising blood glucose levels. Because acarbose's effects center on inhibiting dietary carbohydrate absorption, the drug's effects will not occur in the absence of those foodstuffs. Indeed, effects are better when the drug is taken with or right before meals, and it seems to be more efficacious as the amount of carbohydrate in the meal increases.

Metformin does not directly increase or decrease insulin secretion. In contrast with the sulfonylureas, which are correctly classified as hypoglycemic drugs (i.e., they drive blood glucose levels down), the biguanides are antihyperglycemic, tending instead to keep blood glucose levels from going up.

Pioglitazone (a thiazolidinedione or "glitazone" for short) sensitizes parenchymal cells (mainly adipocytes) to insulin and so reduces insulin resistance. (The glitazones apparently activate a nuclear peroxisomal proliferator-activated receptor, PPAR-γ that participates in the cellular response to insulin.)

Because of the insulin-dependency of their actions, the intensity of the effects of a glitazone increases when insulin levels are high (e.g., postprandial) and diminish as insulin levels fall (e.g., fasting). Regardless, and unless a glitazone is prescribed with insulin or a sulfonylurea (common), the incidence of drug-induced hypoglycemia is very low.

Repaglinide, a meglitinide, seems to trigger pancreatic insulin release in the presence of sufficient (and high) blood glucose levels. However, when blood glucose levels are sufficiently low (as can occur during fasting or meal-skipping), that effect wanes and so the drug is not likely to cause or worsen hypoglycemia.

362. The answer is e. *(Brunton, pp 1666–1668; Craig, pp 758–760; Katzung, pp 721, 727–730.)* Whether used for osteoporosis (prevention or management, men or women, idiopathic or drug-induced) or Paget's disease of the bone, bisphosphonates exert their effects on osteoclasts and osteoblasts. The drug is incorporated into bone. When drug-containing bone is resorbed by the osteoclasts, osteoclast function (and, so, subsequent bone resorption) is inhibited. The bisphosphonates also recruit osteoblasts, which then produce a substance that further inhibits osteoclast activity.

363. The answer is d. *(Brunton, p 1668; Craig, pp 758–760; Katzung, p 730.)* You should be able to deduce hyperparathyroidism as the answer by recalling that the bisphosphonates ultimately affect bone Ca^{2+} metabolism, and the parathyroid gland is the main regulator of serum Ca^{2+} levels. When a bisphosphonate is given to a patient with Paget's disease of the bone, after about a week the dramatic inhibition of bone resorption dramatically lowers serum Ca^{2+} levels (because an important portion of serum Ca^{2+} arises from bone that is being resorbed). When serum Ca^{2+} falls considerably, parathyroid hyperfunction can develop. The easiest way to prevent this is to administer dietary calcium supplements along with the bisphosphonate.

364. The answer is d. (*Brunton, pp 1610–1611; Craig, pp 699–700; Katzung, pp 655–656.*) Metyrapone, because it decreases serum levels of cortisol by inhibiting the β-hydroxylation of steroids in the adrenal, can be used to assess function of the pituitary-adrenal cortical axis. When metyrapone is given to normal persons, the adenohypophysis secretes more ACTH. This causes a normal adrenal cortex to synthesize increased amounts of 17-hydroxylated steroids, which can be measured in the urine. However, patients who have disease of the hypothalamico-pituitary axis do not produce ACTH in response to metyrapone. As a result, we find no increased levels of the steroids in the urine. Before administering metyrapone, we need to test responsiveness of the adrenal cortex to respond to administration of ACTH.

365. The answer is e. (*Brunton, pp 1603–1604; Craig, pp 693–694; Katzung, p 650.*) These findings are characteristic of what one would expect with long-term (and high-dose) systemic glucocorticoid therapy (i.e., prednisone and many others, but not beclomethasone, which is given by oral inhalation and is not absorbed appreciably). Psychoses, peptic ulceration with hemorrhage (coffee-grounds stool, indicative of gastric bleeding) or without (possibly causing guaiac-positive stools), increased susceptibility to infection, edema, osteoporosis, myopathy, and hypokalemic alkalosis can occur. Other adverse reactions include cataracts, hyperglycemia, slowed lineal growth in children, and iatrogenic Cushing's syndrome.

Hydrochlorothiazide (and other thiazide and thiazide-like diuretics, such as chlorthalidone or metolazone) can increase blood glucose levels. However, they typically lower blood pressure (as evidenced by their widespread use as antihypertensives) and tend to raise, not lower, serum calcium levels (which would be inconsistent with the decreased bone density described in this man). None of the other drugs listed would cause a collection of findings consistent with what we described here.

366. The answer is e. *(Brunton, pp 920–921, 1527, 1532t; Craig, pp 187–188; Katzung, pp 232–234, 630, 633.)* Amiodarone, an iodine-rich drug, has several actions that can lead to clinical hypothyroidism (or, less often and mainly in persons with iodine-deficient diets, hyperthyroidism). It inhibits a deiodinase (an enzyme that removes iodine on both the 5 and 5' positions) that converts thyroxine to triiodothyronine (T_3), mainly in the liver. This process is the main contributor to the production of endogenous (circulating) T_3 that is used by most target tissues in the body. Inhibit this enzyme and the peripheral tissues have less T_3 to utilize, and signs and symptoms of hypothyroidism can ensue.

The excess iodine derived from metabolism of amiodarone may also contribute to the hypothyroidism. The mechanism is analogous to the way in which administering large doses of iodide are clinically useful for suppressing thyroid function in hyperthyroid individuals: iodide limits its own transport into follicular cells, and, acutely at least, high circulating levels of iodide inhibit thyroid hormone synthesis.

367. The answer is a. *(Brunton, pp 1635t–1637; Craig, p 772; Katzung, pp 705–706.)* Chlorpropamide is one of the older sulfonylurea oral hypoglycemic drugs and is one of the biggest offenders in terms of the frequency and severity of disulfiram-like reactions it can cause (by inhibiting oxidation of acetaldehyde, an intermediate in ethanol metabolism, by aldehyde dehydrogenase). Chlorpropamide differs from the rest—older or newer sulfonylureas—in some other important ways. It has the longest half-life (duration of action between 1 and 3 days, usually toward the longer). It seems to pose the highest risk of causing hypoglycemia. And it tends to enhance the effects of ADH on the collecting ducts of the nephron and/or enhance ADH release from the posterior pituitary. Greater effects (or levels) of ADH impair renal conservation of water. This leads to formation of large volumes of dilute urine; the extra free water loss may cause weight loss and tends to cause hypernatremia, not the opposite. Chlorpropamide (and the other sulfonylureas) cause no frequent or significant alterations of thyroid hormone status or thyroid function.

368. The answer is b. *(Brunton, pp 665, 1561–1562; Craig, pp 701, 709; Katzung, pp 656, 680.)* Mifepristone is a synthetic drug used as an abortifacient or postcoital contraceptive. Although the drug blocks glucocorticoid receptors, that effect does not account for its use or effects in the context described here. Here the actions arise from blocking uterine progesterone receptors. They include detachment of the conceptus from the uterine wall, softening and dilation of the cervix, and increased myometrial contraction that expels the conceptus. (The latter arises from both a drug-induced increase of local prostaglandin synthesis and greater myometrial responsiveness to them.) If mifepristone fails to induce expulsion of the fetus, misoprostol is usually given to increase uterine contractions further. (Estrogens used alone or in combination with progestins have also proven effective in postcoital contraception.)

Ergonovine and methylergonovine are ergot compounds that cause uterine contraction, and are used postpartum to control bleeding by increasing uterine tone. They are abortifacient drugs, but not used for postcoital contraception. Ralxoifene and tamoxifen are estrogen receptor agonists or antagonists (which effects occurs depends on the tissue) that are used to treat certain estrogen-dependent breast cancers.

Ritodrine is a β_2-adrenergic agonist used to slow uterine contractions and reduce uterine tone in premature labor.

369. The answer is e. (*Brunton, pp 1533–1535; Craig, pp 750–752; Katzung, p 637.*) Hypothyroidism is the most common disadvantage or limitation of using ^{131}I to treat hyperthyroidism. No matter how accurately the dose is calculated, according to some studies about 8 of 10 treated patients develop symptomatic hypothyroidism (that needs to be treated) by 10 or more years after treatment. It results, of course, from excessive thyroid cell destruction.

Substantive symptom relief from ^{131}I takes from several weeks to a couple of months to develop (although blood chemistries change somewhat faster). Until a euthyroid state develops, drugs such as β-adrenergic blockers or oral antithyroid drugs may be needed for symptom control. Oral antithyroid drugs can be given before ^{131}I treatment, but they should be stopped for a couple of days before radiotherapy so as not to prevent radioiodine uptake into the gland. Cancers, metastatic or not, occurring in the thyroid or elsewhere, are rare after ^{131}I therapy.

370. The answer is a. (*Brunton, pp 1384, 1555–1557; Craig, pp 649–650, 707, 709–710; Katzung, pp 679–680, 916–917.*) Tamoxifen is often referred to as a selective estrogen receptor modifier (SERM). It blocks estrogen receptors in some tissues and stimulates them in some others. The drug can be used to prevent or treat estrogen-dependent breast cancers, and it works as an estrogen receptor antagonist there. A receptor-agonist action also accounts for one of the drug's more distressing and common side effects, hot flashes. In contrast, the drug activates estrogen receptors in the uterus, increasing the risk of endometrial cancers. Other estrogen-activating (estrogen-like) consequences include a reduced risk of osteoporosis, desirable changes in serum cholesterol profiles (reduced LDL and total cholesterols; increased HDL), and an increased risk of thromboembolic events. The related drug, raloxifene, is largely tamoxifen-like with one main exception: it does not activate uterine estrogen receptors, and so does not increase the risk of endometrial cancers.

371. The answer is c. (*Brunton, pp 1638–1639; Craig, pp 773–774; Katzung, p 708.*) Metformin, classified as a biguanide, "sensitizes" peripheral cells to insulin, thereby facilitating glucose uptake and utilization, and suppresses release of glucose from the liver and into the blood. It is largely ineffective in the absence of insulin and so is approved only for Type 2 diabetes, used alone or in conjunction with such other drugs as a sulfonylurea or insulin.

Most patients taking metformin lose weight. This is probably due to an appetite-suppressing effect (leading to reduced caloric intake), rather than because of a specific effect on some metabolic reaction(s) or anorexia secondary to GI side effects.

The drug seldom causes hypoglycemia. Rather than actively driving down blood glucose levels (as, say, insulin does), metformin acts as if it caps physiologic rises of glucose concentrations. (Thus, it has been described as being an antihyperglycemic drug, rather than a hypoglycemic agent.)

Metformin is not metabolized by the liver, but liver dysfunction is one contraindication. That's mainly because of the risks of the drug's most important adverse effect, lactic acidosis, which is rare but often fatal when it does occur: impaired liver function impairs lactate elimination and favors its accumulation to toxic levels.

However the main primary cause of the lactic acidosis is renal insufficiency (serum creatinine > 1.5 mg/dL in men, 1.4 mg/dL in women), whether caused by renal disease or by renal hypoperfusion (ischemia, as might occur with heart failure and/or hypotension).

372. The answer is c. (*Brunton, pp 268, 272, 1582–1583; Craig, p 732; Katzung, pp 688, 1030.*) Finasteride competitively inhibits steroid 5-reductase, the enzyme necessary for synthesis of the active form of testosterone (dihydrotestosterone) in the prostate. Testosterone synthesis and circulating testosterone levels don't fall in response to the drug. PSA titers will, however. (Recall, by the way, that the α-adrenergic blockers [e.g., prazosin] provide symptomatic relief in some men with BPH by relaxing smooth muscle in the urethra, bladder neck, and prostate capsule. Their effects do not involve testosterone synthesis or cellular responses to the hormone.)

373. The answer is c. (*Brunton, pp 1622–1624; Craig, p 768; Katzung, p 703.*) Serum glucose reacts nonenzymatically with hemoglobin to form glycated hemoglobin products (e.g., Hb A_{1C}). The rate of Hb A_{1C} formation is related to ambient glucose levels, and the amount of Hb A_{1C} measured in any given blood sample reflects the average blood glucose levels over the last 2–3 months. Thus, although the patient's serum glucose levels may be acceptable after a couple of days' fast, Hb A_{1C} measurements give the big picture about how good glycemic control was on a more long-term (and more important) timeline. Note that although measuring Hb A_{1C} gives important information about the long-term, it does not provide any information about day-to-day fluctuations in glucose levels or what's happening "right now," and such information is important to optimal control of diabetes and its symptoms. Nonetheless, regular, periodic checks of Hb A_{1C} should be part of the monitoring for every patient with diabetes (Type 1 or 2), not so much as a way to assess for noncompliance as to make sure that the current treatment plan with which the patient is complying is working. It is a common and relatively inexpensive assay.

Having the clinical lab measure glucose in a venous blood sample won't give any additional or meaningful information: handheld glucometers, used properly, are remarkably accurate. Glucose tolerance tests, even those done with oral glucose, will provide little historic information, and they are expensive. Few clinical labs are set up to measure serum concentrations of most oral antidiabetic drugs, and the cost for these nonstandard tests would be quite expensive. Measuring urine ketone levels are of no benefit for our purposes. All that they might prove is that our patient has fasted for several days. Urine glucose monitoring is not very enlightening either. Recall that glucose appears in the urine only when serum concentrations exceed a renal threshold for reabsorption (around 180 mg/dL or so). A glucose-free urine sample, then, would only indicate that serum glucose levels are below the threshold: they still could be unacceptably high, or normal, or low, and you would never know just by urine testing.

374. The answer is c. (*Brunton, pp 1624–1630; Craig, pp 765–766, 768–770; Katzung, pp 696–701.*) Insulin modifications, whether by rDNA technology or by physical means (e.g., modification with zinc or NPH) alter onsets and durations of action.

(Recall that regular insulin, given by SC injection, has an onset of about 30 min, peaks in about 3 h, and has a duration of about 7–8 h. Lispro and aspart insulins work faster, peak earlier, and have the shortest durations [rapid/short]; lente and NPH insulins ["intermediate-acting"] have onsets, times to peak, and durations longer than regular insulins; and ultralente insulin and insulin glargine have the slowest onsets [4–6 h], with durations that are on par with lente and NPH.)

In general, the modified human insulins rarely cause allergic responses (not the case with porcine lente and NPH insulins), but the problem is not prevented altogether, particularly with NPH insulins: the protamine used to modify either the human or porcine insulins, which are then called NPH insulins, is a large (and potentially antigenic) protein. Beyond that, however, the modifications yield clinically useful pharmacokinetic—not biochemical—changes.

375. The answer is a. (*Craig, pp 774–775; Brunton, p 1640; Katzung, pp 710–711.*) Acarbose, and the newer related drug, miglitol, act in intestinal brush border cells to inhibit monosaccharide formation from complex carbohydrates and oligosaccharides. They do so by inhibiting alpha glucosidases in the brush border of intestinal cells. The effect is optimal, of course, when carbohydrates are present in the gut: that is, during and right after a meal. Thus, the drug should be taken with meals. Its main effect will be a slowing of carbohydrate absorption and a blunting of typical postprandial rises of blood glucose. GI side effects, mainly those described in the question, are the most common ones with acarbose. Used alone, hypoglycemia is rare; however, the drug is often used as an adjunct to a sulfonylurea, and their propensity for causing hypoglycemia is not reduced by acarbose. Very high doses of acarbose may raise serum transaminases, usually reflecting some hepatic dysfunction caused by the drug.

376. The answer is d. (*Brunton, pp 1563–1566; Craig, p 713; Katzung, p 1119.*) Combination oral contraceptives (presumably the estrogen component) can impair the hepatic metabolism of several drugs, prednisone and several glucocorticoids among them. The most likely outcome is an increase in the number and/or severity of expected corticosteroid-associated side effects, including weight gain and alterations of carbohydrate, lipid, and protein metabolism. Thus, we need to monitor for this and reduce corticosteroid doses downward as needed. Because we have centered this patient scenario on asthma, we should add that oral contraceptives also inhibit clearance and increase the risk of toxicity from, theophylline.

377. The answer is a. *(Brunton, pp 1624–1630; Craig, p 769; Katzung, p 700.)* Insulin glargine is a genetically engineered insulin that is poorly (but adequately) soluble at physiologic pH values. The drug dissolves and enters the bloodstream slowly and in such a way that there is more of a stable plateau than a well-defined spike in blood levels and effects. This plateau is rather, and remarkably, consistent over the typical 24-h duration following a SC injection. Thus, the drug is better able than most other insulins for maintaining round-the-clock control of blood glucose levels, but less able to suppress the postprandial elevation of glucose that is necessary for some patients. Insulin glargine's onset and duration of action are comparable to such preparations as NPH insulins or lente insulins. It is what happens in between, temporally, that distinguishes this drug from the rest.

378. The answer is c. *(Brunton, pp 1521–1524; Craig, pp 749–750; Katzung, pp 636–639.)* Tachycardia, palpitations, tachyarrhythmias, and the possibility of acute myocardial ischemia, are among the hallmarks of thyrotoxicosis or thyroid hormone overdoses. Thyroid hormone levels regulate the "responsiveness" of β-adrenergic receptors to epinephrine and norepinephrine (or exogenous β-agonists), and this probably contributes to the clinical picture. Although excesses of thyroid hormone are the cause of the problems, management is symptomatic and aimed at suppressing β-mediated responses. Hence the use of propranolol or some other suitable β-adrenergic blocker for immediate and quite possibly lifesaving symptom control. Sulfonylureas (a) would not cause the signs or symptoms noted above, and β-blocker therapy for overdoses of one of those drugs would do more harm than good. The same applies to insulin (b); β blockers might control increases of cardiac rate, but they are more likely to further lower blood glucose levels and slow or otherwise blunt rises of blood glucose levels when appropriate therapy to render the patient euglycemic is started. Overdoses of prednisone (c) or propylthiouracil (e) are not likely to present as described, and they are not properly managed with a β blocker.

379. The answer is c. *(Brunton, pp 123, 829–830; Craig, pp 738–740; Katzung, p 189.)* This is the interaction (and one that can be fatal) between the popular ED drugs sildenafil, tadalafil, or vardenafil, and organic nitrovasodilators (e.g., and perhaps especially, immediate-nitroglycerin). It occurs because both interactants cause vasodilation through a nitric oxide–cGMP-dependent mechanism, and the combination causes greater than additive effects of each agent alone. It is also an interaction that should be foremost in the mind of any physician who prescribes one of these wildly popular drugs for erectile dysfunction. For more complete comments on the mechanisms and manifestations of the interaction, check the answer to Question 254 (cardiovascular chapter).

380. The answer is a. *(Brunton, pp 1524–1525; Craig, pp 748–749; Katzung, pp 630, 634–636.)* Levothyroxine is usually considered the first choice for long-term maintenance therapy of hypothyroidism, such as that which occurs after thyroidectomy or radiation therapy of the thyroid. Once absorbed, we get the slow-onset and rather steady, long-lasting effects of the T_4. In addition, much of the administered T_4 is deiodinated in the tissues to T_3, "automatically" providing usually adequate levels and effects of this more rapidly and shorter-acting hormone without the need to administer T_3 (liothyronine) separately.

If the patient develops profound hypothyroidism (e.g., myxedema), some clinicians may still prefer T_3 for its prompt effects. However, in this instance too, T_4 is generally regarded as the preferred way to replace both hormones and reestablish a euthyroid state (administered with corticosteroids for myxedema coma). Desiccated thyroid products (e) are outmoded for managing hypothyroidism. Protirelin (d) is a synthetic tripeptide, chemically identical to thyrotropin-releasing hormone (TRH) that is used to diagnose some thyroid disorders.

381. The answer is b. *(Brunton, p 1663; Craig, pp 754–756; Katzung, p 724.)* We're dealing with hypocalcemia in this patient with tetany postthyroidectomy, because the parathyroid gland was damaged or removed during the surgery. Administration of intravenous calcium gluconate would immediately correct the tetany. Parathyroid hormone (d) could be considered appropriate for long-term management of hypocalcemia, but it has a slower onset of action that would not be of much help in a tetanic state. We would then probably use vitamin D (e) and dietary modifications for long-control of serum calcium levels. Calcitonin (a) is a hypocalcemic antagonist of parathyroid hormone. (Note that calcitonin or calcitriol will raise serum calcium levels faster than vitamin D, but in this emergent situation they will not work fast enough, which is why we need direct administration of ionic calcium.) Plicamycin (c; mithramycin) is used to treat Paget's disease and hypercalcemia. The dose employed is about one-tenth the amount used for plicamycin's cytotoxic action when it is used as a chemotherapeutic drug.

382. The answer is d. *(Brunton, pp 1526–1529; Craig, p 750; Katzung, pp 631–632.)* Propylthiouracil, a thioamide use to manage many patients with hyperthyroidism, has three main actions. It inhibits peroxidase, and in doing so inhibits oxidation of inorganic iodide to iodine, and the iodination of tyrosine. It also blocks coupling of iodotyrosines and inhibits deiodination of T_4 to T_3 in the periphery.

383. The answer is c. *(Brunton, pp 1565–1567; Craig, p 710; Katzung, pp 673–678.)* Thromboembolism associated with OC administration is attributed to the estrogen component in these products. If thromboembolism is a concern, then one approach to reducing the risk would be selecting a product with a lower—not higher—estrogen dose. Even that may not be sufficient, long term. Progestins seem to have little impact on the development of thrombotic/embolic disorders during OC therapy, and so increasing or decreasing progestin content will do little more than nothing for most patients. Smoking is a major risk factor for thromboembolism, especially for women taking an oral contraceptive, so it's essential to encourage the patient to quit (or not start) smoking. There are no OCs that contain estrogen only (unlike the case with progestin-only OCs—the so-called minipills [see Question 388]).

384. The answer is f. *(Brunton, pp 240t, 253; Craig, p 720; Katzung, pp 135–138.)* Ritodrine is a predominantly β_2-selective adrenergic agonist, much like the prototype albuterol. In addition to causing bronchodilation—arguably the main use for drugs in this class—β_2 agonists slow uterine contractions. And that use, applied to suppression of preterm labor (a tocolytic effect), is the main clinical use of this "bronchodilator" drug. Terbutaline is also used for tocolysis. The sequence of events following binding of ritodrine to its receptor includes increased myometrial cAMP formation, activation of cAMP-dependent protein kinase, and extrusion of Ca^{2+} from smooth-muscle cells such that contractile force is reduced. There are no effects on oxytocin synthesis or release, nor on hypothalamic or pituitary function. Ritodrine's effects are not at all like those of ergot compounds (e.g., methylergonovine), which induce uterine contraction by a mechanism that involves α-adrenergic receptor activation. Be sure to understand that despite the classification of ritodrine as a "β_2-selective adrenergic agonist," or as a uterine relaxant, the drug can activate all β-adrenergic receptors and cause a host of unwanted side effects or adverse responses that include tachycardia (direct and reflexly, in response to reduced blood pressure), pulmonary edema, and myocardial ischemia. This very effective drug is contraindicated in eclampsia or severe eclampsia. In these situations the goal is to deliver the fetus (the definitive cure for eclampsia), not prolong labor.

385. The answer is a. (*Brunton, pp 1603, 1610; Craig, pp 692, 693; Katzung, pp 647, 649–650.*) Of the drugs listed, dexamethasone is by far the most potent in terms of relative glucocorticoid effects. The dexamethasone suppression test has several uses: it allows not only complete suppression of pituitary ACTH production, but also accurate measurement of endogenous corticosteroids, such as 17-ketosteroids, in the urine. The small amount of dexamethasone present contributes minimally to this measurement. None of the other drugs listed would be suitable for this test, and all are less potent than dexamethasone.

386. The answer is d. (*Brunton, pp 1582, 1610–1611; Craig, pp 700–701; Katzung, pp 687–688.*) Ketoconazole, traditionally used as an antifungal agent (see the chapter, "Anti-Infectives"), is one of the most efficacious inhibitors of corticosteroid synthesis. It is not a primary therapy for pituitary tumors/Cushing's syndrome, but is a useful adjunct. The main problem associated with this drug is the risk of hepatotoxicity and the potential for interactions with some other drugs. An alternative to ketoconazole is aminoglutethimide, which also interferes with synthesis of all the adrenal steroids.

Cimetidine, the H_2 histamine blocker that is well known as an inhibitor of P450-mediated metabolism of many drugs, would be of no benefit. Massive doses of cortisol, although theoretically "reasonable" (feedback suppression of pituitary function), would be of little help in terms of regulating the pituitary's activity and clearly would aggravate signs and symptoms of adrenal corticosteroid excess that we already have. Fludrocortisone has intense mineralocorticoid activity and is the only drug indicated for replacement therapy in chronic mineralocorticoid deficiencies. Spironolactone blocks aldosterone receptors; it would counteract only the aldosterone-related responses to corticosteroid excess and would not have any effects on adrenal corticosteroid synthesis.

387. The answer is e. (*Brunton, pp 121, 509–510, 523–524; Craig, pp 36–37, 378, 713; Katzung, pp 1119, 1122.*) Phenytoin is one of several agents that can enhance the hepatic metabolism of oral contraceptives (especially the estrogen component), leading to reduced contraceptive levels and unintended pregnancy (contraceptive failure). It is also one that interacts by inducing synthesis of hormone-binding globulins: more hormone molecules are bound to the protein, and so less free (active) drug is in the circulation. Several other common anticonvulsants interact with the same potential outcome, especially barbiturates (including phenobarbital, mephobarbital, and primidone), carbamazepine, and oxcarbazepine. Be sure to recall that rifampin (and rifabutin) and protease inhibitors (ritonavir, others) are also important interactants with OCs via a metabolism-inducing mechanism. Finally, some antibiotics (e.g., tetracyclines) interact with OCs, but here the mechanism differs: the antibiotics suppress gut flora that participate in enterohepatic recycling of the OCs. When the bacteria are suppressed, OCs that are secreted into the gut are lost in the feces, rather than being reabsorbed.

388. The answer is c. (*Brunton, p 1564; Craig, pp 706–712; Katzung, pp 673–679.*) Progestin-only oral contraceptives ("minipills") are associated with a higher risk of menstrual irregularities than the more common estrogen-progestin preparations. That is largely due to the lack of estrogen. However, the absence of estrogen also lowers the risk of thromboembolic disorders. Progestin-only formulations are, overall, less effective in terms of preventing pregnancy than combination products; like combination products they lack definitive spermicidal effects (but they thicken cervical mucus, retard sperm motility in that way, and reduce the likelihood of nidation), and their administration schedule is continuous—every day, rather than the cyclic schedule used for combination products.

389. The answer is b. (*Brunton, pp 1564–1566; Craig, pp 709–711; Katzung, p 675.*) Hypertension, which may occur (and usually transiently) in response to OCs, is mainly due to estrogen excess. Fatigue (a), weight gain (e; usually triggered by increased appetite), and infrequent or missed menses (c) are mainly associated with progestin excess. Hypomenorrhea (c) may also be due to inadequate estrogen levels in the combination product. Unusually frequent menses—hypermenorrhea—tends to be related to too little progestin in the product.

390. The answer is c. *(Brunton, pp 1638–1639; Craig, pp 773–774; Katzung, p 708.)* Metformin, a common drug for managing many patients with Type 2 diabetes mellitus, is a very well-tolerated and effective drug. This biguanide not only lowers circulating glucose levels, but suppresses appetite, thereby lowering dietary caloric intake. One of the main problems associated with metformin is the development of lactic acidosis—admittedly rare but potentially fatal adverse response to this drug and associated with none of the other drugs listed as answer choices.

391. The answer is c. *(Brunton, pp 1639–1640; Craig, p 774; Katzung, pp 704–707.)* Tolbutamide and the older sulfonylureas (e) have been associated with an increased risk of sudden death. The glitazones, however, have been associated with an increased risk of heart failure, which is why patients taking these drugs should be monitored for weight gain, edema, and other expected signs and symptoms of heart failure. Acarbose (a), an inhibitor of gastrointestinal carbohydrate uptake, is relatively free of any serious toxicity. Biguanides (b), of which metformin (d) is an example, are widely used antidiabetic drugs. The major toxicity or adverse response is a risk of lactic acidosis.

392. The answer is b. *(Brunton, p 1609; Craig, p 696; Katzung, p 650.)* We would give betamethasone to enhance fetal surfactant synthesis and suppress airway inflammation, thereby lessening the chance or severity of fetal respiratory distress syndrome at birth. (The action probably involves stimulating synthesis of fibroblast pneumocyte factor, which then stimulates surfactant synthesis by pneumocytes in the fetus. Recall that surfactant lowers alveolar surface tension, thereby reducing the likelihood of alveolar collapse and its consequences on gas exchange.)

Note: Other corticosteroids, especially dexamethasone, could be used. However, betamethasone is preferred because it binds less to plasma proteins than cortisol and most other glucocorticoids, allowing more steroid to cross the placenta.

Even though albuterol is used as a bronchodilator (e.g., for asthma or COPD), it is classified, pharmacologically, precisely as we classify ritodrine, a relatively selective β_2 agonist. With the ritodrine being given already, administering albuterol would be pointless. In obstetrics, ergonovine or methylergonovine are given postpartum; their strong uterine contracting effects are used to reduce postpartum bleeding. Aside from being contraindicated before delivery, they have no pulmonary effects of the sort we want. Indomethacin is sometimes used to slow premature labor. It works by blocking synthesis of prostaglandins that have oxytocic activity, but prostaglandin synthesis inhibition also causes closure of the ductus arteriosus (which, in this setting, would be unwanted). Magnesium sulfate would not cause the desired pulmonary effects; it is used in obstetrics to prevent seizures in preeclampsia/eclampsia. The drug has tocolytic activity, but the jury is out on just how effective and safe the drug is when used to suppress uterine contractions.

Note: Three pharmaceutical preparations of surfactant are now available: calfactant, beractant, and poractant alfa. They are given to neonates with respiratory distress syndrome by direct intratracheal instillation.

393. The answer is b. (*Brunton, p 1668; Craig, pp 758–760; Katzung, p 721.*) Esophagitis, sometimes with esophageal ulcers, is the most worrisome adverse response to bisphosphonates such as etidronate. It is not due to any specific metabolic alteration caused by the drug, but rather by direct, prolonged contact of the drug with the esophagus if the oral dose lodges there without passing quickly enough to the stomach. This is why the drug should not be administered to patients with esophageal disease, difficulty swallowing, or an inability to sit or stand up for at least 30 min (to help gravity bring the tablet to the stomach) after taking the drug. Otherwise, overall, the bisphosphonates cause remarkably few side effects in the vast majority of patients.

394. The answer is c. (*Brunton, pp 1387–1388; Craig, pp 650, 732; Katzung, pp 615, 687, 926.*) Leuprolide is a peptide that is related to GnRH or luteinizing hormone-releasing hormone (LHRH), and it is used to treat metastatic prostate carcinoma. By inhibiting gonadotropin release it induces a hypogonadal state; testosterone levels in the body fall significantly, and this appears to be the mechanism for suppression of the cancer. Aminoglutethimide (a) is an aromatase inhibitor mainly used to treat

Cushing's disease (it inhibits synthesis of adrenal corticosteroids), and some patients with metastatic breast carcinoma. Fludrocortisone (b) is a mineralocorticoid used for chronic adrenal insufficiency (along with gluco-corticoids) or congenital adrenal hypoplasia. Mifepristone (d) is an abortifacient/oxytocic drug. Spironolactone (e) is an aldosterone receptor blocker that is used mainly as for patients with primary or secondary hyperaldos-teronism, and as an adjunct to the management of severe heart failure. It is also classified as a potassium-sparing diuretic.

395. The answer is e. (*Brunton, pp 1634–1637; Craig, pp 771–772; Katzung, pp 704–706.*) Glyburide is one of several sulfonylureas antidiabetic drugs. Recall that the sulfonylureas simplistically fall into two main classes, based largely on how long they have been used: the so-called first-generation agents, such as tolbutamide and chlorpropamide, and the newer second-generation drugs, glipizide, glyburide, and glimepiride. Whether older or newer, these drugs mainly lower blood glucose levels by enhancing insulin release from the β cells of the pancreas. The mechanism involved binding to and blocking an ATP-sensitive K^+ channel on β cell membranes. This depolarizes the membrane, and resulting Ca^{2+} influx triggers insulin release. The mechanistic dependence on insulin release, of course, explains why these drugs are ineffective in Type 1 diabetes.

Other probable actions of the sulfonylureas include reduced serum glucagon level and increased binding of insulin to parenchymal tissue cells. These drugs have no direct effects on renal handling of glucose (b) or insulin synthesis (c). Unlike some other oral antidiabetic drugs, such as the glita-zones (thiazolidinediones), they do not increase parenchymal cell respon-siveness to insulin (d) or do so in any other ways that might be described as "insulin sensitizing." They do not decrease "insulin resistance" (a), which is a common problem for many patients with Type 2 diabetes mellitus, whether by lowering body weight or appetite or by other mechanisms.

396. The answer is b. (*Brunton, pp 1634–1637; Craig, p 772; Katzung, pp 704–707.*) Glyburide is a second-generation sulfonylurea oral hypo-glycemic. Of the main groups or chemical classes of oral antidiabetic agents, these are the ones typically associated with causing hypoglycemia, whether from overdose or as a rather expected response in some patients, particularly before meals. Sulfonylureas release insulin from the β cells of the pancreas (see Question 395 for more on this), even if blood glucose levels already are low. Normally carbohydrates from a meal trigger insulin release; when blood glucose levels are low, as after the 18-h fast this patient experienced, physiologic insulin release would be low too. However, even in a fast-induced hypoglycemic state a sulfonylurea will release insulin and drive blood glucose down even further, with a likely outcome being hypoglycemia.

The elderly are particularly susceptible to sulfonylurea-induced hypoglycemia. Part of this may relate to diet. However, expected age-related falls of renal and/or hepatic function can reduce elimination of these drugs, thereby increasing their serum levels and their effects unless dosages are reduced accordingly.

This propensity for preprandial hypoglycemia is shared by the meglitinides—repaglinide and nateglinide—because they, too, increase pancreatic insulin release.

The thiazolidinediones (glitazones) seldom cause symptomatic hypoglycemia because they do not release insulin. The same applies to metformin, the biguanide; and acarbose (with, along with miglitol, is an α-glucosidase inhibitor). Because of a longer half-life, compared with glipizide, a sulfonylurea is more likely to cause preprandial hypoglycemia. Glipizide is contraindicated in patients with liver disease because it is metabolized in the liver. Care should be taken in the elderly because of their propensity to develop hypoglycemia, which is perhaps due to decreased hepatic and renal function that is evident in this patient population.

397. The answer is a. (*Brunton, p 1640; Craig, pp 774–775; Katzung, p 710.*) Acarbose, classified as an α-glucosidase inhibitor, slows the rate and extent of carbohydrate absorption from the intestines. (The related drug, miglitol, does the same.) The consequence of this for the hypoglycemic patient is that attempts to restore blood glucose levels by consuming sugar or sucrose-containing foods or beverages (e.g., orange juice is a popular choice, as are products such as the one our patient took) will be less effective, if effective at all—and certainly slower in terms of symptom relief. None of the other oral diabetes drugs have this mechanism of action and so will not hinder attempts to restore euglycemia when sugar is consumed.

398. The answer is a. (*Brunton, p 1528; Craig, p 750; Katzung, p 633.*) The incidence of agranulocytosis due to propylthiouracil, or the related thio[n]amide, methimazole, is not rare. In addition, it may develop within the first few weeks of starting therapy, and so a "routine" blood test scheduled for several months or more after starting the drug may not catch it. However, if it is detected early (e.g., the patient promptly reports a sore throat or other flu-like symptoms) and the drug is stopped, it is usually spontaneously reversible. The most common side effect with the thioamides is urticaria. It may abate spontaneously or require symptomatic management with an antihistamine (either first or second generation) or with a corticosteroid.

None of the other responses listed are recognized as being associated with thioamides.

399. The answer is e. *(Brunton, pp 1639–1640; Craig, p 774; Katzung, pp 709–710.)* Pioglitazone, like all the glitazone oral antidiabetic drugs, works by increasing parenchymal cell responsiveness to insulin. The mechanism seems to involve activation of peroxisome proliferator-activated receptors. This apparently increases transcription of insulin—responsive genes that control glucose (and lipid) metabolism and cellular glucose uptake via glucose transporters. The net effects include not only lowered plasma levels of glucose, but also fatty acids and (indirectly) of insulin. Given the necessary involvement of insulin in the drug's effects, it will not work (alone) for patients with Type 1 diabetes. When used for patients who have Type 2 diabetes, and who nonetheless require insulin, a thiazolidinedione can be a valuable adjunct that helps lower daily insulin requirements.

400. The answer is b. *(Brunton, pp 1578f, 1581; Katzung, pp 680–681.)* Danazol is a testosterone derivative used to treat endometriosis, and some of the side effects and adverse responses are those you would expect from testosterone itself: liver dysfunction, virilism (acne, hirsutism, oily skin, reduced breast size), and reductions in HDL cholesterol levels. Other reported adverse reactions include amenorrhea, weight gain, sweating, vasomotor flushing, and edema.

Nonetheless, danazol appears to be just as effective as an estrogen-progesterone combination for managing endometriosis, and relatively few patients have stopped (or have had to stop) danazol treatment because of side effects or adverse reactions.

401. The answer is d. *(Craig, pp 773–774; Brunton, pp 1638–1639; Katzung, p 708.)* Metformin (a biguanide) poses the greatest risk, of all the antidiabetic drugs, of causing lactic acidosis. Although the overall risk of lactic acidosis from this drug is low, should it occur, mortality is quite common. Alcohol consumption or renal or hepatic disease increase the risk of lactic acidosis associated with metformin.

Acarbose, an α-glucosidase inhibitor (blocks starch uptake from the gut), the sulfonylureas (older ones such as tolbutamide or newer ones such as glipizide and glyburide), and rosiglitazone (and other glitazones, e.g., pioglitazone) are not associated with lactic acidosis (unless they are coadministered with metformin).

402. The answer is a. (*Brunton, pp 1654–1656, 1663–1665; Craig, p 760; Katzung, pp 717, 726, 728–729.*) Recall that vitamin D_3 is hydroxylated to 25-OH D_3 (calcifediol). Calcifediol is then hydroxylated in the kidney to the most active form of vitamin D, which is 1,25-dihydroxyvitamin D (calcitriol).

Given as a drug, calcitriol rapidly elevates serum Ca levels by enhancing the intestinal absorption of Ca. It is indicated in vitamin D deficiency, particularly in patients with chronic renal failure or renal tubular disease, hypoparathyroidism, osteomalacia, and rickets. Serum phosphate levels usually increase with prolonged treatment.

403. The answer is c. (*Brunton, pp 1521–1524; Craig, pp 749–750; Katzung, p 656.*) Cardiovascular and related hemodynamic changes, mostly arising from or related to tachycardia, increased ventricular contractility, and potentially leading to acute myocardial ischemia, are among the hallmarks of thyroid hormone excess, whether drug-induced or idiopathic (e.g., thyrotoxicosis of other causes). Increased thyroid hormone levels "up-regulate" the β-adrenergic receptors, leading to heightened and potentially lethal responses that involve overactivation of those receptors. β–Blockade provides important and prompt symptom relief, and may be lifesaving in situations such as this. Other interventions aimed at lowering thyroid hormone synthesis or release ultimately will be important, but saving the patient's life with administration of propranolol or a suitable alternative is the most important first step.

404. The answer is d. (*Brunton, pp 1563–1564; Craig, pp 704–707; Katzung, pp 673–675.*) There are two main mechanisms by which OCs exert their main effects. Arguably the most important is inhibition of ovulation.

This prevents (or reduces the risk of) fertilization, a process that must come before such others as impairing nidation which implicitly means the ovum has been fertilized. The other is thickening of cervical mucus. That effect, mainly caused by the progestin component, provides a physical (rather than metabolic or pH-dependent) barrier that slows or stops sperm motility. It is not a spermicidal effect, per se.

405. The answer is e. *(Brunton, pp 1660–1661, 1666; Craig, pp 459–460; Katzung, pp 717–718.)* Overmedication with vitamin D may lead to a toxic syndrome called hypervitaminosis D. The initial symptoms can include weakness, nausea, weight loss, anemia, and mild acidosis. As the excessive doses are continued, signs of nephrotoxicity can develop, such as polyuria, polydipsia, azotemia, and eventually nephrocalcinosis. In adults, osteoporosis can occur. Also, there is CNS impairment, which can result in mental retardation and convulsions.

406. The answer is c. *(Brunton, pp 1610–1611; Craig, pp 700–701; Katzung, pp 56, 687, 796–797, 926.)* Ketoconazole is typically remembered as an azole antifungal drug, and a common cause of drug interactions due to its powerful cytochrome P450 inhibitor effects. At doses higher than those used when the drug is prescribed as an antifungal, it inhibits corticosteroid synthesis and is one of the preeminent drugs for nonoperable Cushing's disease. Alternatives are metyrapone and aminoglutethimide, not listed here. Dexamethasone (a) is a synthetic corticosteroid with powerful glucocorticoid effects and little or no mineralocorticoid activity. Hydrocortisone (b) is cortisol; an efficacious glucocorticoid with useful (but slight) mineralocorticoid activity. The same applies to prednisone (d), predominately a glucocorticoid used as an oral anti-inflammatory drug for asthma, some arthritides, and other steroid-responsive conditions. Spironolactone (e) is an aldosterone receptor antagonist, used mainly for primary or secondary hyperaldosteronism, for heart failure, and for its potassium-sparing diuretic effects.

407. The answer is c. *(Brunton, pp 309t, 1500; Craig, pp 369, 769; Katzung, pp 275, 277, 452.)* Primary amenorrhea is associated with hyperprolactinemia. Women who are amenorrheic from hyperprolactinemia also often present with galactorrhea and infertility. Bromocriptine, a dopamine receptor agonist, inhibits prolactin release. The site of action is the pituitary, and it involves the same site and mechanism by which dopamine, released from the hypothalamus, normally suppresses prolactin release. Some causes of hyperprolactinemia, in both men and women, include pituitary cancer, hypothalamic dysfunction, and some drugs (e.g., antipsychotics, estrogens). Recall that bromocriptine, by virtue of its central dopaminergic activity, is sometimes used to help correct the dopamine-ACh imbalance that underlies Parkinson's disease.

408. The answer is e. *(Brunton, pp 1649–1658; Craig, pp 755–756; Katzung, pp 716–717.)* Parathyroid hormone's main role is to maintain normal serum Ca^{2+} levels. When serum Ca^{2+} concentrations become sufficiently low, parathyroid hormone synthesis and release increase, and it helps restore a normocalcemic state by promoting (in concert with vitamin D) Ca^{2+} absorption from the intestines, promotes renal tubular Ca^{2+} reabsorption and phosphate excretion, and increases mobilization of Ca^{2+} and phosphate from bone (i.e., bone resorption).

Anti-Infectives

Antibacterials
Antimycobacterials
Antifungals

Antivirals
Antiprotozoals

Questions

DIRECTIONS: Each item contains a question or incomplete statement that is followed by several responses. Select the **one best** response to each question.

409. A patient on antimicrobial therapy develops the following signs and symptoms that ultimately are found to be drug-induced: cough, dyspnea, and pulmonary infiltrates; neutropenia and bleeding tendencies; and paresthesias. Which of the following is the most likely cause of this patient's symptoms?

a. Amoxicillin
b. Azithromycin
c. Ciprofloxacin
d. Isoniazid
e. Nitrofurantoin

410. A patient with an opportunistic infection with *Pneumocystis carinii* is receiving a combination of sulfamethoxazole (SMZ) and trimethoprim (TMP). Which of the following statements describes best the mechanism by which this combination exerts its desired effects—and does so better than if just one of the drugs was administered?

a. The combination exerts significant antiviral activity, thereby reducing the risk of opportunistic *P. carinii* infections during antiviral therapy with other medications
b. The SMZ permeabilizes bacterial cell walls, allowing better penetration of the TMP
c. They inhibit sequential steps in bacterial synthesis of tetrahydrofolic acid
d. TMP inhibits production of resistance factors ("R-factors") directed against SMZ
e. TMP kills gut flora that otherwise would reduce oral bioavailability of the SMZ

411. Ticarcillin is relatively unique among all the penicillins because it poses a greater risk of a relatively unique side effect or adverse response. Which of the following best summarizes what that unique unwanted effect is?

a. Acute renal failure
b. Bronchoconstriction, bronchospasm, asthma
c. Fever, arthralgia, and other signs of a lupus-like syndrome
d. Hypertension, hypervolemia, and bleeding
e. Inducing penicillinase and causing resistance

412. A 39-year-old man with aortic insufficiency and a history of multiple antibiotic resistance is given a prophylactic intravenous dose of antibiotic before surgery to insert a prosthetic heart valve. As the antibiotic is being infused, the patient becomes flushed over most of his body. Which of the following antibiotics is most likely responsible?

a. Erythromycin
b. Gentamicin
c. Penicillin G
d. Tetracycline
e. Vancomycin

413. A patient develops antibiotic-associated pseudomembranous colitis (AAPMC) in response to drug therapy. Which of the following was the most likely cause of this severe problem?

a. Amoxicillin
b. Azithromycin
c. Clindamycin
d. Metronidazole
e. Trimethoprim plus sulfamethoxazole (TMP-SMZ)

414. A 35-year-old woman complains of itching in the vulval area. Hanging-drop examination of the urine reveals trichomonads. Which of the following is the preferred treatment for the trichomoniasis?

a. Doxycycline
b. Emetine
c. Metronidazole
d. Pentamidine
e. Pyrimethamine

415. A 75-year-old man has a fever of 104°F. He develops a cough that produces blood-tinged sputum with gram-positive cocci in clusters. A chest x-ray shows increased density in the right upper lobe. Which of the following penicillins is likely to fail to treat this infection adequately?

a. Cloxacillin
b. Dicloxacillin
c. Nafcillin
d. Oxacillin
e. Ticarcillin

416. A patient will be started on primaquine to treat active *Plasmodium vivax* malaria, specifically to target the hepatic forms of the parasite. Before you administer the drug you should screen the patient to assess their relative risk of developing a relatively common and severe adverse response to the drug. Which of the following best summarizes what that risk is?

a. Cardiac conduction disturbances
b. Hemolytic disease
c. Nephrotoxicity
d. Retinopathy
e. Seizures, convulsions

417. A 50-year-old man with Type 2 diabetes develops an otitis from which *Pseudomonas* organisms are cultured. Topical therapy with polymyxin B is effective. Which of the following best explains the drug's mechanism of action?

a. Disrupts membrane permeability
b. Forms reactive products that interfere with DNA replication
c. Inactivates bacterial protein sulfhydryl groups
d. Inhibits cell-wall synthesis
e. Inhibits protein synthesis by binding to tRNA

418. A 27-year-old woman has just returned from a trip to Southeast Asia. Over the past 24 h she has developed shaking, chills, and a temperature of 104°F. A blood smear reveals *Plasmodium vivax*. Which of the following agents should be used to eradicate the extraerythrocytic phase of the organism?

a. Chloroguanide
b. Chloroquine
c. Primaquine
d. Pyrimethamine
e. Quinacrine

419. A jaundiced 1-day-old premature infant with elevated free bilirubin is seen in the premature baby nursery. The mother had received an antibiotic combination for a urinary tract infection (UTI) 1 week before delivery. Which of the following is the most likely cause of the baby's kernicterus?

a. A fourth-generation cephalosporin
b. An aminopenicillin (e.g., amoxicillin)
c. Azithromycin
d. Erythromycin
e. A sulfonamide
f. A tetracycline

420. A sputum culture of a 65-year-old man with pneumonia is positive for β-lactamase-positive staphylococci. Which of the following is the best choice for penicillin therapy in this patient?

a. Ampicillin
b. Carbenicillin
c. Oxacillin
d. Penicillin G
e. Ticarcillin

421. A young boy presents with an infestation of *Taenia saginata* (tapeworm). Which of the following is the most appropriate drug to administer for treating this helminth problem?

a. Ceftriaxone
b. Chloroquine
c. Mebendazole
d. Niclosamide
e. Primaquine

422. A 40-year-old man is HIV-positive with a cluster-of-differentiation-4 (CD4) count of 200/mm^3. Within 2 months he develops a peripheral white blood cell count of 1000/mm^3 and hemoglobin of 9.0 mg/dL. Which of the following drugs most likely caused the hematologic abnormalities?

a. Acyclovir
b. Dideoxycytidine
c. Foscarnet
d. Rimantadine
e. Zidovudine

423. An 86-year-old man complains of cough and blood in his sputum for the past 2 days. On admission, his temperature is 103°F. Physical examination reveals rales in his right lung, and x-ray examination shows increased density in the right middle lobe. A sputum smear shows many gram-positive *cocci*, confirmed by sputum culture as penicillinase-producing *Staphylococcus aureus*. Which of the following antibiotics would be best to administer?

a. Ampicillin
b. Carbenicillin
c. Mezlocillin
d. Oxacillin
e. Ticarcillin

424. When considering all the main antibacterial drugs that work by inhibiting protein synthesis in one way or another, virtually every one exerts bacteriostatic actions. Which of the following drugs differs from all the rest because the usual consequence of therapeutic serum levels is bactericidal, rather than mere inhibition of bacterial growth and replication?

a. Aminoglycosides
b. Clindamycin
c. Erythromycins
d. Linezolid
e. Tetracyclines

425. A patient with AIDS is treated with a combination of agents, one of which is zidovudine. Which of the following enzymes or replicative processes is the main target of this antiviral drug?

a. Nonnucleoside reverse transcriptase
b. Nucleoside reverse transcriptase
c. RNA synthesis
d. Viral particle assembly
e. Viral proteases

426. A 39-year-old woman with a history of recurrent urinary tract infections develops a new infection. Culture of a urine sample indicated that the offending organism is *Escherichia coli*. She receives therapeutic doses of ciprofloxacin. Symptoms disappear as the offending bacteria are destroyed. Which of the following is the main bacterial process or enzyme that was inhibited by levofloxacin?

a. Cell-wall synthesis
b. Protein synthesis
c. Folic acid synthesis
d. Topoisomerase II (DNA gyrase)
e. DNA polymerase

427. Chloramphenicol is an effective antibiotic, but significant toxicity limits use of the drug, particularly in newborns and infants. Which of the following is the major and most common toxic reaction to this drug, and is the one that severely restricts its use, regardless of the patient's age?

a. Aplastic anemia
b. Hepatotoxicity
c. Interstitial nephritis
d. Pulmonary fibrosis
e. Torsades de pointes or ventricular fibrillation

428. A patient with AIDS, being treated with multiple antiviral and immunosuppressive drugs, develops an opportunistic infection caused by *P. carinii*. Which of the following drugs are we most likely to use to treat the pulmonary infection caused by this protozoan?

a. Carbenicillin
b. Metronidazole
c. Nifurtimox
d. Penicillin G
e. Pentamidine

429. A 25-year-old woman with an upper respiratory tract infection caused by *Haemophilus influenzae* is treated with trimethoprim-sulfamethoxazole. She responds well in a matter of days after starting this TMP-SMZ therapy. Which of the following bacterial processes is inhibited by this combination, and accounts for the antibacterial effects?

a. Cell-wall synthesis
b. Protein synthesis
c. Folic acid synthesis
d. Topoisomerase II (DNA gyrase)
e. DNA polymerase

430. A man who has been at the local tavern, drinking alcohol heavily, is assaulted. He is transported to the hospital. Among various findings is an infection for which prompt antibiotic therapy is indicated. Given his high blood alcohol level, which of the following antibiotics should be avoided because of a high potential of causing a serious disulfiram-like reaction that might provoke ventilatory or cardiovascular failure? (Assume that were it not for the alcohol consumption, the antibiotic prescribed would be suitable for the infectious organisms that have been detected.)

a. Amoxicillin
b. Cefoperazone or cefotetan
c. Erythromycin ethylsuccinate
d. Linezolid
e. Penicillin G

431. Members of the rifamycin antibiotic family (e.g., rifampin) are involved in a significant number of drug interactions. Which of the following summarizes best the pharmacodynamic or pharmacokinetic mechanism by which the rifamycins cause these problems?

a. Displace other drugs from their plasma protein-binding sites
b. Induce resistance to many other drugs by stimulating antibody formation
c. Induce the hepatic microsomal drug-metabolizing enzymes
d. Markedly increase glomerular filtration rates and excretion of the interactants
e. Reduce oral absorption and bioavailability of many drugs via a pH-dependent action in the stomach

432. A 43-year-old woman is recovering from major surgery, following discharge from the hospital, in an assisted-care facility. She develops fever, rales, dyspnea, cough, and purulent sputum. Results of a chest radiograph indicate bilateral pulmonary infiltrates. We send blood and sputum samples to the clinical pathology lab for culturing, but now must turn our attention to what we believe is community-acquired pneumonia caused by antibiotic-resistant pneumococci. We want to start empiric antibiotic therapy until culture results are available. Which of the following drugs would be best for this initial therapy?

a. Amoxicillin
b. Cefazolin
c. Erythromycin
d. Levofloxacin
e. Penicillin G
f. Vancomycin

433. Blood and sputum cultures taken in a critically ill 26-year-old woman indicate the presence of MRSA—methicillin-resistant *Staphylococcus aureus*. Which of the following drugs is most likely to be effective in treating this infection?

a. Amoxicillin plus clavulanic acid
b. Clindamycin
c. Erythromycin
d. Trimethoprim-sulfamethoxazole (TMP-SMZ)
e. Vancomycin

434. Compared with most other cephalosporins, the administration of cefmetazole, cefoperazone, or cefotetan is associated with a higher incidence of an adverse response that is particularly dangerous for some patients. Which of the following states best what that rather unique adverse response is?

a. Acute heart failure
b. Acute renal failure
c. Bleeding tendencies in patients taking warfarin
d. Hypertension
e. Ototoxicity
f. Severe allergic reactions in patients with mild penicillin allergies

435. A patient with an infectious disease routinely takes their antimicrobial medication with milk or other dairy products in an attempt to reduce stomach upset from the drug. The antibiotic fails to work adequately because calcium in the milk chelates the drug and reduces its oral bioavailability. Which of the following antimicrobial drugs or drug classes was the patient most likely taking?

a. Aminoglycoside
b. Antimycobacterial drug, specifically isoniazid
c. Cephalosporin, first generation
d. Cephalosporin, third generation
e. Penicillin
f. Tetracycline

436. A patient develops profuse, watery diarrhea, fever, abdominal pain, and leukocytosis in response to antibiotic drug therapy. *C. difficile* infection in the gut is confirmed. Which of the following drugs is the preferred agent for therapy of this antibiotic-associated pseudomembranous colitis?

a. Amoxicillin
b. Azithromycin
c. Clindamycin
d. Metronidazole
e. Trimethoprim plus sulfamethoxazole

437. Ampicillin and amoxicillin are in the same group of penicillins. However, there are important differences. Which of the following best states how amoxicillin differs from ampicillin?

a. Has better oral bioavailability, particularly when taken with meals
b. Is effective against penicillinase-producing organisms
c. Is a broad-spectrum penicillin
d. Does not cause hypersensitivity reactions
e. Has great antipseudomonal activity

438. A patient's history notes a documented severe (anaphylactoid) reaction to penicillin. What other antibiotic or class is likely to cross-react and so should be avoided in this patient?

a. Aminoglycosides
b. Azithromycin
c. Cephalosporins
d. Erythromycin
e. Linezolid
f. Tetracyclines

439. A 30-year-old woman develops a severe *P. aeruginosa* infection. The physician chooses to treat it with amikacin, not with gentamicin. Which of the following statements best describes how amikacin differs from gentamicin?

a. Does not require monitoring of blood levels during therapy
b. Exerts significant bactericidal effects against anaerobes too
c. Has broader spectrum against gram-negative bacilli
d. Lacks ototoxic potential
e. Protects against typical aminoglycoside nephrotoxicity

440. A 19-year-old being treated for leukemia develops a fever. You give several agents that will cover bacterial, viral, and fungal infections. Two days later, he develops acute renal failure. Which of the following drugs was most likely responsible?

a. Acyclovir
b. Amphotericin B
c. Ceftazidime
d. Penicillin G
e. Vancomycin

441. Penicillins, cephalosporins, and amphotericin B are quite different structurally, and the antimicrobial spectrum of amphotericin B is decidedly different from that of the other agents. Which of the following properties or actions is shared by all three of these drugs or drug groups?

a. Act, though various mechanisms, on cell walls or membranes of susceptible organisms
b. Contraindicated in immunocompromised patients
c. Interact with many drugs by inducing their hepatic metabolism
d. Leukopenia (increased white cell counts) is a common side effect
e. Nephrotoxicity precludes use in patients with impaired renal function

442. A patient with a *P. aeruginosa* infection is receiving intravenous gentamicin. The aminoglycoside blood levels are well above the minimum inhibitory concentration (MIC), but the clinical response is not satisfactory. A new medication order calls for adding a penicillin, administered in a separate IV line to avoid a physical incompatibility. If this order is carried out, which of the following is most likely to occur?

a. The aminoglycoside will inactivate the penicillin
b. The aminoglycoside will chemically neutralize and abolish the effects of the penicillin
c. The patient is likely to develop *Clostridium difficile* colitis (superinfection)
d. The penicillin will act synergistically with the aminoglycoside
e. The penicillin will increase the risk of aminoglycoside nephrotoxicity
f. The risk of inducing resistance to both drugs increases dramatically

443. Narrow spectrum penicillins, both penicillinase-sensitive and -resistant, have relatively poor activity against gram-negative bacteria. Which of the following is the main property or characteristic that explains why these microorganisms do not respond well to the penicillins?

a. Actively transport any absorbed penicillin back to the extracellular space
b. Have an outer membrane that serves as a physical barrier to the penicillins
c. Lack a surface enzyme necessary to metabolically activate the penicillins
d. Lack penicillin-binding proteins
e. Metabolically inactivate these penicillins by mechanisms not involving β-lactamase

444. A 30-year-old man with a 2-year history of chronic renal failure requiring dialysis consents to transplantation. A donor kidney becomes available. He is given cyclosporine to prevent transplant rejection. Which of the following is the most likely adverse effect of this drug?

a. Bone marrow depression
b. Nephrotoxicity
c. Oral and GI ulceration
d. Pancreatitis
e. Seizures

445. Amantadine, sometimes used in the management of parkinsonism, is also used prophylactically against influenza A infections. Which of the following statements best summarizes this drug's antiviral mechanism of action?

a. Causes lysis of infected host cells by release of intracellular lysosomal enzymes
b. Inhibits production of viral capsid protein
c. Prevents virion release
d. Prevents penetration of the virus into the host cell
e. Prevents uncoating of viral DNA

446. Streptomycin and other aminoglycosides cause their antimicrobial effects in susceptible organisms by inhibitng protein synthesis. Which of the following is the primary target of these drugs?

a. 30S ribosomal subunits
b. DNA
c. mRNA
d. Peptidoglycan units in the cell wall
e. RNA polymerase

447. We have a patient with an intraabdominal infection, and *Bacteroides fragilis* is the main organism found upon culture. Which of the following cephalosporins has the greatest activity against anaerobic bacteria such as *B. fragilis*?

a. Cefaclor
b. Cefoxitin
c. Cefuroxime
d. Cephalexin
e. Cephalothin

448. You are taking an initial health history from a 22-year-old woman who just moved to your town. She is remarkably fit and healthy, but is wearing two hearing aids for binaural (bilateral) high-frequency hearing loss. You inquire about the possible reason(s) for this. She says she lost most of her hearing after receiving an antibiotic for a severe infection when she was 19, but cannot recall the specific drug. Which of the following drugs was most likely responsible for her hearing loss?

a. Aminoglycoside (e.g., gentamicin)
b. Cephalosporin, first-generation
c. Cephalosporin, third-generation
d. Fluoroquinolone (e.g., ciprofloxacin)
e. Penicillin

449. A 26-year-old woman with acquired immunodeficiency syndrome (AIDS) develops cryptococcal meningitis. She refuses intravenous medication. Which of the following antifungal agents is the best choice for oral therapy of the meningitis?

a. Amphotericin B
b. Fluconazole
c. Ketoconazole
d. Metronidazole
e. Nystatin

450. An adult patient is being treated with a parenteral aminoglycoside for a serious *Pseudomonas aeruginosa* infection. He requires immediate surgery. He is premedicated with midazolam. A dose of succinylcholine is given for intubation, with skeletal muscle paralysis maintained during surgery with pancuronium. Balanced anesthesia is provided with nitrous oxide, isoflurane, and oxygen. Which of the following is the most likely outcome of having the aminoglycoside "on board" in the perioperative setting along with all these other drugs?

a. Acute hepatotoxicity from an aminoglycoside-isoflurane interaction
b. Antagonism of midazolam's amnestic and sedative effects
c. Enhanced aminoglycoside toxicity to host cells
d. Increased or prolonged response to neuromuscular blockers
e. Reduced risk of catecholamine-induced cardiac arrhythmias

451. A patient with tuberculosis is started on isoniazid (INH) as part of a multidrug regimen. The physician also starts therapy with vitamin B₆ at the same time. Which of the following is the main reason for giving the vitamin B₆ prophylactically?

a. Facilitates INH renal excretion, thereby protecting against nephrotoxicity
b. Inhibits metabolism of INH, thereby increasing INH blood levels
c. Is a cofactor required for activation of the INH to its antimycobacterial metabolite
d. Potentiates the antitubercular activity of the INH
e. Prevents some adverse effects of INH therapy

452. One antibiotic is considered very effective in treatment of *Rickettsia*, *Mycoplasma*, and *Chlamydia* infections. It is also used to mange some patients with acne vulgaris lesions. To which of the following drugs does this description apply?

a. Bacitracin
b. Gentamicin
c. Penicillin G
d. Tetracycline
e. Vancomycin

453. A 45-year-old man with recurrent asthma is being treated with oral theophylline and prednisone, supplemented with an adrenergic bronchodilator (e.g., albuterol), inhaled "as needed." He has been exposed to *Haemophilus influenzae* by a family member and is started on rifampin for prophylaxis against getting the infection himself. Which of the following is the most likely outcome of adding the rifampin?

a. Failure of rifampin prophylaxis due to induction of its metabolism by the theophylline
b. Increased risk of theophylline toxicity
c. Loss of asthma control, onset of asthma signs and symptoms
d. Rapid development of cholestatic jaundice and liver failure from acute rifampin toxicity
e. Sudden sodium and fluid retention, weight gain, from impaired prednisone metabolism

454. A 55-year-old man has an infection with *Legionella*. Assuming no contraindications, which of the following is the drug of choice?

a. Chloramphenicol
b. Erythromycin
c. Lincomycin
d. Penicillin G
e. Streptomycin

455. We are starting therapy for an established HIV infection in a 28-year-old man. The drugs are ritonavir, saquinavir, zidovudine, and didanosine. We are obviously using two protease inhibitors and two nucleoside reverse transcriptase inhibitors (NRTIs). Which of the following is the main purpose of using the ritonavir?

a. Help maintain adequate saquinavir levels by inhibiting its metabolism
b. Induce the metabolic activation of the NRTIs, which are prodrugs
c. Prevent the likely development of hypoglycemia
d. Reduce, or hopefully eliminate, saquinavir-mediated host toxicity
e. Serve as the main, most active, inhibitor of viral protease in this combination

456. As part of a multidrug attack on a patient's infection with *Mycobacterium* tuberculosis, a physician plans to use an aminoglycoside antibiotic. Which of the following is most active against the tubercle bacillus and seems to be associated with the fewest problems with resistance or typical aminoglycoside-induced adverse effects?

a. Amikacin
b. Kanamycin
c. Neomycin
d. Streptomycin
e. Tobramycin

457. Such agents as clavulanic acid, sulbactam, or tazobactam are often added to some proprietary (manufactured) penicillin combination products. Which of the following is the main reason for including them, or best describes their action?

a. Add antibiotic activity against *Pseudomonas* and many *Enterobacter* species
b. Facilitate antibiotic penetration into the central nervous system and cerebrospinal fluid
c. Inhibit cell wall transpeptidases
d. Inhibit inactivation of penicillin by β-lactamase-producing bacteria
e. Inhibit the normally significant hepatic metabolism of the penicillin
f. Reduce the risk and/or severity of allergic reactions in susceptible patients

458. A patient with active tuberculosis is being treated with isoniazid (INH) and ethambutol as part of the overall regimen. Which of the following is the main reason for including the ethambutol?

a. To facilitate entry of the INH into the mycobacteria
b. To facilitate penetration of the blood-brain barrier
c. To retard the development of organism resistance
d. To slow renal excretion of INH to help maintain effective blood levels
e. To retard absorption after intramuscular injection

459. A patient has a severe infection caused by anaerobic bacteria. The first-year house officer writes an order for gentamicin. This approach is doomed to fail because aminoglycosides have no activity against anaerobes. Which of the following best explains why anaerobes will be resistant?

a. Cannot metabolize the aminoglycosides, which are all prodrugs, to their bactericidal free radical forms
b. Cannot oxidatively metabolize aminoglycosides to moieties that are nontoxic to host cells
c. Lack molecular oxygen that is a prerequisite for drug binding to the 50S subunit of bacterial ribosomes
d. Lack the ability to transport aminoglycosides from the extracellular milieu in the absence of oxygen
e. Synthesize more and more active resistance factors than do aerobic bacteria

460. In patients with hepatic coma, or portal-systemic encephalopathy, decreasing the production and absorption of ammonia from the gastrointestinal (GI) tract will be beneficial. Which of the following is the antibiotic of choice in this situation and this purpose?

a. Cephalothin
b. Chloramphenicol
c. Neomycin
d. Penicillin G
e. Tetracycline

461. A child who previously was healthy develops bacterial meningitis. Assuming no specific contraindications, which of the following is the drug of choice?

a. Ceftriaxone
b. Erythromycin
c. Penicillin G
d. Penicillin V
e. Procaine penicillin

462. A patient is being treated with an antibiotic for a vancomycin-resistant enterococcal infection. They consume an over-the-counter medication containing ephedrine and develop a significant spike of blood pressure that leads to a pounding headache. They are transported to the hospital. As part of the workup, blood tests indicate some bone marrow suppression. Which of the following antibiotics is most likely associated with this clinical picture?

a. Azithromycin
b. Ciprofloxacin
c. Erythromycin estolate
d. Gentamicin
e. Linezolid

463. A 59-year-old woman is diagnosed with tuberculosis (TB). Before prescribing a multidrug regimen, you take a careful medication history because one of the drugs commonly used to treat TB induces some of the microsomal cytochrome P450 enzymes in the liver. Which is the most likely drug?

a. Ethambutol
b. Isoniazid
c. Pyrazinamide
d. Rifampin
e. Vitamin B$_6$

464. A patient requires an antibiotic that is most effective against *P. aeruginosa*. Which of the following is the quinolone of choice?

a. Ciprofloxacin
b. Enoxacin
c. Lomefloxacin
d. Norfloxacin
e. Ofloxacin

465. A patient has a severe bacterial infection that normally would respond to an oral penicillin or a cephalosporin. However, his chart documents anaphylactoid reactions to both drugs. Which of the following would be the best choice for treating the infection and poses the least risk of cross-reactivity and an allergic response?

a. Clotrimazole
b. Gentamicin
c. Metronidazole
d. Tetracycline
e. Vancomycin

Anti-Infectives

Answers

409. The answer is e. *(Brunton, pp 1123–1124; Craig, pp 64, 521; Katzung, p 829.)* Although several of the antimicrobial agents listed here can cause one (or perhaps two) of the adverse responses noted here, nitrofurantoin is the most likely cause. GI side effects (anorexia, nausea, vomiting) are the most common side effects caused by this drug, which is still widely used for managing acute lower urinary tract infections (e.g., from many strains of *E. coli, staphylococci, streptococci, Neisseria, Bacteroides*). However, the drug can also cause acute or subacute pulmonary reactions such as those described, various hematologic reactions (in particular, leukopenia and thrombocytopenia), and peripheral sensory and motor neuropathies.

Amoxicillin—and most other penicillins—may cause central neurotoxicity if present at extraordinarily high serum levels. Beyond that, allergic reactions are the most important adverse responses. Pulmonary, hematologic, and peripheral neuropathic adverse responses are not associated with these drugs.

Azithromycin's profile of adverse effects is quite similar to that of erythromycin and other macrolides, and that profile does not include the signs and symptoms noted here (GI upset, mild to severe, are the most common complaints, and azithromycin may be ototoxic, a property not shared by other macrolides).

Ciprofloxacin (or other fluoroquinolones) is not likely to cause any of the adverse responses noted. They are quite well tolerated and cause a variety of side effects that, in general, are mild. If one were to recall one "unique" toxicity, it would be alterations of collagen metabolism that may lead to tendon rupture.

Isoniazid can cause peripheral neuropathy (mainly from a drug-induced pyridoxine deficiency) and hepatotoxicity. Pulmonary and bleeding problems are not at all common in terms of drug-induced problems.

410. The answer is c. *(Brunton, pp 1104, 1111–1115; Craig, pp 518–519; Katzung, pp 775–776.)* SMZ and TMP act on sequential steps in the synthesis of tetrahydrofolic acid in susceptible bacteria. Sulfamethoxazole and sulfonamides in general inhibit incorporation of para-aminobenzoic acid (PABA) into folic acid. Trimethoprim then inhibits dihydrofolate reductase, the enzyme that (in the presence of NADPH) converts dihydrofolate into tetrahydrofolate. This leads to the bacteriostatic effect in susceptible organisms, and a clinical response that is better than with either drug used alone. Note that this mechanism accounts for the selectively toxic effect on microbes, as opposed to host cells, because (a) mammalian cell dihydrofolate reductases are largely insensitive to the effects of TMP and (b) host cell viability is not dependent on tetrahydrofolate synthesis (they use "preformed" folic acid, i.e., folate from the diet) and so they are unaffected by the sulfonamide.

Neither SMZ nor TMP, alone or in combination, exerts antiviral activity. Moreover, none of the other mechanisms listed apply.

411. The answer is d. (*Brunton, p 1143; Craig, pp 530–531; Katzung, pp 741–742.*) There are several main reasons for the greater propensity for cardiovascular and bleeding problems with ticarcillin. The drug is available as a disodium salt and we often need to administer large doses of the drug. The added sodium load can increase blood volume and blood pressure. In addition, ticarcillin seems to have antiplatelet activity. This, alone, can cause a slight increase in the risk of spontaneous or excessive bleeding, and it appears that the risks are much greater if the ticarcillin is given to a patient already taking antiplatelet drugs or drugs that impair coagulation or platelet function by other mechanisms.

Ticarcillin is no more nephrotoxic than other penicillins (low). It is not contraindicated for asthmatics, nor does it (or other penicillins) cause signs or symptoms of asthma other than those that would be expected with allergic responses to any penicillin. None of the penicillins induce penicillinase (β-lactamase).

412. The answer is e. (*Brunton, pp 632, 1196; Craig, pp 553–554; Katzung, p 749.*) This "red man" syndrome is characteristically associated with vancomycin. It is thought to be caused by histamine release. The risk or severity can be reduced dramatically by infusing the drug more slowly, and by pretreatment with antihistamines (H_1 receptor blockers, e.g., diphenhydramine).

413. The answer is c. (*Brunton, pp 1188–1190; Craig, p 549; Katzung, pp 760–761.*) More so than just about any other antibiotic, clindamycin is associated with the highest risk of AAPMC (*C. difficile* superinfection). Thus, it is mainly reserved for certain anaerobic infections located outside the CNS (susceptible anaerobes include *B. fragilis*, *Fusobacterium*, and *Clostridium perfringens*, plus anaerobic *streptococci*).

414. The answer is c. *(Brunton, pp 1050, 1058–1060; Craig, pp 607–608; Katzung, pp 877–878.)* Metronidazole penetrates all body fluids and tissues and fluids. Its spectrum of activity is limited largely to anaerobic bacteria—including *B. fragilis*—and certain protozoa. It is considered to be the drug of choice for trichomoniasis in females and carrier states in males, as well as for intestinal infections with *Giardia lamblia*.

415. The answer is e. *(Brunton, pp 1131t, 1133; Craig, pp 529–530.)* Ticarcillin, which is quite similar to carbenicillin in many clinically relevant ways, has a high degree of potency against Pseudomonas and Proteus organisms, but is inactivated by penicillinase produced by various bacteria, including most staphylococci. Oxacillin, cloxacillin, nafcillin, and dicloxacillin are all penicillinase-resistant and are effective against staphylococci.

416. The answer is b. *(Brunton, pp 101–102, 1040–1045; Craig, p 614; Katzung, pp 871–882.)* Hemolysis is the most common and serious adverse response to primaquine. The risk is clearly highest in patients who have red cell deficiencies in glucose-6-phosphate dehydrogenase, a heritable trait and one that can be screened for before giving the drug. (This G6PD deficiency is more common in blacks, and whites with darker skin [e.g., some from certain regions of the Middle East or the Mediterranean countries]) Regardless of the results of pretreatment screening, periodic blood counts should be done, and the urine checked for unusual darkening (indicating the presence of hemoglobin from lysed red cells), during treatment.

Note: If you answered "retinopathy," you were probably thinking about chloroquine, because that adverse response (accompanied by visual changes) is associated with that other commonly used antimalarial drug.

417. The answer is a. *(Brunton, pp 1193–1194; Craig, p 554; Katzung, pp 829, 1016.)* Polymyxins disrupt the structural integrity of the cytoplasmic membranes by acting as cationic detergents. On contact with the drug, the permeability of the membrane changes. Polymyxin is often applied in a mixture with bacitracin and/or neomycin for synergistic effects. Bacitracin, cycloserine, cephalothin, and vancomycin inhibit cell-wall synthesis.

418. The answer is c. (*Brunton, pp 1025t, 1040–1045; Craig, p 614; Katzung, pp 864–867.*) Primaquine is effective against the extraerythrocytic forms of *P. vivax* and *P. ovale*. It is used to eradicate plasmodia from the liver, and in doing so it not only provides a cure but also helps prevent relapse. Chloroquine would not be used because it is effective only in the erythrocytic phase of the malarial parasites' life span: it will not work against the exoerythrocytic forms of malaria parasites, nor can it serve as primary prevention. This 4-aminoquinoline derivative is a weak base that selectively concentrates in infected red blood cells. There it probably interferes with the ability of *plasmodia* to convert heme—a toxin to the parasite—to nontoxic metabolites.

419. The answer is e. (*Brunton, pp 1102, 1116; Craig, p 517; Katzung, p 775.*) Sulfonamides cross the placenta and enter the fetus in concentrations sufficient to produce toxic effects. They compete with and displace bilirubin from plasma protein binding sites, raising free bilirubin levels and causing the jaundice and other manifestations of kernicterus. For the same reason, sulfonamides should also not be given to neonates, especially premature infants. This woman should not have been given the sulfonamide, whether alone or in combination with trimethoprim.

420. The answer is c. (*Brunton, pp 1129t, 1333–1343; Craig, pp 528–531; Katzung, pp 736, 740–741.*) Oxacillin is classified as a penicillinase-resistant penicillin that is relatively acid-stable and, therefore, is useful for oral administration. Major adverse reactions include penicillin hypersensitivity and interstitial nephritis. With the exception of methicillin, which is no longer used, all penicillinase-resistant penicillins are highly bound to plasma proteins. Oxacillin has a very narrow spectrum and is used primarily as an antistaphylococcal agent.

421. The answer is d. (*Brunton, pp 1077, 1088; Craig, pp 622, 625; Katzung, p 892.*) Niclosamide exerts its effect against cestodes by inhibition of mitochondrial oxidative phosphorylation in the parasites. The mechanism of action is also related to its inhibition of glucose and oxygen uptake in the parasite.

422. The answer is e. (*Brunton, pp 1280, 1284–1285, 1440; Craig, pp 586–587; Katzung, pp 810–813.*) One of zidovudine's major adverse effects is bone marrow depression that appears to be dose- and length-of-treatment-dependent. The severity of the disease and a low CD4 count contribute to the bone marrow depression.

423. The answer is d. (*Brunton, pp 1129–1133; Craig, pp 529–530.*) Unlike the other listed drugs, oxacillin is resistant to penicillinase. The other four agents are broad-spectrum penicillins, whereas oxacillin is generally specific for gram-positive microorganisms. Use of penicillinase-resistant penicillins should be reserved for infections caused by penicillinase-producing *staphylococci*.

424. The answer is a. (*Brunton, pp 1156–1158, 1159t; Craig, pp 538–539; Katzung, pp 764–767.*) Of all the protein synthesis inhibitors, only the aminoglycosides routinely cause bacterial death, not just suppression of growth or replication.

425. The answer is b. (*Brunton, pp 1283–1284, 1290; Craig, pp 586–587; Katzung, pp 810–813.*) Zidovudine competitively inhibits HIV-1 nucleoside reverse transcriptase. It is also incorporated in the growing viral DNA chain to cause termination. Each action requires activation via phosphorylation of cellular enzymes. Zidovudine decreases the rate of clinical disease progression and prolongs survival in HIV-infected patients.

426. The answer is d. (*Brunton, pp 1119–1121; Craig, pp 519–521; Katzung, pp 777–780.*) Bacterial DNA gyrase is composed of four subunits. Ciprofloxacin (a quinolone) binds to the strand-cutting subunits and in doing so inhibits bacterial growth and replication. The quinolones, the original member of which was nalidixic acid, have a broad spectrum of antibiotic activity and are relatively free from common or serious side effects (some members associated with significant toxicities were withdrawn from the market), and tend not to be associated with rapidly developing antibiotic tolerance to their actions.

427. The answer is a. (*Brunton, pp 1179–1182; Craig, pp 59, 546–547; Katzung, p 755.*) Hematologic toxicity is by far the most important adverse effect of chloramphenicol. The toxicity consists of two types: (1) bone marrow depression (common) and (2) aplastic anemia (rare). Chloramphenicol can produce a potentially fatal toxic reaction, the "gray baby" syndrome, caused by diminished ability of neonates to conjugate chloramphenicol, leading to high serum concentrations of the drug.

428. The answer is e. *(Brunton, pp 1064–1066; Craig, p 609; Katzung, pp 879–881.)* Both trimethoprim-sulfamethoxazole (not listed) and pentamidine are effective in pneumonia caused by *P. carinii.* This protozoal disease usually occurs in immunodeficient patients, such as those with AIDS. Nifurtimox is effective in trypanosomiasis and metronidazole in amebiasis and leishmaniasis, as well as in anaerobic bacterial infections. Penicillins are not considered drugs of choice for this particular disease.

429. The answer is c. *(Brunton, pp 1104, 1111–1115; Craig, pp 517–518; Katzung, pp 775–777.)* Trimethoprim inhibits dihydrofolic acid reductase. Sulfamethoxazole inhibits *p*-aminobenzoic acid (PABA) from being incorporated into folic acid by competitive inhibition of dihydropteroate synthase. Either action inhibits the synthesis of tetrahydrofolic acid, but by giving the combination we inhibit two essential and *sequential* steps in the formation of folate-dependent metabolites that are necessary for bacterial viability and replication. (See the answer to Question 410 for more information.)

430. The answer is b. *(Brunton, pp 1145t, 1149; Craig, p 533; Katzung, pp 375, 1112.)* Cefoperazone (third-generation cephalosporin) or cefotetan (second-generation) inhibit aldehyde dehydrogenase and cause accumulation of acetaldehyde (as does disulfiram), and so can cause all the typical and potentially serious consequences of a disulfiram-like reaction. Cefmetazole, a second-generation cephalosporin, also causes a similar adverse interaction with alcohol. (Note that these three cephalosporins are also the ones that are associated with vitamin K–related bleeding problems, as addressed in Question 434.)

Erythromycin (whether administered as the base or one of the common salts, e.g., ethylsuccinate, estolate, or stearate) can inhibit the hepatic P450 system sufficient to cause adverse interactions with (excessive effects of) such drugs as warfarin, carbamazepine, and theophylline. However, based on current evidence there is no specific inhibition of aldehyde dehydrogenase, nor resulting accumulation of acetaldehyde, that would correctly qualify as a disulfiram-like interaction.

Amoxicillin, penicillin G, and other penicillins do not participate in disulfiram-like reactions.

Linezolid inhibits monoamine oxidase (MAO), albeit weakly, and so can trigger potentially significant adverse interactions in persons receiving such sympathomimetics as cocaine, ephedrine, or pseudoephedrine. However, the drug does not inhibit alcohol metabolism or cause the adverse responses noted in this question.

431. The answer is c. *(Brunton, pp 121, 1209; Craig, pp 37, 559; Katzung, pp 551, 785, 1123.)* Rifampin and other rifamycins are noteworthy for their ability to induce the hepatic P450 enzyme system, increasing the metabolism of other drugs. The main cytochromes that are affected are CYP3A4, 1A2, 2C9, and 2C19. Because most of the documented interactants with rifampin are inactivated by metabolism, the consequence of that interaction is a reduced response to the interactant. None of the other answers given are correct, because rifampin does not possess those properties.

432. The answer is d. *(Brunton et al., pp 1119–1121, 1146; Craig, pp 562–563; Katzung, pp 777–779.)* Levofloxacin or another quinolone would be a good choice, not only because of their antibiotic spectrum of activity, but also because our working hypothesis is that we're dealing with a community-acquired respiratory infection caused by resistant bacteria. The resistance is likely to render penicillins (a, e), cephalosporins (b), and even erythromycin or other macrolides (c) ineffective. Resistance to fluoroquinolones has not become that much of a problem yet. Note that cefazolin (b), a first generation cephalosporin, is ineffective against pneumococci, and is mainly suitable only for infections with *S. aureus* or streptococci that are not resistant to penicillins. Vancomycin (f) might ultimately be needed, but since it must be given parenterally (and we never mentioned that the patient was unable to take oral medications) it would be premature to use this otherwise "last resort" antibiotic.

433. The answer is e. *(Brunton, pp 1096, 1098, 1131–1132, 1146–1147, 1194–1196; Craig, pp 529–530, 553–554; Katzung, pp 768–770.)* The only suitable drug listed for this potentially fatal infection is vancomycin. The finding of MRSA is not uncommon, particularly in hospitals, rendering therapy with penicillins (including amoxicillin with clavulanate, the β-lactamase inhibitor; a) ineffective. Macrolides (including clindamycin, b; and erythromycin, c) are also unsuitable, in part because of a growing resistance problem. Resistance to the trimethoprim-sulfamethoxazole (d) combination is also a major problem, regardless of the infections for which this folate reductase inhibitor therapy is prescribed.

434. The answer is c. (*Brunton, pp 1145, 1149; Craig, p 533.*) Cefmetazole and cefotetan, both second-generation cephalosporins, and cefoperazone (third generation) can interfere with hepatic vitamin K metabolism, leading to what amounts to a deficiency of vitamin K–dependent clotting factor activity. Because this is the general mechanism by which warfarin exerts its anticoagulant effects, combined use of one of these cephalosporins can cause further (and potentially dangerous) prolongations of the International Normalized Ratio (or prothrombin time); the clinical consequence can be spontaneous, prolonged, or excessive bleeding. One should also be cautious when these cephalosporins are given to patients taking aspirin or other antiplatelet drugs (e.g., clopidogrel) or thrombolytics.

Although most cephalosporins are excreted unchanged by the kidneys, renal failure (especially severe and acute) seldom occurs with these or other cephalosporins. There is no link between administration of even high doses of these cephalosporins (or others) with the development of acute heart failure. Hypertension or other substantial changes of blood pressure are not associated with cephalosporins, nor are these drugs ototoxic.

Although a history of severe allergic reactions to penicillins requires caution when considering a cephalosporin (indeed, cephalosporins should be avoided, if possible, in such patients), there is nothing unique about cefmetazole, cefoperazone, or cefotetan in this context. None of the cephalosporins are contraindicated for patients with mild allergic reactions due to penicillins.

435. The answer is f. (*Brunton, pp 121, 1175–1176; Craig, p 545; Katzung, p 756.*) Tetracyclines interact with many polyvalent metal cations such that their absorption from the gut (i.e., bioavailability) is reduced. The extent of this reduction can be clinically significant, that is, leading to inadequate blood levels and effects of the antibiotic.

Calcium is, of course, abundant in dairy products, some OTC antacid products, and in supplements touted for "bone health." Other metals that can interact with tetracyclines by this mechanism include iron, magnesium, aluminum, and zinc. Note that one or several of these interactants are typically found in antacid products, multivitamin/mineral supplements, and even (the trend is growing) in some (mineral-) fortified foods, such as cereals, and citrus juices.

Although foods (in general) may interfere with the oral absorption of several other antibiotics, the cation-antibiotic interaction is specific for and important to the tetracyclines. You might want to remember that aminoglycosides are not effective when given orally.

436. The answer is d. *(Brunton, pp 1058–1060; Craig, p 608; Katzung, pp 828, 877–878.)* Among the indications for metronidazole is management of *C. difficile* (and other *clostridia*) infections, including AAPMC. Many other obligate anaerobes will respond, as will various types of intestinal or systemic amebiasis infections (the drug is generally used adjunctively with iodoquinol for gut infections—symptomatic amebiasis—and for giardiasis and *Trichomonas vaginalis* infections [generally the drug of choice]).

An alternative (or adjunct) to metronidazole in the setting of AAPMC would be vancomycin.

None of the other drugs listed would be suitable. As noted in the previous question, clindamycin would be wholly inappropriate as it is the most likely cause of the AAPMC to begin with.

437. The answer is a. *(Brunton, pp 1139–1140; Craig, pp 528–531; Katzung, p 756.)* Amoxicillin and ampicillins are aminopenicillins. Amoxicillin absorption is affected less by the presence of food, so the bioavailability is better. Amoxicillin is inactivated by β-lactamases and has a narrow spectrum of activity toward certain gram-positive and gram-negative organisms, but not *Pseudomonas*. Because it is a penicillin, hypersensitivity reactions are possible.

438. The answer is c. *(Brunton, pp 1143–1150; Craig, pp 530–531, 533; Katzung, p 747.)* Unless there are no reasonable alternatives, cephalosporins should be avoided for patients with prior severe responses to penicillins because of their cross-reactivity. None of the other drugs or drug groups listed here cross-react in penicillin-sensitive patients. "Mild" allergic reactions to penicillins do not necessarily contraindicate cephalosporin use.

439. The answer is c. *(Brunton, pp 1155–1159, 1166–1167; Craig, pp 539–541; Katzung, p 770.)* Amikacin stands out among all the aminoglycosides in two main ways: it has the broadest spectrum against gram-negative bacilli, and it is least susceptible to bacterial enzymes that inactivate aminoglycosides and lead to resistance. (Recall that among gram-negative bacteria, genetic information that codes for the production of these inactivating enzymes is transferred via R factors.)

440. The answer is b. *(Brunton, pp 1228–1229; Craig, pp 597–598; Katzung, pp 792–794.)* Amphotericin B, given intravenously, often alters kidney function. The most common and most easily detected manifestation of this is decreased creatinine clearance. If this occurs, the dose must be reduced. Amphotericin B also commonly increases potassium (K^+) loss, leading to hypokalemia; and can cause anemia and neurologic symptoms. A liposomal preparation of amphotericin B may reduce the incidence of renal and neurologic toxicity. Vancomycin may cause renal damage, but the overall incidence is lower, the severity less.

441. The answer is a. *(Brunton, pp 1128–1132, 1225–1229; Craig, pp 527, 531, 596–597; Katzung, pp 734, 742, 793.)* Penicillins, cephalosporins, and amphotericin B exert their desired clinical effects by altering the structure or function of cell walls of susceptible organisms. Penicillins interfere with bacterial cell wall synthesis: their β-lactam structures bind to and inhibit enzymatic function of transpeptidases that normally provide susceptible bacteria with cell walls that are capable of maintaining an osmotically stable intracellular milieu. Cephalosporins, by virtue of their β-lactam ring, work in essentially the same way. Amphotericin B (a polyene antifungal drug) binds to ergosterol in the fungal cell membrane; the ultimate outcome is increased cell permeability. Nonetheless, the ultimate effect is osmotic instability of the organism, leading to cell death.

Neither penicillins, cephalosporins, or amphotericin B are contraindicated in patients with immunodeficiencies. Indeed, they may play a key role in managing opportunistic infections in such patients.

They do not induce the metabolism of other drugs, or interact in most of the typical pharmacokinetic ways. They do not trigger leukopenia.

Amphotericin B can cause decreased platelet counts and leukopenia, but this is rare. The most common hematologic adverse response to this drug is a normochromic, normocytic anemia. Penicillins and cephalosporins do not share these properties.

Finally, you should know that amphotericin B is clearly nephrotoxic. When given intravenously, renal dysfunction is the most serious and most common long-term manifestation of this antifungal drug's toxic spectrum. Penicillins and cephalosporins are not nephrotoxic.

(You might also want to recall that the new lipid formulations of amphotericin B—amphotericin B colloidal dispersion, liposomal amphotericin B, and a lipid complex of the drug—apparently cause much less nephrotoxicity than conventional amphotericin B formulations. That is probably because these newer formulations alter distribution of the antifungal drug such that renal concentrations, and so the nephrotoxic potential, are lower.)

442. The answer is d. (*Brunton, pp 1104, 1155–1159; Craig, p 540; Katzung, p 768.*) The rationale behind this combination is that penicillins essentially weaken the cell walls of susceptible bacteria, which in turn facilitates access of the aminoglycoside to its site of action, the bacterial ribosomes. This usually provides better antibiotic response than with either antibiotic used alone, and with the aminoglycoside, serum levels aren't necessarily so high that they are more likely to cause ototoxicity, nephrotoxicity, or other adverse responses.

You should also recall at least two other things: (1) the penicillin in this combination is usually an extended-spectrum penicillin, such as ticarcillin, and (2) as we have specifically noted in the question, the administration of these drugs is by separate IV lines. That is because if the two drugs were mixed together in sufficiently high concentrations, the penicillin may chemically inactivate the gentamicin.

443. The answer is b. (*Brunton, pp 1134–1138; Craig, pp 527–530; Katzung, pp 734–736.*) Both susceptible and resistant gram-negative and gram-positive bacteria have penicillin-binding proteins (PBPs). Resistance to the narrow spectrum penicillins by gram-negative bacteria arises from the presence of an outer membrane with pores that are too small to allow adequate penetration of the drug and access to the PBPs. Thus, we are dealing with what amounts to a physical barrier to the drug.

Most penicillins (with few exceptions, such as bacampicillin) are active in the form in which they are administered (i.e., they are not prodrugs), and so no subsequent metabolic activation is required.

444. The answer is b. (*Brunton, p 1695; Craig, p 659; Katzung, pp 589, 941.*) Nephrotoxicity may occur in almost three-quarters of patients treated with cyclosporine. Regular monitoring of blood levels can reduce the incidence of adverse effects.

445. The answer is e. (*Brunton, pp 1256–1258; Craig, p 575; Katzung, p 824.*) Amantadine's mechanism of action involves inhibition of uncoating of the influenza A viral DNA. The primary target is the membrane M2 protein. The drug does not affect penetration and DNA-dependent RNA polymerase activity. Amantadine both reduces the frequency of illness and diminishes the serologic response to influenza infection. The drug has no action, however, on influenza B. As a weak base, amantadine buffers the pH of endosomes, thus blocking the fusion of the viral envelope with the membrane of the endosome. (Amantadine is, indeed, a useful drug for some patients with parkinsonism. How it works is unclear, but reasonable hypotheses include facilitation of dopamine release, blockade of neuronal dopamine reuptake, and/or central antimuscarinic actions.)

446. The answer is a. (*Brunton, pp 1156–1159, 1164–1165; Craig, pp 538–539; Katzung, p 764.*) The bactericidal activity of streptomycin and other aminoglycosides involves a direct action on the 30S ribosomal subunit, the site at which these agents both inhibit protein synthesis and diminish the accuracy of translation of the genetic code. Proteins containing improper sequences of amino acids (known as nonsense proteins) are often nonfunctional.

447. The answer is b. (*Brunton, pp 1143–1150; Craig, pp 531–533; Katzung, p 745.*) Cefoxitin or cefmetazole (not listed) are suitable for treating intraabdominal infections caused by many aerobic and anaerobic gram-negative bacteria, including and especially *B. fragilis.* Cefoxitin alone has been shown to be as effective as the traditional therapy of clindamycin plus gentamicin. The other cephalosporins have much lower antibiotic activity against these organisms, and so generally are not appropriate.

448. The answer is a. (*Brunton, pp 1160–1163; Craig, pp 541–542; Katzung, pp 767–768.*) Aminoglycosides (gentamicin, tobramycin, others) are classic examples of ototoxic drugs, and they can affect both branches of the eighth cranial nerve.

The risks of aminoglycoside-induced ototoxicity (and nephrotoxicity) are among the reasons why it is important to keep an eye on peak and trough drug levels during therapy, adjust dosages accordingly, and avoid concomitant use of other ototoxic drugs. That is because the hearing loss is blood level–dependent (as opposed to being an idiosyncratic or allergic reaction). Aminoglycoside-induced ototoxicity is usually irreversible. The risk and severity of hearing loss from aminoglycosides are increased if they are administered with other ototoxic drugs.

Recall that there are two main forms of drug-induced ototoxicity. Cochlear toxicity includes hearing loss, tinnitus ("ringing in the ears"), or occasionally both. Hearing loss may also occur with loop diuretics (particularly ethacrynic acid), cis-platinum, and the vinca alkaloids (anticancer drugs). These drugs are intrinsically ototoxic; use one or more of them together or with an aminoglycoside and the risk of ototoxicity increases greatly.

Tinnitus (usually reversible) is typically associated with such drugs as aspirin (and, possibly, some other NSAIDs) and quinidine.

The other main form of ototoxicity is vestibular toxicity, which is typically manifest as balance and gait problems, vertigo, and nausea resulting from vestibular apparatus dysfunction.

Nephrotoxicity may develop during or after the use of an aminoglycoside. It is generally more common in the elderly when there is preexisting renal dysfunction. In most patients, renal function gradually improves after discontinuation of therapy. Aminoglycosides rarely cause neuromuscular blockade that can lead to progressive flaccid paralysis and potential fatal respiratory arrest. Hypersensitivity and dermatologic reactions occasionally occur following use of aminoglycosides.

None of the other antibiotics listed are linked to ototoxicity, whether from excessive blood levels or due to a hypersensitivity or true allergic reaction. Azithromycin (not an answer choice) is, however, another antibiotic for which there is growing evidence of a link to sudden onset hearing loss. The mechanism is unknown, and the incidence is neither dose-dependent nor predictable.

449. The answer is b. (*Brunton, pp 1233–1234; Craig, pp 598–599; Katzung, p 797.*) Fluconazole penetrates into cerebrospinal fluid, where it exerts good antifungal activity against *Cryptococcus neoformans*. When it is given orally, blood levels are almost as high as when it is given parenterally. Amphotericin is administered intravenously and even when given intrathecally does not appear to be highly effective in fungal meningitis.

450. The answer is d. (*Brunton, pp 227, 1164; Craig, pp 541–542; Katzung, pp 440, 767–768.*) Aminoglycosides, at sufficiently high serum levels, can cause skeletal neuromuscular blockade in their own right. This probably arises from a combination of effects: inhibition of neuronal ACh release and perhaps direct blockade of nicotinic receptors on skeletal muscle. This would add to and prolong the effects of both neuromuscular blockers the patient has received. In addition, isoflurane and other halogenated hydrocarbon volatile liquid anesthetics have some neuromuscular blocking effects in their own right—but not to a degree that is sufficient to obviate the need for succinylcholine and/or nondepolarizing blockers when skeletal muscle paralysis is indicated. So here we have a combination of drugs that affect skeletal muscle activation.

The greatest concern, of course, would be the prolongation of neuromuscular blockade. A "greater degree" of paralysis is largely inconsequential, so long as ventilation is supported. It is the prolonged blockade—and especially the return of skeletal muscle weakening and ventilatory insufficiency after mechanical ventilation has been discontinued and additional doses of aminoglycoside are given—which poses the greatest risk if the patient had already been taken off ventilatory support.

(Note, too, in your studies, that some other antimicrobials seem to have some skeletal neuromuscular blocking activity, including polymyxin B and clindamycin.)

You should recall that although such agents as isoflurane and other halogenated hydrocarbon volatile liquid anesthetics may potentiate the effects of a neuromuscular blocker, once they are eliminated (that occurs rather rapidly when inhalation is stopped) there is no added risk of prolonged or greater skeletal muscle weakness or paralysis.

We should add that in settings (e.g., hospitals) where the overall incidence of aminoglycoside resistance is low (or in the absence of documented resistance to a particular aminoglycoside in a particular patient), tobramycin or gentamicin is usually the aminoglycoside of choice. Amikacin should be reserved for situations where there is proven resistance to the alternatives.

As with other aminoglycosides, periodic monitoring of peak and trough serum levels is essential to help insure optimal antibiotic effects while reducing the risk of ototoxicity and nephrotoxicity—both of which can be caused by any aminoglycoside (although with varying relative risks). No aminoglycoside has "nephroprotective" effects.

Finally, no aminoglycoside can kill anaerobes.

451. The answer is e. (*Brunton, pp 1102, 1206–1207, 1451; Craig, pp 558–559; Katzung, pp 782–784.*) Isoniazid (INH) inhibits cell-wall synthesis in mycobacteria. Increasing vitamin B_6 levels prevents some common and potentially significant complications associated with this inhibition, including peripheral neuritis, insomnia, restlessness, muscle twitching, urinary retention, convulsions, and psychosis, without affecting the antimycobacterial activity of INH.

452. The answer is d. (*Brunton, pp 1173–1174, 1178, 1690; Craig, pp 545–546; Katzung, pp 755–758.*) Tetracycline is one of the drugs of choice in the treatment of *Rickettsia, Mycoplasma,* and *Chlamydia* infections. The antibiotics that act by inhibiting cell-wall synthesis have no effect on *Mycoplasma* because the organism does not possess a cell wall; penicillin G (c), vancomycin (e), and bacitracin (a) will be ineffective. Gentamicin (b) also has little or no antimicrobial activity against these organisms.

453. The answer is c. (*Brunton, pp 121, 1209; Craig, pp 37, 559; Katzung, p 1123.*) Rifampin is an excellent example of a drug that induces the hepatic metabolism of many other drugs, thereby lowering blood levels (and effects) of its interactants. Theophylline and corticosteroids are among them. Thus, as a result of the interaction we would expect decreases—not increases—in the effects of theophylline and/or of the prednisone. Both are susceptible to the metabolizing-inducing effects of rifampin.

With the expected decline in blood levels of both the oral bronchodilator (theophylline) and the anti-inflammatory drug (prednisone), it is likely that control of the patient's asthma will be lost and symptoms will appear.

Absorbed rifampin is rapidly eliminated in the bile and undergoes enterohepatic recirculation. However, there is no reason to suspect that either the theophylline, the corticosteroid, or their combination would have effects on rifamycin elimination. Likewise, these drugs do not increase the risk of rifampin-induced hepatotoxicity, which is quite rare unless the patient is taking other hepatotoxic drugs or has preexisting liver disease.

454. The answer is b. (*Brunton, pp 1182–1183, 1185–1186; Craig, p 548; Katzung, pp 758–760.*) Erythromycin, a macrolide antibiotic, was initially designed to be used in penicillin-sensitive patients with streptococcal or pneumococcal infections. Erythromycin has become the drug of choice for the treatment of pneumonia caused by *Mycoplasma* and *Legionella*.

455. The answer is a. (*Brunton, pp 1297, 1301–1302; Craig, pp 590–592; Katzung, pp 816–819.*) Ritonavir is a powerful inhibitor of the liver's P450 system. Ritonavir is used in combination with saquinavir solely to inhibit saquinavir's metabolism, thereby keeping serum concentrations in a therapeutic range longer. Ritonavir does have protease inhibitory activation, but in this combination it is the saquinavir that is causing the main therapeutic effect. The protease inhibitors do not cause hypoglycemia, nor does ritonavir reduce the ability of saquinavir to alter serum glucose levels. In fact, whether used alone or in combination, the protease inhibitors typically cause hyperglycemia (and may cause clinical diabetes mellitus), and quite often raise serum cholesterol and triglycerides levels too.

The NRTIs (zidovudine, didanosine) are, indeed, prodrugs that must be metabolically activated to the triphosphate form in order to serve as a substrate for reverse transcriptase. However, the protease inhibitors do not facilitate that metabolism.

456. The answer is d. (*Brunton, pp 1158–1159, 1164–1165, 1211; Craig, pp 541, 560; Katzung, p 786.*) Streptomycin is bactericidal for the tubercle bacillus organism. Other aminoglycosides (e.g., gentamicin, tobramycin, neomycin, amikacin, and kanamycin) have activity against this organism but are seldom used clinically because of toxicity or development of resistance.

457. The answer is d. (*Brunton, pp 1132–1133, 1151–1152; Craig, p 530; Katzung, pp 747–788.*) These agents are inhibitors of penicillinase (β-lactamase) and are used in conjunction with β-lactamase-sensitive penicillins to potentiate their activity. These drugs are found in several brand-name fixed-dose penicillin combination products (amoxicillin and clavulanic acid; sulbactam with ampicillin; tazobactam with piperacillin). Clavulanic acid is an irreversible inhibitor. These agents do not, per se, add activity against *Pseudomonas* or *Enterobacter* (an activity already possessed by piperacillin but not by ampicillin or amoxicillin). Likewise, they have no intrinsic effect to facilitate entry into the CNS or CSF. They do not inhibit hepatic metabolism of the penicillins, and you should recall that renal excretion (not metabolism) is the main pathway for penicillin elimination. Importantly, the penicillinase inhibitors have absolutely no impact on the risks or severities of allergic reactions to penicillins.

458. The answer is c. (*Brunton, pp 1203–1204, 1210, 1214–1215; Craig, p 560; Katzung, pp 785–786.*) An important problem in the chemotherapy of TB is bacterial drug resistance. For this reason, concurrent administration of two or more drugs should be employed to delay the development of resistance. Ethambutol is often given along with INH for this purpose. Streptomycin or rifampin may also be added to the regimen to delay even further the development of drug resistance.

459. The answer is d. *(Brunton, pp 1097, 1155–1158; Craig, pp 539–540; Katzung, pp 764–767.)* Aminoglycosides, which are mainly used for parenteral therapy of severe infections from aerobic gram-negative bacilli (e.g., *E. coli, Serratia, Klebsiella*), require oxygen in order for the drug to be transported across the bacterial cell membrane. Such incorporation is necessary for these drugs to exert their bactericidal effects, which arise from binding to the 30S subunit of susceptible bacteria. Ultimately the aminoglycoside-ribosomal binding leads to premature termination of bacterial protein synthesis and the formation of abnormal bacterial proteins. Such abnormal proteins ultimately insert into the bacterial cell membrane, causing leakiness and cell death.

The aminoglycosides are not prodrugs, and so metabolism (whether aerobic or otherwise) is not necessary for activity; formation of an oxygen free radical or an aminoglycoside free radical has nothing to do with their antibiotic effects. Moreover, metabolism by host cells is not an important process in the elimination of aminoglycosides, nor of reducing host cell toxicity (e.g., to the kidneys or auditory nerve). Renal excretion is the main route of elimination for these drugs, which explains why renal function is such an important consideration in dosing adjustments.

Clearly, both aerobic and anaerobic bacteria can elaborate resistance factors (or develop resistance in other ways) to a variety of antibiotic classes. From a clinical viewpoint, the presence or absence of molecular oxygen is not a crucial or even relevant issue in this matter, however.

460. The answer is c. *(Brunton, pp 1167–1168; Craig, pp 539, 540; Katzung, p 770.)* Neomycin, an aminoglycoside, is not significantly absorbed from the GI tract. After oral administration, the intestinal flora is suppressed or modified and the drug is excreted in the feces. This effect of neomycin is used in hepatic coma to decrease the coliform flora, thus decreasing the production of ammonia and reducing levels of free nitrogen in the bloodstream. Other antimicrobial agents (e.g., tetracycline, penicillin G, chloramphenicol, and cephalothin) do not have the potency of neomycin in causing this effect.

461. The answer is a. *(Brunton, p 1150; Craig, pp 531–533; Katzung, pp 745–746.)* Penicillins were used in the treatment of meningitis because of their ability to pass across an inflamed blood-brain barrier. The third-generation cephalosporin, ceftriaxone, is preferred because it is effective against β-lactamase producing strains of *H. influenzae* that may cause meningitis in children.

462. The answer is e. *(Brunton, pp 1992–1993; Katzung, p 762.)* There are several pieces of information you should link together to help arrive at the answer, for which a relatively new drug is the correct answer. (1) Although linezolid has several uses, it is best reserved for vancomycin-resistant enterococci (VRE) and methicillin-resistant *S. aureus* (MRSA) infections. (It's seldom a first-line antibiotic because of the risk of resistance.) (2) Linezolid is occasionally linked to bone marrow suppression that is usually reversible upon discontinuation of the drug. (Granted, such other antibiotics as chloramphenicol pose greater risks of bone marrow suppression, but this property is nonetheless associated with linezolid.) (3) The third piece of evidence is the rise of blood pressure in response to ephedrine, a mixed-acting sympathomimetic (adrenomimetic) that works, in part, by releasing neuronal norepinephrine. Linezolid has monoamine oxidase inhibitory activity (albeit relatively weak compared with traditional MAO inhibitors). Piece these three lines of evidence together and the only reasonable choice is linezolid.

463. The answer is d. *(Brunton, pp 121, 1209; Craig, pp 37, 559; Katzung, p 1123.)* Rifampin induces cytochrome P450 enzymes, which causes a significant increase in elimination of drugs, such as oral contraceptives, anticoagulants, ketoconazole, cyclosporine, and chloramphenicol. It also promotes urinary excretion of methadone, which may precipitate withdrawal. See also the explanation for Question 431.

464. The answer is a. *(Brunton, pp 1119–1122; Craig, pp 519–520; Katzung, pp 777–780.)* Ciprofloxacin is highly effective against *P. aeruginosa*. Other members of the fluoroquinolone class have less activity against this organism, although they are effective against many other common gram-negative bacteria.

465. The answer is e. *(Brunton, pp 1194–1196; Craig, pp 553–554; Katzung, pp 768–770.)* Vancomycin, which must be given intravenously, has an antimicrobial spectrum closest to those of penicillins and cephalosporins, and it does not cross-react in immunologically susceptible patients. Like penicillins and cephalosporins, there is a growing risk of resistance to vancomycin (particularly in hospital settings, where the drug is mainly used), but it nonetheless is considered the best (if not the last resort) drug for these patients. Clotrimazole (a) is an antifungal drug, mainly used for such fungal infections as those involving *Candida*. Metronidazole (c) is also used mainly for systemic or urinary tract fungal infections, although it does have some antibacterial activity. Gentamicin (b) would be inappropriate, in part because its spectrum of activity is not likely to include organisms killed or inhibited by penicillins, cephalosporins, or vancomycin. The same applies to tetracyclines (d).

Cancer Chemotherapy and Immunosuppressants

Cell cycle, cell cycle specificity
Alkylating agents
Anticancer hormones and their
antagonists
Antitumor antibiotics

Antimetabolites
Plant alkaloids
Immunomodulaters

Questions

DIRECTIONS: Each item contains a question or incomplete statement that is followed by several responses. Select the **one best** response to each question.

466. A 47-year-old woman with choriocarcinoma is treated with very high doses of methotrexate (MTX). You anticipate significant host cell toxicity in response to the high MTX dose. Which of the following drugs would you give to limit toxic effects of the MTX on normal host cells?

a. Deferoxamine
b. Leucovorin
c. N-acetylcysteine
d. Penicillamine
e. Vitamin K

467. We administer vincristine, the prototype of the vinca alkaloids, to a patient with a tumor that is likely to be responsive to this drug. Which of the following is the most likely adverse response to this drug?

a. Nephrotoxicity, renal dysfunction or failure
b. Neutropenia
c. Peripheral sensory and motor neuropathy
d. Pulmonary damage
e. Thrombocytopenia, bleeding

468. A cancer patient develops severe irreversible cardiomyopathy because the maximum lifetime dose of an anticancer drug was exceeded. Which of the following is most likely responsible for this patient's symptoms?

a. Asparaginase
b. Bleomycin
c. Cisplatin
d. Cyclophosphamide
e. Doxorubicin
f. Vincristine

469. A patient with Wilms' tumor is receiving a chemotherapeutic agent that is described as working by intercalating into DNA strands, and that is efficacious regardless of which stage of the cell cycle the tumor cells are in. Which of the following agents best fits this description?

a. Anastrozole
b. Cytarabine
c. Dactinomycin (actinomycin D)
d. Fluorouracil
e. Tamoxifen

470. A 42-year-old woman is diagnosed with metastatic breast cancer. You consider use of tamoxifen, raloxifene, toremifene, or fulvestrant. Why might fulvestrant be the best choice, all other factors being equal?

a. Exerts antiplatelet, rather than thrombotic, effects
b. Lacks ability to cause hot flashes or other disturbing side effects
c. Lower risk of causing endometrial cancer
d. Provides clinical cure, rather than palliation, in all patients
e. Significantly improves mineral density in, strength of, long bones

471. A patient with chronic myelogenous leukemia (CML) is being treated with imatinib (STI571), a relatively new drug for this disorder. Which of the following side effects should you anticipate in response to imatinib therapy?

a. A high rate of therapeutic failure and the need to switch to interferons α-2a and -2b
b. Hypotension and hypovolemia due to significant drug-induced diuresis
c. Interactions with other drugs that depend on or affect the cytochrome P450 system
d. Significant toxicity to normal host cells due to profound inhibition of tyrosine kinase
e. Thrombocytosis, with a high risk of intravascular clotting

472. As a rule, large (and older) solid tumors are more difficult to eradicate when chemotherapy is started. Which of the following tumor-based properties explains best the reason for this chemotherapeutic limitation?

a. Growth fraction slows, more cells enter G_0
b. Higher tumor blood flow washes away anticancer drugs faster
c. P-glycoprotein activity decreases as tumors get older
d. Their higher metabolic rate makes them less vulnerable to chemotherapeutic agents
e. Topoisomerase activity (ability to self-repair DNA strand damage) increases with tumor size

473. A man has prostate cancer that will be treated with leuprolide. Which of the following drugs are we most likely to use adjunctively when we start chemotherapy?

a. An aromatase inhibitor (e.g., anastrozole)
b. Flutamide
c. Prednisone or another potent glucocorticoid
d. Tamoxifen
e. Testosterone

474. A 45-year-old woman has had a heart transplant. She receives cyclosporine as part of the immunosuppressant regimen. Which of the following is the main mechanism of cyclosporine's immunosuppressant effects?

a. Blocks the CD3 site on T lymphocytes, blocks all T cell functions
b. Directly destroys proliferating lymphoid cells
c. Directly inhibits B and T lymphocyte proliferation
d. Inhibits calcineurin and resulting IL-2 synthesis that is necessary for B and T cell proliferation
e. Lyses antigen-activated lymphocytes, reduces responsiveness of T lymphocytes to IL-1, reduces IL-2 production by lymphocytes and monocytes

475. The oncology team has treated many patients with acute lymphocytic leukemia using a combination of drugs. One drug tends to cause a high incidence of lumbar and abdominal pain, significant increases of serum amylase and transaminase activity, and other symptoms of hepatic and/or pancreatic dysfunction. Some patients developed serious hypersensitivity reactions upon drug administration, and there have been occasional sudden deaths. Which of the following drugs best fits this description?

a. 6-Mercaptopurine
b. Asparaginase
c. Doxorubicin
d. Methotrexate
e. Vincristine

476. A 30-year-old woman being treated for ovarian cancer develops high frequency hearing loss and declining renal function in response to anticancer drug therapy. Which of the following drugs is the most likely cause?

a. Bleomycin
b. Cisplatin
c. Doxorubicin
d. 5-Fluorouracil
e. Paclitaxel

477. A 41-year-old woman is admitted to the outpatient area of the hematology-oncology center for her first course of adjuvant chemotherapy for metastatic breast cancer following a left modified radical mastectomy and axillary lymph node dissection for infiltrating ductal carcinoma of the breast. Two biopsies were positive for cancer.

Following premedication with dexamethasone and ondansetron, she will receive combination chemotherapy with doxorubicin, cyclophosphamide, and fluorouracil. Premedications include intravenous ondansetron and dexamethasone. Twenty-four hours after the first course of chemotherapy, she will start a 10-day regimen with filgrastim. Which of the following is the most likely reason for administering the filgrastim?

a. Control of nausea and emesis
b. Potentiate the anticancer effects of the chemotherapeutic agents
c. Prevent doxorubicin-induced cardiotoxicity
d. Reduce the risk/severity of chemo-induced neutropenia and related infections
e. Stimulate the gastric mucosa to repair damage caused by the chemotherapy drugs

478. While reviewing charts in a general medicine clinic you see that a patient, 55-years-old and with no history of cancer at all, is taking methotrexate. What is the most likely condition for which this "anticancer drug" is being given?

a. Asthma or emphysema
b. Hyperthyroidism
c. Hyperuricemia or clinical gout
d. Myasthenia gravis
e. Rheumatoid arthritis or psoriasis

479. A cancer patient receives prophylactic allopurinol before a course of chemotherapy. Which of the following is the main reason for which the allopurinol is given?

a. Facilitate host cell detoxification of the chemotherapeutic drug, thereby reducing host cell toxicities
b. Inhibit the potential for DNA repair, by topoisomerases, that otherwise might lead to chemotherapy failure
c. Potentiate the action of a nitrogen mustard or nitrosourea to bind to (cross-link) purine moieties in DNA strands
d. Prevent myelosuppression and related blood dyscrasias
e. Reduce the risk of hyperuricemia and its main consequences (renal damage, gout) that can occur with a massive cell kill

480. We have a 48-year-old patient who was in renal failure, but fortunately she received a kidney transplant. We start her on cyclosporine to reduce the risk of graft rejection. Which of the following is or are the most common and worrisome adverse responses associated with this immunosuppressant?

a. Cardiotoxicity and hepatotoxicity
b. Hepatotoxicity and nephrotoxicity
c. Hypotension and pulmonary fibrosis
d. Nephrotoxicity and infection risk
e. Thrombosis and pulmonary embolism or ischemic stroke

481. Most of the common cancer chemotherapeutic drugs work only, or best, on cells that are in an active growth or replication phase. Given that information, which of the following stages of the normal cell cycle are most resistant to these anticancer drugs?

a. G_0
b. G_1
c. G_2
d. M
e. S

482. Our patient has advanced Hodgkin's disease. One of the drugs we administer is vincristine, as part of the so-called MOPP regimen (vincristine, mechlorethamine, procarbazine, and prednisone).

Which of the following is the most likely mechanism by which the vincristine is exerting its intended cytotoxic effects?

a. Alkylates DNA, causing cross-links between parallel DNA strands
b. Blocks microtubular assembly and mitosis during M-phase
c. Inhibits topoisomerase, preventing repair of DNA strand breaks
d. Intercalates in DNA strands, thereby preventing DNA replication by mRNA
e. Stabilizes microtubular arrays, thereby preventing mitosis

483. As part of the treatment plan for the Hodgkin's patient described in Question 482, we have given mechlorethamine. Which of the following statements best describes the anticancer mechanism of action of this drug?

a. Alkylates DNA, causing cross-links between parallel DNA strands
b. Blocks microtubular assembly and mitosis during M-phase
c. Inhibits topoisomerase, preventing repair of DNA strand breaks
d. Intercalates in DNA strands, thereby preventing DNA replication by mRNA
e. Stabilizes microtubular arrays, thereby preventing mitosis

484. Allopurinol is commonly administered before initiating chemotherapy of leukemias and other blood-based cancers to prevent hyperuricemia and its consequences. It is also important in preventing hyperuricemia in response to chemotherapy of some solid tumors. However, it may potentiate the host toxicity of certain anticancer drugs by inhibiting their metabolic inactivation and detoxification. With which of the following drugs should concomitant use of allopurinol be avoided, or be used with extra caution?

a. Bleomycin
b. Cisplatin
c. Cyclophosphamide
d. Doxorubicin
e. Mercaptopurine

485. As part of a comprehensive cancer chemotherapy regimen for metastatic breast carcinoma, we treat our patient with ondansetron. Which of the following is the most likely purpose for administering this drug?

a. Activate cancer cells to move out of G_0 and into a more responsive, actively replicating cell cycle phase
b. Block estrogen receptors, thereby enhancing the efficacy of the cyclophosphamide
c. Prevent cardiotoxicity caused by one of the anticancer drugs in the combination
d. Prevent metabolism of adrenal cortical androgens to estrogens, which would facilitate breast tumor growth
e. Suppress chemotherapy-induced nausea and vomiting

Cancer Chemotherapy and Immunosuppressants

Answers

466. The answer is b. (*Brunton, pp 1335, 1339, 1694; Craig, pp 643–644; Katzung, pp 907–908.*) This essential technique to reduce host cell toxicity in response to MTX therapy is known as leucovorin rescue. Methotrexate, a folic acid analog/antimetabolite, can be curative for women with choriocarcinoma and is also useful for non-Hodgkin's lymphomas and acute lymphocytic leukemias in children. The drug kills responsive cancer cells by inhibiting dihydrofolate reductase, an enzyme necessary for forming tetrahydrofolic acid (FH_4). The FH_4, in turn, is critical for eventual synthesis of DNA, RNA, and proteins. Inhibition of thymidylate synthesis is probably the single most important consequence in the overall reaction scheme.

Some cancer cells are resistant to MTX because they lack adequate mechanisms for transporting the drug intracellularly. These include some head and neck cancers and osteogenic sarcomas. In such cases we need to give very large doses of MTX to establish a high concentration gradient that essentially "drives" it into the cells. Unfortunately, normal host cells depend on folate metabolism, they take up MTX well, and they will be affected.

To protect normal cells we administer leucovorin (also called citrovorum factor or folinic acid) right after giving the MTX. It is taken up by the normal cells, bypasses the block induced by the MTX, and so spares normal cell metabolism. The leucovorin does not spare cancer cells: just as they cannot take up MTX well, they cannot take up the rescue agent and save themselves from cytotoxicity.

Leucovorin rescue is not done "automatically" in every case when MTX is given. When low MTX doses are used leucovorin may be withheld until and unless blood counts show evidence of MTX-induced bone marrow suppression. However, it is quite usually given along with MTX when MTX doses are very high (as in severe or MTX-resistant cases), and host toxicity is very probable.

The main adverse responses to MTX, regardless of the purpose for which it is given, include bone marrow suppression, pulmonary damage (infiltrates, fibrosis), stomatitis, and lesions elsewhere in the GI tract. High doses can be nephrotoxic (risk reduced by maintaining adequate hydration and alkalinizing the urine). MTX is also teratogenic.

Recall that deferoxamine is used to treat iron poisoning (it is an iron chelator). N-acetylcysteine is mainly used either as a mucolytic (mucus-thinning) drug for certain pulmonary disorders (e.g., COPD) or as an antidote for acetaminophen poisoning. Penicillamine is mainly a copper chelator, used for copper poisoning or Wilson's disease. Vitamin K is used for deficiency states, for combating excessive effects of warfarin, or for managing bleeding disorders in newborns of mothers who have been taking certain drugs (e.g., anticonvulsants such as phenytoin) during pregnancy.

467. The answer is c. *(Brunton, pp 1350–1354; Craig, p 648; Katzung, p 911.)* Vincristine is one of relatively few cytotoxic anticancer drugs that does not cause bone marrow suppression (and all the potential consequences of that) as its main toxicity. Rather, it causes neuropathies involving both sensory and motor nerves. Paresthesias are a common example of the former (hearing loss can also occur); muscle weakness and obtunded reflexes are examples of the latter. Important note: Vincristine differs from the other two vinca alkaloids, vinblastine and vinorelbine, which do cause bone marrow suppression (and not neuropathies) as their main dose-limiting toxicity.

468. The answer is e. *(Brunton, pp 1357–1360; Craig, p 646; Katzung, pp 913–914.)* Doxorubicin, an antitumor antibiotic, is cardiotoxic, and the risk for and severity of cardiomyopathy is dose-related. (There is a maximum recommended lifetime [cumulative] dose for this drug, and if it is exceeded the risk of cardiac damage rises significantly.)

Asparaginase, used only for acute lymphocytic leukemia, tends to cause mainly pancreatitis, hepatic dysfunction, and allergic/hypersensitivity reactions. The main organ-specific toxicity of bleomycin, also an antitumor antibiotic, is pulmonary damage that presents initially usually as pneumonitis. It occurs in about 1 of 10 patients treated with this drug. In some cases the pulmonary damage will progress to pulmonary fibrosis that is, of course, irreversible.

Cisplatin's main dose-limiting toxicity is renal damage, which can be prevented somewhat by ensuring that the patient is adequately hydrated and producing adequate amounts of urine. Diuretics may be used as adjuncts. The goal is to minimize accumulation of the nephrotoxic drug in the renal tubules and urine. (A related drug, oxaliplatin, tends to cause peripheral sensory neuropathies and does so in most patients who receive this drug.)

Cyclophosphamide has no particular organ-specific toxicity. Rather, main manifestations of toxicity involve rapidly growing cells such as those in the bone marrow, intestinal tract mucosae, and hair follicles.

Vincristine's major dose-limiting toxicity is peripheral nerve damage: motor, sensory, and in some cases autonomic. It probably arises in a manner related to the drug's anticancer effect:· inhibition of microtubular function—or, in the case of nerves, neurotubules—as a result of drug binding to tubulin.

469. The answer is c. *(Brunton, pp 1356–1357; Craig, pp 647–648; Katzung, pp 913–914.)* Dactinomycin intercalates between and eventually binds to DNA base pairs. This distortion of the DNA chains makes the DNA an unsuitable template for RNA polymerase, and ultimately RNA and protein synthesis is inhibited. Dactinomycin is phase-nonspecific.

Anastrozole is a relatively new aromatase inhibitor. This is an oral agent used for postmenopausal women with early or advanced breast cancer. In postmenopausal women, the major source of estrogen (which supports growth and replication of estrogen-dependent tumors) is adrenal androgens. Those androgens are metabolized by aromatase to estrogens. As a result, anastrozole depletes estrogens and can arrest tumor cell growth.

Cytarabine (also called cytosine arabinoside) is a pyrimidine analog (antimetabolite) that is metabolized to the active moiety, ara-CTP. The ara-CTP becomes incorporated into DNA, with the main ultimate effect being suppression of DNA synthesis. It is highly specific for cells in S-phase.

Fluorouracil, also an antimetabolite, inhibits thymidylate synthetase through its active metabolite, 5-fluoro-2'-dxoyuridine-5'-monophosphate (FdUMP). It is not phase-specific, but its activity depends on cells not being in the G_0 stage.

Tamoxifen is used for breast cancers. It blocks estrogen receptors on the breast cancer cells (for which the main physiologic agonist is estradiol). Recall that tamoxifen is classified as a selective estrogen receptor modifier (SERM). Although it blocks estrogen receptors on responsive breast cancer cells and is therapeutic for them, it acts as an estrogen receptor agonist in the uterus. Thus, one of the main risks of therapy with tamoxifen is endometrial hyperplasia that may lead to endometrial cancer. Because the drug acts as an estrogen receptor agonist in some tissues and an antagonist in others, risk-benefit ratios must be considered carefully. The beneficial effects in active breast carcinoma may outweigh the risks of inducing endometrial disease. However, the preventative use in the absence of breast cancer has a much lower benefit-to-risk ratio.

470. The answer is c. *(Brunton, pp 1383–1384, 1556–1557; Craig, pp 649, 707, 711–712; Katzung, pp 917, 926, 961.)* Fulvestrant is associated with a much lower risk of causing endometrial pathology, including cancer. It is a "pure" estrogen antagonist. That effect, in breast tissue, is what accounts for the drug's beneficial effects in some patients with metastatic, estrogen-supported, breast cancer. In contrast, tamoxifen, raloxifene, and toremifene are classified as selective estrogen receptor modifiers (SERMs). Although they block estrogen receptors in breast tissue (just as fulvestrant does), they also have estrogenic (agonist) activity in some other tissues, notably the uterus. There they can cause endometrial proliferation, hyperplasia, and (apparently) an increased risk of endometrial cancer. (For more information, see the answer to Question 370 in the chapter "Endocrine System.")

Because fulvestrant lacks estrogen agonist activity, it will not enhance bone mineralization nor favorably modify cholesterol profiles, as the SERMs tend to do. The SERMs slightly increase the risk of thromboembolism. Fulvestrant may too, but it also lacks any ability to prevent platelet aggregation or thromboembolism. Hot flashes are fairly common with any of these drugs.

471. The answer is c. *(Brunton, pp 1366–1368; Craig, p 653; Katzung, pp 841–842, 948, 970, 978–979.)* One of several problems with imatinib therapy is that it is a substrate and rather powerful inhibitor of several cytochromes (CYP3A4, 2C9, and 2D6), which are important for the metabolism of many other drugs—warfarin, theophylline, and many others—whose actions can be increased excessively if dosages are not adjusted accordingly. Conversely, imatinib is a target of interactions by this mechanism. Phenytoin, carbamazepine, barbiturates, and rifampin are examples of drugs that can induce imatinib metabolism and reduce the clinical response to it; and such drugs as azole antifungals and erythromycin can reduce imatinib's clearance and increase the risk of toxicity.

Because of the issue of drug interactions, a high frequency of adverse responses, limited use (see below), and even cost, imatinib is generally reserved for use after a trial of interferons has proven inadequate. The reverse—using imatinib first—usually isn't done.

Hypotension and hypovolemia are not what one would expect with this drug. Rather, we see a rather high incidence of fluid retention that may not only affect blood pressure, but also cause such other problems as ascites, pericardial and pleural effusions, and possibly pulmonary edema. Likewise, thrombocytosis is the opposite of what typically occurs: thrombocytopenia and bleeding problems, plus neutropenia and an increased risk of infection are fairly common.

You should recall that chronic myelogenous leukemia cells do synthesize an abnormal constitutively active tyrosine kinase (Bcr-Abl) that is involved in (abnormal) protein phosphorylation. It is that aberrant tyrosine kinase—not ones found in normal host cells—that is affected by the drug and that confers selectivity for the drug's actions. Thus, tyrosine kinase inhibition does not seem to account for the adverse effects of this drug on host cells.

472. The answer is a. (*Brunton, pp 1315–1322; Craig, pp 631–632; Katzung, pp 900–901.*) Gompertzian analysis (a plot of the log of the number of cancer cells in a tumor vs. time) shows that after a tumor has reached a certain size, the rate of tumor growth (and "overall metabolic rate") slows: lower growth fraction or, stated differently, the longer it takes for the tumor to double in size. This slowed growth is partially due to more cells entering the G_0 (resting) phase of the cell cycle, where responsiveness to many chemotherapeutic agents is low. (One reason for this is the sheer size of the tumor as related to blood flow and the delivery of nutrients that the rapidly dividing cells need. Reduced nutrient and oxygen delivery not only reduces cell replication, but also delivery of the chemotherapeutic agents.)

P-glycoprotein activity does not necessarily decrease with time or tumor size. However, even if it did, that would predict increased responsiveness to most anticancer drugs, because it is P-glycoprotein that normally pumps drugs out of the cancer cell. Self-repair mechanisms, as by topoisomerase, is not a factor in explaining reduced vulnerability of very large tumors.

473. The answer is b. (*Brunton, pp 1387–1390; Craig, pp 650, 732; Katzung, pp 688, 917, 926.*) Flutamide, one of a small number of androgen receptor blockers used for managing prostate cancer, is used as an adjunct to leuprolide. Leuprolide acts like gonadotropin-releasing hormone (GnRH; or luteinizing hormone-releasing hormone). When leuprolide therapy is started, it stimulates release of interstitial cell–stimulating hormone from the pituitary, thereby increasing testosterone production and supporting tumor growth. It is only with continued exposure to leuprolide that GnRH receptors become desensitized, and the eventual inhibition of testosterone production (and, thereby, support of tumor growth) occurs. Flutamide, by blocking androgen receptors, prevents the potential worsening of the tumor in the early phase of leuprolide therapy when testosterone levels rise. Even when leuprolide's pituitary-desensitizing effects occur, androgens that can support prostate tumor growth will come from the adrenal gland. Their effects, too, are blocked by the flutamide.

474. The answer is d. *(Brunton, pp 1409–1411; Craig, p 659; Katzung, pp 940–941.)* Cyclosporine acts on helper T lymphocytes. First it binds to cyclophilin and then inhibits calcineurin, which is important in the synthesis of cytokines, including IL-2. These cytokines are necessary for proliferation of B cells and cytolytic T cells (also called cytotoxic T cells, or CD8 cells). Tacrolimus works by a mechanism that is largely similar to that of cyclosporine, but its initial intracellular binding site is not cyclophilin, but rather another protein.

Muromonab-CD3 is the immunosuppressant that blocks the CD3 site on T lymphocytes. Cyclophosphamide exerts direct toxic effects on proliferating lymphoid cells. Azathioprine, which is metabolically activated to mercaptopurine, inhibits B and T lymphocyte proliferation by inhibiting DNA synthesis. Glucocorticoids, at high doses, lyse antigen-activated lymphocytes and reduce IL-2 production by lymphocytes and macrophages.

475. The answer is b. *(Brunton, pp 1363–1364; Craig, pp 639, 649; Katzung, p 918.)* Asparaginase is an enzyme that catalyzes the hydrolysis of serum asparagine to aspartic acid and ammonia. Major toxicities from asparaginase are related to antigenicity (it is a foreign protein, and some fatal anaphylactic reactions have occurred), pancreatitis, and a 50% incidence of some hepatic dysfunction based on the presence of elevated serum transaminases. The drug, which is largely G_1 phase-specific, is not cytotoxic to cells other than leukemic lymphoblasts. Host (and other cells) can synthesize and replace asparagine that has been hydrolyzed by the drug; the lymphoblasts cannot, and so they are killed.

476. The answer is b. (*Brunton, pp 1326t, 1334; Craig, pp 651–652; Katzung, pp 905–907.*) Cisplatin, which is sometimes classified along with traditional alkylating agents, is unique among all the common anticancer agents in terms of the relative incidence of hearing loss and nephrotoxicity. (You are correct in associating vincristine with hearing loss, but nephrotoxicity is very rare; in contrast, you may have recalled that methotrexate can cause nephrotoxicity, but it does not cause hearing loss, and it is indicated for a variety of cancers, but not ovarian.)

Bleomycin's main targeted toxicity is the lungs (pulmonary infiltrates, fibrosis, etc.). Doxorubicin, as noted, is cardiotoxic. The drug is mainly used for testicular carcinomas, squamous cell cancers, and lymphomas. 5-FU, a pyrimidine antimetabolite, is used for a variety of solid tumors. However, peripheral neuritis or neuropathy (and, especially, hearing loss) or renal damage are uncommon; rather, we are faced with a relatively high incidence of bone marrow suppression and oral and GI mucosal damage. Paclitaxel is a microtubular stabilizing drug (and plant alkaloid). It is considered first-line for some patients with advanced ovarian cancer or non-small-cell lung cancers, causes dose-dependent bone marrow suppression and peripheral neuropathy, and a fairly high incidence of acute infusion-related hypersensitivity reactions (probably due to the vehicle in which the drug is delivered).

477. The answer is d. (*Brunton, pp 1440–1441; Craig, pp 639, 653; Katzung, pp 539, 919.*) Filgrastim, also known as granulocyte colony-stimulating factor (GCSF), enhances neutrophil production. One use, therefore, is to prevent neutropenia and infection associated with bone marrow depression from cancer chemotherapy. (Hint: Look at the generic name, filgrastim: *g*ranulocyte *stim*ulating.) The drug lacks antiemetic effects, potentiates the chemotherapeutic actions of no drug, and has no effect on the gastric mucosa or on doxorubicin-mediated cardiotoxicity.

478. The answer is e. (*Brunton, pp 690, 706, 1339; Craig, pp 432–433; Katzung, p 588.*) The main uses of MTX for conditions other than responsive cancers are management of rheumatoid arthritis (RA) and psoriasis. Doses and dosage schedules differ from those typically used for cancers.

MTX is one of many disease-modifying antirheumatic drugs (DMARDs), which are often called slow-acting antirheumatic drugs (SAARDs) because their onset of symptom relief is much slower than traditional NSAIDs (salicylates and other first-generation COX-1/-2 inhibitors, or second-generation/COX-2 inhibitors, i.e., the "coxibs").

Nonetheless, although the onset is considered slow, meaningful symptom relief usually occurs with as little as 3–4 weeks of therapy—faster than the other DMARDs. (Other typical first-choice DMARDs are sulfasalazine and hydroxychoroquine, which unlike MTX, have no cancer-related uses.) All the potential side effects, adverse responses, and contraindications that apply to using MTX for cancer apply to the drug's use for RA or psoriasis (see also Question 310).

479. The answer is e. *(Brunton, pp 708–709, 1015–1016, 1414; Craig, pp 445–446; Katzung, pp 598–599.)* Hyperuricemia is associated with many cancers and is a common outcome of massive cell kills induced by chemotherapeutic drugs. The uric acid is derived from cellular purine degradation, eventually formed from hypoxanthine and xanthine via xanthine oxidase, the enzyme that is inhibited by allopurinol. Recall that renal damage (and other damage, such as gout) is due to uric acid's poor solubility in body fluids, especially at low pH.

Allopurinol has no effect on the P450 system or on cellular transitions from one phase of the cell cycle to another. There is no effect on DNA synthesis or repair, or any direct cytoprotective effect on myeloid or other tissues.

Be sure you remember that the metabolic detoxification of azathioprine and 6-mercaptopurine depends in part on xanthine oxidase. Inhibiting that enzyme with allopurinol, therefore, may increase the risk of toxicity to host cells.

480. The answer is d. *(Brunton, p 1695; Craig, p 659; Katzung, p 941.)* Nephrotoxicity, or at least some clinically significant degree of renal dysfunction, occurs in about 8 of 10 patients receiving cyclosporine. It is typically dose-dependent and, particularly in renal transplant patients, could be due to either the drug (too much) or to rejection. Infection occurs about as often as renal dysfunction. Cyclosporine can cause hepatotoxicity, but the incidence is far lower than that of renal responses or infection. Blood pressure changes can occur, but with cyclosporine the change usually involves increased pressure, and it is common. Cardiac or pulmonary toxicities and thromboembolism due to the drug itself are extremely uncommon.

481. The answer is a. (*Brunton, pp 1316–1318, 1320f; Craig, pp 630–631; Katzung, pp 900–902.*) The G_0 phase is the resting or dormant stage of the cell cycle. No cell division takes place. This phase is, overall, the most resistant to most chemotherapeutic agents because most of the anticancer drugs (called phase-specific) produce their lethal effects quickest and best on cells that are actively proliferating, whether synthesizing or preparing to synthesize DNA, or undergoing mitosis. Good examples of drugs that are reasonably effective against cells in G_0 (or any other phase) are the alkylating agents (e.g., cyclophosphamide) and several of the antitumor antibiotics (e.g., dactinomycin, doxorubicin).

Obviously, not all cancer cells present in a solid tumor will be in a more vulnerable stage of the cell cycle (i.e., not in G_0), but some will be. This provides one rationale for combining a cycle-nonspecific agent with a cycle-specific one: attack as many cancer cells as possible, no matter where in the cell cycle they may be. This concept also provides a reason why cycle-specific agents are often administered in repeated courses over an extended time (as opposed to a single dose): repeating the dose increases the chance that we will eventually catch more cells as they enter into a more responsive or vulnerable part of the cycle.

482. The answer is b. (*Brunton, pp 1327, 1351; Craig, pp 639, 648; Katzung, p 911.*) Vincristine and the other vinca alkaloids bind to tubulin and impair microtubular assembly, preventing mitosis (M-phase-specific).

483. The answer is a. (*Brunton, pp 1320, 1322f, 1325, 1327; Craig, p 640; Katzung, pp 926–930.*) Mechlorethamine, like cyclophosphamide (and carmustine and several others), is an alkylating agent. They are called bifunctional alkylating agents because they can covalently bind to DNA in two places ("nucleophilic attack"), thereby forming cross-links between two adjacent strands or between two bases in one strand. This ultimately disrupts DNA and RNA synthesis or may cause strand breakage. Cyclophosphamide (which can be considered the prototype of the alkylating agents) is actually a prodrug—it requires metabolic activation in order for its effects to occur. Cyclophosphamide (and other alkylating agents) is cell cycle-nonspecific, although their efficacy is greater when cells are not in G_0.

Bleomycin, dactinomycin, and doxorubicin are good examples of drugs that intercalate in DNA strands. Thus, the altered DNA no longer serves as an adequately precise template for eventual synthesis of more functional DNA and RNA. They are classified as antitumor antibiotics.

Etoposide and topotecan are examples of drugs that inhibit topoisomerase II. The consequence is inhibited ability of affected cells to repair DNA strand breaks. This stops the cell cycle in G_2.

The taxoids (e.g., paclitaxel) impairs mitosis, but by stabilizing assembled microtubules rather than by exerting a vinca alkaloid-like inhibition of microtubular assembly.

484. The answer is e. *(Brunton, pp 708–709, 1015–1016, 1414; Craig, pp 446, 644; Katzung, p 909.)* Mercaptopurine is a (thio)purine antimetabolite that is metabolically inactivated (detoxified) by xanthine oxidase. This purine degradation pathway of metabolism not only leads to formation of uric acid, but also is important to reducing host cell toxicity to the thiopurines. Thus, concomitant use of allopurinol increases the risk of host cell toxicity. Note that azathioprine (an inhibitor of B and T lymphocyte proliferation, and typically used as an immunosuppressant) is metabolized to mercaptopurine. As a result, its metabolism is also inhibited by allopurinol.

The metabolism of the other drugs listed is not xanthine oxidase–dependent, and so is not affected by allopurinol.

485. The answer is e. *(Brunton, pp 1001–1004; Craig, p 477; Katzung, pp 271–272, 1049–1052.)* Ondansetron is used to control nausea and vomiting, which are common consequences of chemotherapy. It is a serotonin 5-HT$_3$ receptor antagonist, working primarily in the chemoreceptor trigger zone and afferent vagal nerves in the upper GI tract. It is probable that the dexamethasone, which was also given to our patient, was also given for antiemetic effects.

Note that serotonin antagonists such as ondansetron (and dopamine receptor antagonists such as prochlorperazine) have the broadest antiemetic spectrums (and clinical uses) of all the main antiemetic drug classes. They are useful for controlling not only emesis associated with chemotherapy, but also that which arises in radiation therapy and in many common postoperative settings.

Ondansetron has no effect on the cell cycle or the cytopathology of cancer, nor does it have any effect on estrogen receptors or estrogen metabolism (as from androgens, which is important in postmenopausal women and is a process that can be inhibited by such drugs as anastrozole, an aromatase inhibitor). Ondandsetron has no effect on chemotherapy-induced cardiotoxicity (which, in the drug combination noted here, would be a property of the doxorubicin).

Toxicology

Air pollutants, toxic gases
Alcohols, ethylene glycol
Antidotes for common drugs

Chemical warfare agents
Heavy metals
Poisonings of unknown cause

Questions

DIRECTIONS: Each item contains a question or incomplete statement that is followed by several responses. Select the **one best** response to each question.

486. Your patient developed acute poisoning as a result of inhaling cyanide gas in an industrial accident. In addition to providing symptomatic, supportive care, and other appropriate interventions, administering which of the following would be the most likely to play a crucial role in treating the cyanide poisoning?

a. Ammonium chloride
b. Deferoxamine
c. Dimercaprol (BAL; British anti-Lewisite)
d. N-acetylcysteine
e. Pralidoxime
f. Sodium thiosulfate

487. A patient has taken a potentially lethal dose of acetaminophen. We begin administering repeated doses of oral N-acetylcysteine, which can be lifesaving in many such cases. Which of the following is the main mechanism by which this antidote exerts its beneficial effects?

a. Alkalinizes the urine to facilitate acetaminophen excretion
b. Causes metabolic acidosis to counteract metabolic alkalosis caused by a toxic acetaminophen metabolite
c. Inhibits P450 enzymes, thereby inhibiting formation of acetaminophen's toxic metabolite
d. Inhibits synthesis of superoxide anion radical and hydrogen peroxide
e. Is rich in sulfhydryl (–SH) groups that react with and inactivate a toxic acetaminophen metabolite

488. A patient who receives a rapid IV injection of a drug develops hypocalcemic tetany. Which of the following was the most likely cause?

a. Deferoxamine
b. Dimercaprol
c. Edetate disodium (Na_2EDTA)
d. N-acetylcysteine
e. Penicillamine

489. A patient presents in the emergency department with a drug overdose. Among other things, the physician correctly orders IV infusion of sodium bicarbonate to alkalinize the urine, which increases drug elimination through pH-dependent inhibition of its tubular reabsorption. To which of the following drugs does this description most likely apply?

a. Amphetamine
b. Aspirin (acetylsalicylic acid)
c. Cocaine
d. Morphine
e. Phencyclidine

490. A 3-year-old girl ingests 30 tablets of aspirin, 325 mg each. We've gotten her to the emergency department within 30 min of the poisoning. Which of the following antidotes would be the most rational and effective to administer as part of the initial treatment plan?

a. Activated charcoal
b. Deferoxamine
c. Dimercaprol
d. N-acetylcysteine
e. Penicillamine

491. A 50-year-old man has been consuming large amounts of ethanol on an almost daily basis for many years. One day, unable to find any ethanol, he ingests a large amount of methanol (wood alcohol) that he had bought for his camp lantern. Which of the following is the most likely consequence of his methanol poisoning?

a. Atrioventricular conduction defect (block)
b. Blindness
c. Bronchospasm
d. Delirium tremens
e. Metabolic alkalosis

492. A 15-year-old boy attempts suicide with a liquid that he found in his parents' greenhouse. His dad used it to broken first of "varmints" around the yard. The toxin causes intense abdominal pain, skeletal muscle cramps, projectile vomiting, and severe diarrhea that leads to fluid and electrolyte imbalances, hypotension, and difficulty swallowing. On examination he is found to be volume depleted and is showing signs of a reduced level of consciousness. His breath smells "metallic." Which of the following probably accounts for these symptoms?

a. Arsenic
b. Cadmium
c. Iron
d. Lead
e. Zinc

493. A 60-year-old man has been using a kerosene space heater and candles to keep warm in the winter. He is transported to the hospital with complaints of severe headaches, nausea, dizziness, and a diminution in vision. He has a decreased arterial blood oxygen (O_2)-carrying capacity, but no change of his arteria P_{O_2}. Which of the following most likely accounts for these findings?

a. Carbon monoxide (CO)
b. Methane
c. Nitrogen dioxide
d. Ozone
e. Sulfur dioxide

494. A 5-year-old boy consumed a liquid from a container in the family garage. He presents with central nervous system (CNS) depression, obtunded reflexes, and ventilatory depression. A blood sample indicates profound metabolic acidosis. A check of the urine reveals crystals that are presumed to be oxalate. Which of the following is the most likely cause of the poisoning?

a. A halogenated hydrocarbon from a can of spray paint
b. An insecticide (organophosphate cholinesterase inhibitor)
c. Ethylene glycol
d. Gasoline
e. Paint thinner such as acetone

495. A 22-year-old girl is brought to the emergency department by a friend. They had been at a bar for about an hour, and then the patient suddenly became drowsy but was still conscious. She fell and cut her head, and she says "yes, it hurts." Her ventilatory rate and depth are depressed, but not to a worrisome degree. Her patellar reflexes are blunted and she is ataxic. She responds slowly to questions, but is unable to recall anything that happened after arriving at the bar. Her friend stated that the patient had only one cocktail and hadn't been drinking before they went out.

Based on this information, with which of the following was this patient's drink most likely "spiked?"

a. A barbiturate
b. A benzodiazepine
c. An opioid
d. Chloral hydrate
e. Cocaine
f. Pure (grain) alcohol

496. Recent occupational health studies in several heavily populated urban areas have revealed an astonishingly large number of homes that have lead-based paint and children living in them. However, a number of environmental poisons that could lead to acute or chronic poisoning have also been found there. Which of the following signs and symptoms would be consistent with chronic exposure to toxic levels of inorganic lead?

a. Anorexia and weight loss; weakness, especially of extensor muscles (e.g., wrist drop); recurrent abdominal pain
b. Gingivitis, discolored gums, loosened teeth, or stomatitis; tremor of the extremities; swollen parotid or other salivary glands
c. Hallucinations, insomnia, headache, generalized CNS irritability
d. Hyperventilation in response to metabolic acidosis; hypotension; abdominal pain, diarrhea, brown or bloody vomitus; pallor or cyanosis
e. Severe, watery diarrhea; garlicky or metallic breath; encephalopathy, hypovolemia and hypotension

497. Not long ago, several patients (and a health care provider who is now incarcerated) seeking "relief" from their facial wrinkles nearly died because they received injections of botulinum toxin that was improperly obtained and inadequately diluted. Which of the following is a correct characteristic, finding, or mechanism associated with this toxin?

a. Complete failure of all cholinergic neurotransmission
b. Favorable response to administration of pralidoxime
c. Impairment of parasympathetic, but not sympathetic, nervous system activation
d. Massive overstimulation of all structures having muscarinic cholinergic receptors
e. Selective paralysis of skeletal muscle

498. A terrorist drops a vial of "nerve gas" into a crowded subway at rush hour. The patients are brought to the nearest emergency centers and are given atropine. Which of the following effects of the nerve gas will persist after giving the atropine?

a. Bradycardia
b. Bronchospasm
c. Excessive lacrimal, mucus, sweat, and salivary secretions
d. GI hypermotility, fluid and electrolyte loss from profuse diarrhea
e. Skeletal muscle hyperfunction or paralysis

499. Lab tests conducted by the local health department are positive for chronic lead exposure in a child. Lead levels are significantly elevated, but symptoms fortunately are mild and not at all imminently life-threatening. Which of the following is the most appropriate antidote for reducing his body load of excessive and potentially toxic lead?

a. Ca-Na$_2$-EDTA
b. Deferoxamine
c. Dimercaprol
d. N-acetylcysteine
e. Penicillamine
f. Succimer

500. A young child, wandering through his dad's garage early one winter, finds some antifreeze. It smells sweet, and he drinks enough to become seriously ill. He is brought to the emergency department several hours after signs and symptoms develop. Which of the following is the preferred drug to administer to manage the poisoning?

a. Allopurinol
b. Atropine
c. Ethanol
d. Lorazepam
e. Syrup of ipecac

501. Physostigmine is the antidote for poisoning with antimuscarinic drugs (e.g., atropine). Other common AChE inhibitors, a good example of which is neostigmine, are not suitable because they have virtually no beneficial actions at a key site or structure that can easily be targeted by physostigmine. Which of the following is that site or structure?

a. Central nervous system (e.g., the brain)
b. Exocrine glands
c. Heart
d. Skeletal muscle
e. Smooth muscles, airway and vascular

502. A mother calls to report that her 6-year-old child appears to have swallowed a large amount of an over-the-counter sleep aid about 5 h ago. The product contained only one active drug, and knowing your drugs you suspect the poisoning is due to diphenhydramine. Assuming your reasoned guess about the cause of poisoning was correct, which of the following signs or symptoms would you expect to find, upon physical exam, to confirm your hunch?

a. Fever; clear lungs; absence of bowel sounds; urinary retention, dry, flushed skin; mydriasis and photophobia; bizarre behavior
b. Bradycardia and profuse diarrhea
c. Miosis with little/no papillary response to bright lights; spontaneous micturition; lack of response to painful stimuli
d. Hypothermia; bounding pulse; hypertension
e. Skeletal muscle weakness or paralysis; profound hypermotility of gut and bladder smooth muscle; bronchospasm

Toxicology

Answers

486. The answer is f. *(Brunton, p 885; Craig, p 66; Katzung, pp 190, 992t.)* Whether cyanide poisoning occurs from leakage of gas, the combustion of plastics, nitroprusside overdoses, or other causes, management includes many common elements. Cyanide reacts with Fe(III) in mitochondrial cytochrome oxidase, inhibiting oxidative phosphorylation. The shift in metabolism from aerobic metabolism to glycolysis soon leads to not only ATP depletion, but also severe lactic (anion gap) acidosis.

We manage cyanide poisoning first by dealing with the high reactivity of CN⁻ with Fe(II) in hemoglobin and the subsequent formation of Fe(III) hemoglobin. We do that by first administering sodium nitrite (intravenously) to regenerate active cytochromes and convert hemoglobin to the more cyanide-reactive methemoglobin. Then we administer sodium thiosulfate to form the somewhat less toxic and more readily excreted thiocyanate. Cyanide also normally reacts with endogenous thiosulfate, and under catalysis by the hepatic enzyme rhodanese forms relatively less toxic thiocyanate that is more easily excreted in the urine. In cyanide poisoning, however, those endogenous thiosulfate stores are quickly depleted, so this provides the basis for infusing sodium thiosulfate (f, the correct answer) to lower cyanmethemoglobin levels. In cases of severe methemoglobinemia, we can also give methylene blue intravenously. (Note that large doses of inorganic nitrites can be intrinsically toxic as a result of methemoglobin formation. However, in the context of cyanide poisoning we can capitalize on the reactivity of otherwise toxic inorganic nitrite, in conjunction with thiosulfate administration, to help treat an otherwise fatal toxic scenario.)

Ammonium chloride (a) would be ineffective and may actually make matters worse by exacerbating metabolic acidosis. Deferoxamine (b), an iron chelator, would be of no benefit, nor would dimercaprol (c), a heavy metal (mainly lead) chelator. N-acetylcysteine (d), routinely used as an antidote for acetaminophen poisoning, would not alleviate or shorten signs and symptoms in cyanide poisoning. Pralidoxime (e) is a cholinesterase "reactivator" that is used for poisoning with organophosphate insecticides, nerve gases (sarin, soman), or other drugs that cause profound and "irreversible" inactivation of acetylcholinesterase.

487. The answer is e. *(Brunton, pp 82–83, 693–694, 1741; Craig, pp 66, 314; Katzung, pp 59f, 988.)* We give N-acetylcysteine for acetaminophen poisoning and use it because it is a sulfhydryl-rich drug that, if given soon enough and properly enough, can prevent hepatic necrosis. At safe blood levels, the major pathways of acetaminophen elimination involve glucuronidation and sulfation. When these pathways are overwhelmed, as occurs with acetaminophen poisoning, a cytochrome P450–dependent pathway attempts to handle the metabolic load. The active toxic metabolite, N-acetyl-benzoqinoneimine, is formed in levels that exceed the ability of intrinsic sulfhydryl compounds to inactivate it. So long as ample hepatocyte stores of glutathione (an –SH compound) are available, cytotoxicity will not occur. However, severe poisoning depletes –SH stores, and so the hepatotoxic metabolite attacks key cellular macromolecules. That leads to hepatic necrosis.

N-acetylcysteine acts as a substitute for endogenous glutathione to react with the toxic metabolite, thereby sparing –SH groups on key hepatocyte macromolecules.

Alkalinization of the urine is of no benefit with acetaminophen poisoning, as it can be with severe salicylate poisoning (because raising urine pH reduces tubular reabsorption of salicylate and increases its excretion). Moreover, N-acetylcysteine does not directly change urine pH. Superoxide anion radical or hydrogen peroxide is not directly involved in the cytotoxicity (d).

488. The answer is c. *(Brunton, pp 1660–1663; Katzung, pp 532, 977–979, 994.)* Disodium EDTA (edetate sodium), a calcium chelator that is used to treat severe, acute hypercalcemia, causes hypocalcemic tetany on rapid IV administration. This effect is not observed on slow infusion (15 mg/min) because extracirculatory calcium stores are available and drawn upon to prevent a significant reduction in plasma calcium levels. When Ca-Na$_2$-EDTA is given IV (it is sometimes used to diagnose or treat lead poisoning), hypocalcemia does not develop, even when large doses are required.

The other drugs listed do not cause hypocalcemia. Deferoxamine (a) is used as an iron chelator. Dimercaprol (British anti-Lewisite [BAL; b]), another chelator, is used to treat arsenic and Hg poisoning, as well as in certain cases of lead poisoning in children. (Succimer, a water-soluble dimercaprol analog, is indicated for treating lead poisoning in children, but is commonly used for adults also.) N-acetylcysteine (d) is an antidote used in the treatment of overdosage with acetaminophen to prevent hepatotoxicity.

Penicillamine (e), mainly used as a copper chelator, is the drug of choice in treating Wilson's disease (chronic copper poisoning). It is also used sometimes to chelate mercury and lead.

489. The answer is b. (*Brunton, pp 686, 691–692, 1749–1750; Craig, p 42; Katzung, pp 579, 581–582, 988, 991.*) Alkalinizing the urine interferes with the renal tubular reabsorption of organic acids (such as aspirin and phenobarbital) by increasing the ionized form of the drug in the urine (per the Henderson-Hasselbach equation). This increases their net renal excretion. Conversely, excretion of organic bases (such as amphetamine, cocaine, phencyclidine, and morphine) would be *reduced* by alkalinizing the urine.

Note that another consequence of severe aspirin (salicylate) toxicity is a combined metabolic plus respiratory acidosis. So in addition to enhancing urinary excretion of salicylate, the administration of sodium bicarbonate also tends to counteract the fall of blood pH.

490. The answer is a. (*Brunton, pp 691–692, 1746–1749; Craig, pp 312–313; Katzung, pp 987–988.*) Activated charcoal, a fine, black, powder with a high adsorptive capacity, is considered to be a valuable agent in the treatment of many kinds of oral drug poisonings—primarily if administered early on and followed by gastric lavage. Drugs that are well adsorbed by activated charcoal include primaquine, propoxyphene, dextroamphetamine, chlorpheniramine, phenobarbital, carbamazepine, digoxin, and aspirin. Mineral acids, alkalis, tolbutamide, and other drugs that are insoluble in acidic aqueous solution are not well adsorbed. Charcoal also does not bind Ca, lithium (Li), or Fe.

Deferoxamine, dimercaprol, and penicillamine are polyvalent cation chelators (iron, lead, copper) and play no role in managing aspirin (salicylate) poisoning or poisoning with any substances other than the metals they chelate. N-Acetylcysteine is the preferred antidote for acetaminophen overdoses (Question 485).

(Note the term *adsorb*—to bind; it is decidedly different from the more common pharmacologic/therapeutic term *absorb*.)

491. The answer is b. (*Brunton, p 600; Craig, pp 64, 66; Katzung, pp 375–377, 989, 993.*) Methanol is metabolized by the same enzymes that metabolize ethanol, but the products are different: formaldehyde and formic acid in the case of methanol. Headache, vertigo, vomiting, abdominal pain, dyspnea, and blurred vision can occur from accumulation of these metabolic intermediates. However, the most dangerous (or at least permanently disabling) consequence in severe cases is hyperemia of the optic disc, which can lead to blindness. The rationale for administering ethanol to treat methanol poisoning is fairly simple. Ethanol has a high affinity for alcohol and aldehyde dehydrogenases and competes as a substrate for those enzymes, reducing metabolism of methanol to its more toxic products. Important adjunctive treatments include hemodialysis to enhance removal of methanol and its products and administration of systemic alkalinizing salts (e.g., sodium bicarbonate) to counteract metabolic acidosis. Administration of systemic acidifying substances such as ascorbic acid would aggravate the condition.

492. The answer is a. (*Brunton, pp 1763–1766; Craig, pp 64, 66t, 68; Katzung, pp 974–975, 977–979.*) Arsenic is a constituent of fungicides, herbicides, and pesticides. Symptoms of acute toxicity include tightness in the throat, difficulty in swallowing, and stomach pains. Projectile vomiting and severe diarrhea can lead to hypovolemic shock, significant electrolyte derangements, and death. Chronic poisoning may cause peripheral neuritis, anemia, skin keratosis, and capillary dilation leading to hypotension. Dimercaprol (British anti-Lewisite [BAL]) is the main antidote used for arsenic poisoning.

493. The answer is a. (*Brunton, pp 390–393; Craig, pp 66–67; Katzung, pp 959–961, 992.*) Carbon monoxide has an affinity for hemoglobin that is about 250 times greater than that of O_2. It therefore binds to hemoglobin (forming carboxyhemoglobin) and reduces the O_2-carrying capacity of blood. The symptoms of poisoning are due to tissue hypoxia; they progress from headache and fatigue to confusion, syncope, tachycardia, coma, convulsions, shock, respiratory depression, and cardiovascular collapse. Carboxyhemoglobin levels below 15% rarely produce symptoms; above 40%, symptoms become severe. Treatment includes establishment of an airway, supportive therapy, and administration of 100% (or hyperbaric) O_2. Sulfur dioxide, ozone, and nitrogen dioxide are mucous membrane and respiratory irritants. Methane is a simple asphyxiant.

494. The answer is c. (*Brunton, p 1749; Craig, p 66; Katzung, p 993.*) The question describes some of the classic findings with ethylene glycol (the active osmolyte in most commercial antifreezes) ingestion. Ethylene glycol is initially oxidized by alcohol dehydrogenase and then further metabolized to oxalic acid and other products. Oxalate crystals can be found in various tissues of the poisoned individual's body, but they are eliminated in the urine, which is where they can be detected relatively easily. Renal failure can occur because of tubular blockade by the crystals. There will be a significant anion gap indicative of the metabolic acidosis and the presence of unmeasured anions' accompanying it (anion gap = $[Na^+ + K^+] - [HCO_3^- + Cl^-]$; we would also see this with methanol poisoning).

495. The answer is b. *(Brunton, pp 404–412; Katzung, pp 358, 361–362, 413, 989, 993.)* Arguably the most important tip-off in this presentation is the antegrade amnesia, which (among other things) is rather uniquely associated with benzodiazepines. The most likely benzodiazepine used in this scenario was rohypnol (flunitrazepam, better known as "roofies" on the street and by those who use it as a date rape drug).

Unless this patient were a very atypical responder, it is unlikely that any of the other CNS depressants—a barbiturate, an opioid, chloral hydrate—would cause the same responses. She's had one drink yet still feels pain from her head gash. She apparently hasn't had enough alcohol to be so obtunded that she doesn't feel pain, and a barbiturate is likely to enhance the sensation of pain (hyperalgesic effect).

Chloral hydrate is still used medically, mainly as a sedative for children. However, it is not as readily available as the illicit benzodiazepines; it does not cause antegrade amnesia (important to the perpetrator, because he or she anticipates no recall of what happened by the victim), but it is not readily available, and it simply doesn't have the "reputation" as a preferred date rape drug among those who use such drugs.

496. The answer is a. *(Brunton, pp 1754–1758; Craig, p 68; Katzung, pp 971–974.)* The presentation of chronic lead exposure, as from being exposed to (or even eating) older lead-based paints, differs from the typical presentation of acute organic lead poisoning (answer c), which usually arises from sniffing leaded gasoline (and just about all gasolines nowadays are organic lead-enriched). Answer b, with the predominant gingival/head/neck signs and symptoms, is typical of chronic or acute mercury intoxication. Answer d, with the hyperventilation, GI disturbances (including discolored vomitus) and pallor, is what you are likely to encounter in acute iron poisoning (as from a consuming ferrous sulfate supplements in large doses). A characteristic breath (garlicky or metallic), profuse diarrhea, encephalopathy, and hypotension (answer e) are typical of acute inorganic arsenic poisoning (see Question 490). Knowing more about the patient's history and environment will help immensely in sorting out what the "most likely" cause of intoxication is.

497. The answer is a. (*Brunton, pp 151–152, 171; Craig, pp 66–67, 94, 340–341; Katzung, pp 90, 444, 1107.*) Botulinus (botulinum) toxin prevents release of acetylcholine (from storage vesicles) by virtually all cholinergic nerves. Thus, there is no activation of any cholinergic receptors, whether nicotinic or muscarinic. Noteworthy findings, then, include an inability to activate all postganglionic neurons (sympathetic and parasympathetic), no physiologic release of epinephrine from the adrenal medulla, and flaccid skeletal muscle paralysis due to failure of ACh release from motor nerves. The cause of death is ventilatory failure because the intercostal muscles and diaphragm are nonfunctional.

Pralidoxime is a cholinesterase reactivator, an antidote and adjunct (along with atropine) for poisonings with "irreversible" cholinesterase inhibitors such as soman, sarin, VX ("nerve gases"), and many organophosphorus insecticides. Because no ACh is being released in botulinus poisoning, "reactivation" of the enzyme that normally metabolizes the neurotransmitter is irrelevant (and ineffective).

498. The answer is e. (*Brunton, pp 189–190, 195–197, 209–211; Craig, pp 68–69, 126–130; Katzung, pp 101–107, 989, 992.*) Most of the adverse responses to nerve gases (irreversible ACh esterase inhibitors such as soman and sarin) are due to a buildup of ACh at muscarinic receptors (i.e., ACh released from postganglionic parasympathetic nerves or sympathetic/cholinergic nerves innervating sweat glands). Those responses will be attenuated by atropine, because it is a highly specific competitive muscarinic antagonist. However, skeletal muscle stimulation (or eventual paralysis) involves nicotinic receptor activation. That will not be affected by atropine, and unless other supportive measures are provided, the patient is likely to die from ventilatory arrest/apnea.

499. The answer is f. (*Brunton, pp 1754–1758; Craig, p 66; Katzung, pp 972–974, 979.*) Succimer (a more polar salt of dimercaprol; British anti-Lewisite; BAL) would be the choice, given the proof of lead poisoning, the lack of acute symptoms, and the fact that our patient is a child. Succimer is easy to give orally and is tolerated far better than the alternatives: Ca-Na$_2$-EDTA, penicillamine (traditionally viewed as a copper chelator, but it also chelates lead), or dimercaprol itself. Although the heavy metal chelation profiles for succimer are not drastically different from those of dimercaprol, the fact that succimer is more polar (and, therefore, less likely to enter cells) seems to account for far fewer and milder side effects than those of dimercaprol (especially with respect to risks of tachycardia and hypertension).

500. The answer is c. (Brunton, p 600; Craig, p 66; Katzung, p 993.) Most commercial antifreezes (unless specifically and plainly marked otherwise) contain ethylene glycol. We give ethanol to inhibit the first step in the metabolism of ethylene glycol and, thereby, prevent further formation of oxalate and other products. Muscarinic receptor activation and purine degradation play no role in this poisoning, so atropine (b) or allopurinol (a) is irrational. Lorazepam (d) would be indicated if seizures develop, but giving it (or any other CNS depressant) early on is premature and more likely to aggravate CNS depression than to help. Syrup of ipecac (e), an emetic, would increase the risk of ethylene glycol aspiration, increase absorption, and do more harm than good. Gastric lavage would be indicated, however, if the patient gets treatment soon enough after glycol ingestion. (Note: With the recognition of the serious outcomes from ethylene glycol poisoning—whether in humans or family pets—many manufacturers are replacing that substance with propylene glycol...far less toxic and, in fact, an ingredient in many commercially prepared foods; and fully capable of lowering the freezing point of water.)

501. The answer is a. (Brunton, pp 198, 206–208, 214; Craig, pp 126–130; Katzung, pp 101–102, 105–106, 989–990.) Physostigmine is basically the only clinically useful AChE inhibitor that gets into the brain, a major target of atropine/antimuscarinic poisoning. That is because it lacks the quaternary (charged at virtually all pH values likely to be found in a living person) structure that nearly all the other common alternatives possess, and lacking that structure it can cross the blood-brain barrier.

Alternatives such as neostigmine, pyridostigmine, and others, will combat peripheral effects of atropine poisoning, just as physostigmine will. Unfortunately, some of the CNS manifestations (e.g., severe fever, leading to seizures) contribute greatly to the morbidity and mortality associated with high doses of antimuscarinics, and the quaternary agents simply will not combat them in the CNS.

By the way, basically the only clinical use for physostigmine is for managing poisoning from antimuscarinic ("atropine-like") drugs in a variety of classes. You won't encounter too many patients overdosed on atropine itself, but you'll see many poisoned with older antihistamines (e.g., diphenhydramine); some of the centrally acting antimuscarinics that are used for parkinsonism (e.g., benztropine and trihexyphenidyl); scopolamine (used for motion sickness); and most of the phenothiazine antipsychotics (e.g., chlorpromazine). Owing to the often strong antimuscarinic side effects of these drugs, treating overdoses of most of them probably will involve managing what amounts to "atropine poisoning"—and many other problems too. Note: Older antidepressants—for example, the tricyclics such as amitriptyline and imipramine—have strong antimuscarinic actions. However, because of the multiplicity of their effects (including high efficacy for blocking neuronal reuptake of norepinephrine and dopamine in the periphery and in the CNS) and the complicated clinical picture, physostigmine or other cholinesterase inhibitors should be avoided; they may do more harm than good.

502. The answer is a. (*Brunton, pp 198, 637–642; Craig, pp 138–139, 454–455; Katzung, pp 270–274, 379, 1085t.*) Most OTC sleep aids contain a first-generation antihistamine (sedating agent, almost always an ethanolamine, either diphenhydramine or the very similar drug, doxylamine). The preponderant signs and symptoms of toxicity arise not from any histamine receptor-blocking activity, but from intense antimuscarinic (atropine-like) effects, plus dose-dependent CNS depression that ultimately (and early on, in children) can lead to seizures. The signs and symptoms of this "anticholinergic syndrome" include many, if not all, that you will see in "atropine poisoning." Aside from symptomatic and supportive care, including the use of traditional drugs for status epilepticus, physostigmine (the nonquaternary, centrally and peripherally acting acetylcholinesterase inhibitor) may be lifesaving. It will certainly help reverse many of the central and peripheral signs and symptoms of the overdose.

Index